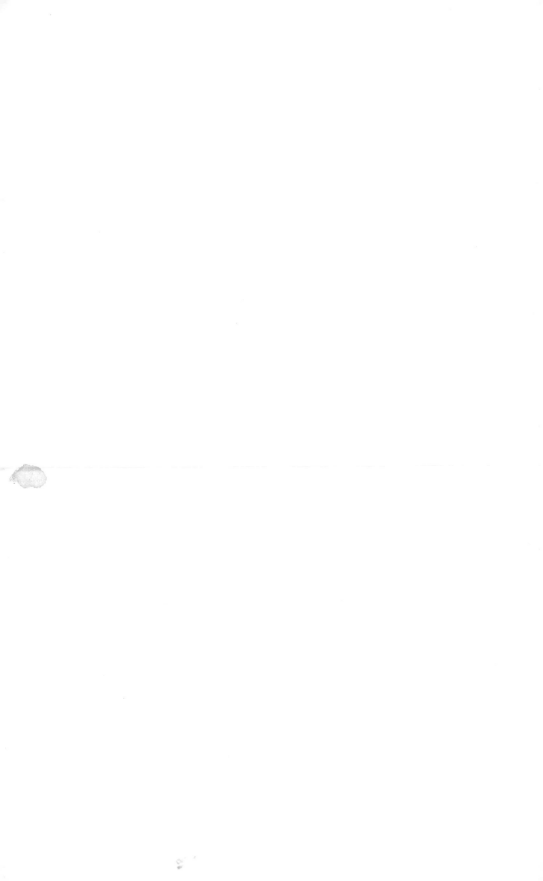

Diagnostic
Dysmorphology

Diagnostic Dysmorphology

Jon M. Aase, M.D.

University of New Mexico
School of Medicine
Albuquerque, New Mexico

Plenum Medical Book Company • New York and London

Library of Congress Cataloging-in-Publication Data

Aase, Jon M. (Jon Morton), 1936-
    Diagnostic dysmorphology / Jon M. Aase.
        p.   cm.
    Includes bibliographical references.
    Includes index.
    ISBN 0-306-43444-X
    1. Abnormalities, Human--Diagnosis. 2. Physical diagnosis.
I. Title.
    [DNLM: 1. Adnormalities--diagnosis.   QS 675 A1154d]
RG628.A27   1990
618.92'0043--dc20
DNLM/DLC
for Library of Congress   90-7897
                                                              CIP

10 9 8 7 6 5 4 3

Illustrations and cover design by Ching Shyu, M.S., Santa Clara, CA.

ISBN 0-306-43444-X

Plenum Medical Book Company is an imprint of Plenum Publishing Corporation

Printed in the United States of America

This book is dedicated to the memory of
Dr. David W. Smith . . .

the best and finest man I ever knew.
                    "The Empty House"

Foreword

Although far less dramatic than legionnaire's disease, toxic shock syndrome, or AIDS, severe congenital birth abnormalities are far more common, affecting two to four infants in every 100 births. Thus, in aggregate and over many years, birth anomalies have a great impact on our economy. And surely they generate considerable emotional erosion. Yet apart from the National Foundation March of Dimes, there have been few large organizations that have supported investigation of birth anomalies, and none has been concerned with the training of dysmorphologists.

The dysmorphologist or syndromatologist is often thought of by other clinicians as being lost in arcane details, obsessed with minutiae, speaking in tongues beyond the realm of professional comprehension, understood by none except those similarly engaged. On the other hand, the consulting family perceives the dysmorphologist as one who knows all, who will provide a diagnosis and answer all questions about prognosis and therapy. In truth, neither of these views is correct.

There is probably no other area of endeavor in which failure to diagnose is accepted as the norm. Could one practice surgery or civil engineering or law and fail so often, yet be considered an expert? Under no circumstances! Nevertheless, it has been demonstrated repeatedly that the best of us has no greater than a 20% overall rate of success. Surely it must be the only field in which one can perform so dismally yet be considered competent.

There is something metaphysical about naming a disorder. All concerned—the patient, the clinician, the parents—seem to experience a certain satisfaction or sense of security when an unknown condition is defined. This is valid, since understanding has its incipience in definition. The unknown is scary. Once the condition has been measured and its extent limned, its recognition is made easier. Thereby, interest and concentration can be more easily focused upon it. This, in turn, may lead to therapy and control.

One has the illusion of power over a disorder or a person if one can use a private designation, that is, the name. To show that this property is universal, I should like to use a few examples. The first is the naming of a power figure. As children, the most powerful figures we know are our parents. We almost invariably call our parents not by their given names, but by an artificial appellation such as "Mama," "Papa," or some other variant. As we grow older, the same applies to our teachers or bosses. They are called "Mr." or "Mrs." or "Dr." or "Professor," the general concept being that familiar speech would cause a loss of respect. These power figures do not generally brook use of their first or private names. Second, to bolster my point, I shall relate a personal experience. While working in Greenland, I met a group of Eskimos. Remembering the names they gave me, almost always long and compounded, was difficult. Upon seeing them next time and again asking, I noted that each time a different name was offered. Explaining the problem, the Danish doctor told me that the Eskimos were given their *true* names by a shaman and that they considered those names to be equivalent to their souls. Under no circumstances were they going to bare their souls to me; therefore, when asked, they would always proffer a false name.

A third point is exemplified when a child is seen at the office with a spurious diagnosis. The parents of the infant wish to know the recurrence risk and something about the disorder. When the clinician candidly says that the patient does not have the erroneously diagnosed condition, that a misdiagnosis has been made, the parents are understandably disturbed. If the clinician does not know what the child actually has, there can be no discussion of recurrence risk and prognosis. The parents leave disappointed, even angry, because the clinician has deprived them of a certain sense of security, false though it was.

Naming is a two-way street, for there is nothing that makes a clinician happier than defining a problem or naming a disorder. At times, the clinician may be all too eager to do this, and hence may commit what I choose to call Procrustean error. Procrustes was a professional robber in ancient Athens. He had a modus operandi, and a relatively simple one at that. Stationing himself at a busy crossroad, he would see a tired traveler on the way to Athens and ply him with drink until the traveler was completely intoxicated. He would then invite the traveler to use his iron bed for the evening saying that he, Procrustes, would sleep on a pallet on the ground. After the traveler was asleep, if his feet stuck over the edge of the bed, Procrustes would slice off his feet, making the body fit the bed. The head could be similarly severed, and if the traveler were too short, he would be stretched until he fit the bed. One might view this as antisocial behavior. But it is not antisocial; it is normal behavior, for Procrustes is indeed Everyperson. If the individual does not fit our chosen diagnosis, then the patient must represent an "atypical" form, a forme fruste, or a "variant of," and so it goes.

Dr. Jon Aase has accomplished a tour de force in leading the reader through a careful step-by-step experience designed to lead to the diagnosis of myriad dysmorphic conditions. He has done this with linguistic grace, explaining the genesis of congenital anomalies by first reviewing the normal sequence of embryologic events, followed by a clear discussion of how anomalies arise in each system of the body. Dr. Aase's analogy to diagnostic detective work is an apt one. While the denouement of a detective story often involves a sleuth who, by her or his "eyeballing" of the evidence, presents an instant solution, in real life the answers are far more likely to come from careful, laborious sifting of signs and symptoms, and Dr. Aase emphasizes this.

Dr. David Smith, his mentor and an inspiration to all dysmorphologists, would have been pleased with Dr. Aase's logical approach to the field. He, like Sherlock Holmes to Dr. Watson, would have said, "Good job, Jon, good job!"

Robert J. Gorlin, D.D.S., M.S., D.Sc. (Athens)
Regents' Professor of Oral Pathology and Genetics
University of Minnesota School of Dentistry
Minneapolis, Minnesota 55455

Preface

*I propose to devote my declining years to the
composition of a textbook which shall focus the
whole art of detection into one volume.*
—"The Abbey Grange"

Reaching a diagnosis in a child with congenital abnormalities bears many similarities to the work of a detective in solving a crime. The physician is confronted with the end product of events that took place weeks or months before, unseen and usually unsuspected. He must use every available physical clue, together with the testimony of "witnesses," to try to reconstruct the crime. If he can solve the mystery and identify the cause of the malformation, he can provide invaluable help for the victim and his family. In some rare instances, the "culprit" can be permanently removed from circulation, as in the case of thalidomide and, it is to be hoped, rubella.

Surely the fictional archetype for observation and deduction is Sherlock Holmes. His uncanny ability to construct logical chains of reasoning from the most obscure evidence has made his name synonymous with the word "detective." I heartily recommend the stories of Arthur Conan Doyle as bedtime reading for anyone interested in the art and science of observation. A number of quotations from these works have been inserted at appropriate places in this text, not so much as "comic relief," as to emphasize the value of certain general principles in the diagnosis of dysmorphic conditions.

While the detective analogy should not be stretched too far, the principles of careful data gathering, minute observation of subtle physical clues, and deductive reasoning do form the basis of dysmorphologic diagnosis, and these techniques are incompletely addressed in textbooks of physical examination and compilations of birth defect "syndromes." This book is intended to describe the methods used by dysmorphologists to gather clues from the history and physical examination and to outline the reasoning processes used to reach a meaningful diagnosis. It is intended primarily for the instruction of house officers, fellows, and practicing physicians, and assumes a background in clinical medicine and, particularly, pediatrics.

Jon M. Aase

Albuquerque, New Mexico

Contents

Appendixes

Diagnostic
Dysmorphology

Introduction

It is my business to know things. Perhaps I have trained myself to see what others overlook.
— "A Case of Identity"

DYSMORPHOLOGY

The word *dysmorphology* was coined by Dr. David Smith in the 1960s to describe the study of human congenital malformations. Literally, it means "the study of abnormal form," emphasizing a focus upon structural abnormalities of development. As a scientific discipline, dysmorphology combines concepts, knowledge, and techniques from the fields of embryology, clinical genetics, and pediatrics (Fig. Intro. 1). As a medical subspeciality, dysmorphology deals with *people* who have congenital abnormalities and with their families. Whenever any physician is confronted by a patient with a birth defect he or she becomes, for the moment at least, a dysmorphologist.

HISTORY

Children with birth defects have appeared in every age, but rarely and unpredictably, and every society has asked the question "Why?" To explain the meaning and cause of such abnormalities, people develop a belief system, often colored by attitudes of the past but incorporating their own cultural values.

In ancient Babylonia, the birth of a malformed baby was thought to be a sign from the gods, predicting future events of great consequence. Priests drew up an elaborate code defining the significance, for good or evil, of each of a variety of anomalies. The child's family or village or even the entire nation might be influenced, depending on the nature of the abnormality. This idea apparently persisted until the time of Classic Rome: the word *monster* is derived from the Latin *monere* ("to warn"), the root for terms such as *premonition* and *admonish*.

By the Middle Ages, religious teachings and the concept of personal guilt had altered perceptions of divine intervention (at least in Europe). The birth of a baby with congenital anomalies was believed to be proof of and punishment for previous sins of the parents, usually the mother. In more remote areas, parents of an affected child were sometimes accused of unnatural union with lower animals, an accusation based on fancied resem-

1

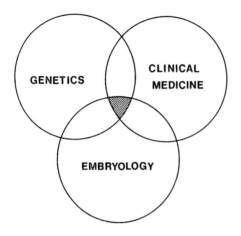

Figure Intro. 1. Diagram showing contributions of various disciplines to the field of dysmorphology.

blances to some beast. In such cases, the baby might be killed and the parents ostracized. Somewhat later, congenital abnormalities were attributed to "demonic possession" of mother or child, and elaborate religious rituals were undertaken to drive out the evil spirits.

Then came the Enlightenment, and attempts to explain the cause of abnormal birth in terms of earthly rather than supernatural influences. "Maternal impressions" were thought to account for many anomalies. If the mother spilled milk during her pregnancy, the baby might be born with a white forelock; if frightened by a rabbit, she could give birth to a child with a "harelip."

As might be expected, many of these beliefs die hard; today, the attitudes of families and society toward children with birth defects still may be shadowed by the prejudices of the past. Some groups remain strongly influenced by the concept of divine punishment, while others retain a firm belief in maternal impressions. This last idea has also undergone mutation toward undue concern that events during the pregnancy must be to blame if a child is born imperfect. This modern "superstition" is reflected in the widespread concern about environmental agents as causes of birth defects. In truth, known teratogens* are responsible for only a handful of congenital anomaly syndromes. We simply do not know the causes of most birth defects; of the remainder, the largest part are genetic in origin and thus are determined at the moment of conception.

In most developed countries, social changes over the last few decades have affected people's reproductive decisions. Women are having children later in life, families are smaller, and there is an understandable (if largely unfounded) expectation that modern medical science can ensure that each child will be perfect. These and many other influences color the attitudes of the present generation toward children with birth defects.

Given the remarkable pace of recent developments in the understanding of human

*The term *teratology* (literally, "the study of monsters") is now applied mainly to the investigation of mechanisms by which external influences (especially chemicals and physical agents such as radiation) cause aberrant embryological development. Beginning in the 1950s, this field received a new injection of interest and vigor from growing public and professional concern with human teratogens, including the rubella virus and thalidomide.

genetics, we may look forward to a time when both diagnosis and treatment of genetic disease become as straightforward and accurate as, say, the antibiotic treatment of bacterial infection. At present, however, the vast majority of congenital abnormalities must be dealt with on the basis of incomplete information, and the clinical skills of the dysmorphologist remain among the most useful tools in our armamentarium.

DYSMORPHOLOGIC DIAGNOSIS

In medicine, the word *diagnosis* has two meanings. First, it means the process of seeking clinical clues, sifting the evidence, forming a hypothesis, and eliminating false suspects. In this sense, *diagnosis* describes the activity of identifying the true nature of a patient's disorder. When this procedure is successful, its product is also called a *diagnosis*; and in this second sense, the word implies that something important is known about the patient that was not known before. On the most superficial level, a diagnosis is only a label, a handy name by which to refer to a complex set of pathological features. At a deeper level, however, the establishment of an accurate diagnosis provides the framework for all subsequent medical decisions.

To be useful, a diagnosis must be both accurate and specific. For example, a child is found to have a rash: this may be an accurate diagnosis, but it provides little information on which to base treatment or prediction of the clinical course and eventual outcome. If the rash can be identified as a viral exanthem, its meaning becomes clearer, and equally important, other causes of skin eruption can be excluded from consideration. When the history, clinical features, and laboratory tests all confirm rubella virus infection, the rash can be seen as part of a larger pattern, with implications not only for the patient but possible risks to other family members as well.

In dysmorphology, a "diagnosis" of "multiple congenital abnormalities" (or, worse, "funny-looking kid") carries virtually no useful information. No conclusions can be reached about the potential for occult abnormalities, the possibility of specific complications, the general outlook for survival, intellectual progress or growth, or the chance of the same abnormalities being found in subsequent members of the family. Without a specific diagnosis, the help that can be offered is limited to piecemeal treatment of individual malformations. Yet it must be understood that achieving a diagnosis, important though it is, is only one necessary step in the process of providing care and counseling for the affected child and the family.

THIS BOOK

Birth defect syndromes number in the thousands, and each condition has its own implications for prognosis, therapy, and recurrence risk. Discriminating among a number of overlapping and often confusing entities requires a systematic approach, well-honed powers of observation, a thorough appreciation of the variations of "normal," and a solid fund of information about human development and its aberrations. This book is devoted solely to the principles of diagnosis, and especially to the attainment of the first three of these qualities. It has been written as a "how to do it" manual, offering a number of techniques and methods of approach to the patient with birth defects, so that the information obtained can be as specific and complete as possible.

Chapter 1 contains a brief review of basic principles of normal and abnormal embryology, along with a classification system for anomalies that has proven to be clinically useful. Chapter 2 outlines a general scheme of approach to dysmorphologic diagnosis. More specific guidelines for obtaining a complete history are contained in Chapter 3. In Chapter 4, the physical examination of the patient is broken down into sections addressing each of 20 anatomic zones. A brief summary of the embryology of each region is followed by a review of its normal anatomy and landmarks and appropriate examination techniques. Finally, normal structural variations and both major and minor abnormalities are discussed and illustrated. Chapter 5 once again addresses the overall scheme of the diagnostic process, with some practical examples and helpful hints.

There are several things that this book is not. First, no attempt has been made to duplicate the contents of the several excellent textbooks that catalog and describe in detail the thousands of birth defect syndromes which have been discovered to date; these sources are listed in References. Second, information about the most recent advances in molecular biology and genetic engineering also are not dealt with. This book purposely steps back a bit from the frontiers of science in order to emphasize the value of classic clinical skills. Last, discussion of the vital topics of therapy, support, counseling, and long-term care for children with birth defects is being set aside for another time.

What follows, then, is one approach to dysmorphologic diagnosis. It draws heavily on the teaching and inspiration of Dr. David W. Smith, and just as was the man, the method seems to be effective, robust, idiosyncratic, and constantly expanding its limits. If the reader comes away with some glints of the enthusiasm and tremendous insight of that master dysmorphology sleuth, this book will have served its purpose.

1

Principles of Normal and Abnormal Embryogenesis

*There are some trees, Watson, which grow to a
certain height and then suddenly develop some
unsightly eccentricity. You will see it often in
humans.*
— "The Empty House"

By definition, the subject matter of dysmorphology is aberrant structural development occurring primarily before birth. Normal embryogenesis is an exceedingly complex and finely orchestrated process whose molecular and biochemical basis is just beginning to be unraveled. This chapter reviews only the most basic principles of embryology as they are understood to influence the production of congenital abnormalities. Further details of the structural development of each body system are provided in Chapter 4, but a much more complete account of human embryology will be found in the texts listed in References.

1.1. EMBRYOLOGY

1.1.1. Developmental Timing

Prenatal development may be conveniently divided into three time periods: the *implantation* stage, extending from the time of fertilization of the egg to the end of the third week of gestation, the *embryonic* stage, from the beginning of week 4 to the end of week 7, and the *fetal* stage, from week 8 until birth.

During the implantation stage, rapid cell proliferation leads to the formation of the hollow blastocyst, within which develops the embryonic plate. The amniotic cavity appears, and primitive circulatory connections with the placenta are established. Early cell differentiation begins late in this period, with somites demarcated in the mesodermal layer, and longitudinal folds of neurectoderm indicating the site of the future brain and spinal cord.

The embryonic stage is the time of primary tissue differentiation and the formation of definitive organs. Neural tissues undergo very rapid proliferation, with closure of the neural tube and flexion of its anterior segments to form the divisions of the developing brain. The heart begins to beat, allowing blood to circulate through the newly formed

5

vascular system even before cardiac structures are fully formed. Primordia of facial structures, limbs, and internal organs appear and gradually assume their final shapes and positions.

By the beginning of the fetal stage, a distinctly human form has been achieved, with differentiation of all organ systems complete. The remainder of gestation is primarily a period of growth in size, with progressive enlargement of skeletal structures, muscle and, especially, brain. Fetal movement is usually perceived by the mother at about week 19 or 20, becoming progressively stronger. Body fat deposition and lung maturation take place during the last 8 weeks of prenatal life.

1.1.2. Embryologic Mechanisms

Early embryonic development involves several distinct phenomena by which cells form various tissues, organs, and body structures. Simple *cell proliferation* occurs at different rates in different parts of the body, both before and after *differentiation* into specific tissues. Some cell types, such as melanocytes, undergo *migration* in relation to their neighbors, eventually arriving at locations far removed from their sites of origin. Programmed *cell death* is an important factor in the formation of many structures, as in the separation of the digits of the hand and the degeneration of the central cellular core of the intestine. *Fusion* between adjacent tissues is also an important mechanism in the formation of such structures as the upper lip and the heart.

There is now clear evidence that many of these developmental processes are brought about by *induction* by neighboring cells. Tissues of different types seem to communicate chemically with each other across intervening cell membranes, and the ensuing "dialogue" seems to be crucial to normal embryonic development.

All of these developmental processes normally take place in a specific *sequence* peculiar to each tissue or structure, and the timing may be quite critical. For this reason, even a brief delay in migration or cell death may result in abnormal formation, not only of the structure in question but of adjoining tissues as well. Sometimes, a seemingly minor interruption of the intricate orchestration of development produces a cascade of widespread developmental abnormalities, as in failure of complete closure of the neural tube (see Section 4.14). On the other hand, abnormal development does not occur backward in time. Once a structure has been formed to a certain point, it cannot be "unformed," although it can be distorted or destroyed by mechanical forces or infection. When a structure can be shown to have reached a certain stage of development before a malformation occurred, the time of the appearance of the defect often can be estimated with considerable accuracy.

Once a tissue has reached a certain stage of differentiation, its eventual form becomes fixed, and this stage seems to be reached quite early in embryogenesis. Thus, a portion of tissue destined to become limb bud will form a recognizable limb, even if it is mechanically displaced to quite a different body site.

1.1.3. Abnormal Embryogenesis

Given the complexity of normal embryonic development, it may seem surprising that it takes place as well as it does. Failure or inadequate completion of any one of the embryonic functions briefly outlined above can give rise to malformation of any tissue or structure. The nature of the resulting abnormality depends on the tissue involved, the exact developmental mechanism at fault, and the time at which it occurs.

During the implantation stage, most aberrations severe enough to damage the embryo at all cause spontaneous abortion. It is estimated that at least 15% of all conceptions are lost in this fashion.

Abnormal developmental mechanisms acting during the embryonic stage may cause a whole gamut of structural anomalies, since organ formation is in progress. Inadequate cellular proliferation usually results in *deficiencies* of body structure, ranging from absence of a limb to mild diminution of the size of the external ear. Abnormal or incomplete differentiation of cells into mature tissues may produce local hamartomatous lesions such as hemangiomas or more widespread anomalies of a single organ system. Failure of cellular induction is probably responsible for abnormalities such as biliary atresia, while aberrant cell migration plays a part in some anomalies of skin pigmentation and probably in certain defects of the central face. Inadequate cell death may lead to problems such as syndactyly or imperforate anus, and incomplete tissue fusion is involved in the various forms of cleft lip and palate.

Obviously, many of these different abnormal mechanisms may occasionally act in concert, producing more complex or widespread anomalies. Most developmental processes are under genetic control, and a single mutant gene may affect several embryonic systems, perhaps through different mechanisms. A few teratogenic agents also interfere with these processes, but unlike aberrant genes, their effects are strongly influenced by the time of their action during the embryonic sequence.

1.2. BIRTH DEFECTS

About 3% of all the children born in any hospital or in any country or in any year will have a significant congenital abnormality—one which is of more than cosmetic concern and which, uncorrected, will interfere with normal functioning (Fig. 1.1A). Although such anomalies occur in only a small fraction of all newborns, they cause a much larger proportion of neonatal and infant deaths, and children with birth defects make up about 30% of all admissions to pediatric hospitals. Furthermore, these problems appear, by definition, at the very start of life, and many affected individuals require chronic care for decades. The burdens imposed on these people, their families, and society at large are enormous. As yet, the great majority of birth defects are neither detectable by prenatal diagnosis nor preventable, and thus the impact of these problems has not decreased despite all the advances in other areas of pediatric medicine.

Almost all birth defect syndromes are exceedingly rare, and a practicing physician would be expected to see only a handful of such cases in his or her professional lifetime, yet there are so many different disorders that even a specialist in the field will never gain experience with all of them. Therefore, the approach set forth here depends not on rote memorization of the features of rare syndromes but on recognition and analysis of their component anomalies.

For purposes of conceptualization as well as for ease of discussion, it is helpful to divide birth defects into those affecting one or several organ systems (Fig. 1.1B). A further

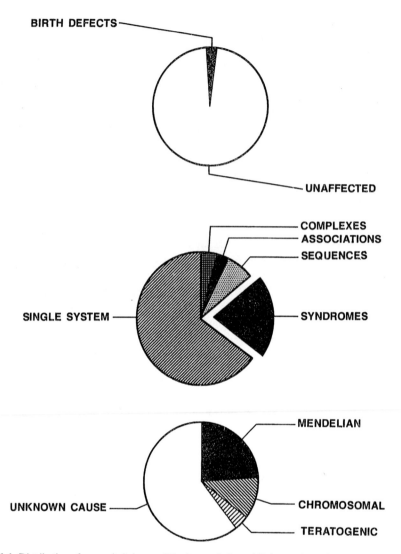

Figure 1.1. Distribution of congenital abnormalities in populations. (A) Approximate incidence of birth defects in all populations. (B) Proportions of single-system abnormalities versus true multiple-malformation syndromes. (C) Approximate distribution of syndromes by etiology.

rough subdivision of congenital syndromes by supposed *etiology* provides perspective on the wide diversity of abnormalities that make up the subject matter of dysmorphology (Fig. 1.1C). This section begins, however, with an outline of the four major types of *pathogenesis* of birth defects, since this classification cuts across all other categories and provides the framework for discussion of specific abnormalities in Chapter 4.

1.2.1. Pathogenetic Mechanisms

1.2.1.1. Deformation

Deformational anomalies are produced by aberrant mechanical forces that distort otherwise normal structures. Deformations usually occur late in gestation and can result in surprisingly severe changes in the configuration of various body structures. Such problems as asynclitism of the skull, tibial bowing, and even micrognathia have been shown to be caused by such extrinsic deforming forces.

Causes of intrauterine constraint include maternal factors such as primigravidity, an unusually small pelvic outlet, or structural abnormalities of the uterus (bicornuate uterus or uterine fibroids). An intra-abdominal pregnancy or the presence of more than one fetus in the uterus obviously can produce crowding. Deformation can also result from such fetal factors as abnormal presentation, oligohydramnios, or even a preexisting malformation or disruption that limits fetal movement. Most deformational abnormalities involve cartilage, bone, and joints, probably because softer tissues yield to intrauterine pressure, but return readily to their original forms.

After the abnormal mechanical stresses are removed, most deformations begin to correct spontaneously. Differential growth often occurs in the affected parts, with the result that the distortion gradually disappears over a course of several months to a few years. Occasionally, however, treatment is necessary to help restore a normal configuration of bones and joints. In these cases, therapy "uses fire to fight fire": casts, braces, or exercises are designed to produce mechanical stress opposite that of the deforming forces, and bone and connective tissue slowly remodels to a more normal form.

1.2.1.2. Disruption

Structural defects also may be caused by actual destruction of previously normal tissue. In contrast to the deformational abnormalities, such disruption is not exclusively the result of mechanical forces but also can be produced by phenomena such as ischemia, hemorrhage, or adhesion of denuded tissues. Disruptional abnormalities commonly affect several different tissue types in a well-demarcated anatomic region, and the structural damage does not conform to the boundaries normally imposed by embryonic development. Thus, an amniotic band may slice across the lower quadrant of the fetus, penetrating skin, muscle, bone, and soft tissue without regard to their embryonic relationships (see Appendix C).

It should be emphasized that both deformations and disruptions usually affect structures that had previously developed normally, and their presence does not imply intrinsic abnormality of the tissues involved. Moreover, there is seldom need for concern about mental deficit or other hidden problems. The recurrence risk is low unless uterine malformation is found in the mother. Further information concerning deformation and disruption is found in *Smith's Recognizable Patterns of Human Deformation,* edited by J. M. Graham (see References).

1.2.1.3. Dysplasia

The third category of pathogenesis important in the production of birth defects is dysplasia. This term refers to abnormal cellular organization or function within a specific tissue type throughout the body, resulting in clinically apparent structural changes. For a few of these disorders, a specific aberration of cellular biochemistry has been defined, usually involving abnormalities of enzyme production or synthesis of structural protein.

Almost all dysplasias seem to be caused by major mutant genes. Examples include metabolic disorders such as the so-called storage diseases, the wide variety of skeletal dysostoses, and the ectodermal dysplasias. Exceptions to the rule of genetic causation may be found among the *hamartomas,* abnormal admixtures of tissue types often producing discrete tumors such as hemangiomas and nevi.

An important feature of most dysplastic conditions is their continuing course. Since the tissue itself is intrinsically abnormal, clinical effects may persist or worsen as long as the tissue continues to grow or function. This contrasts with the three other pathogenetic mechanisms mentioned here. Malformation, deformation, and disruption all have their effects during a distinct interval of development, and although the pathology they produce may be long-lasting, the actions causing it are relatively brief in duration. Dysplasia can continue to produce dysmorphic changes throughout life.

1.2.1.4. Malformation

The term *malformation* is reserved for abnormalities caused by failure or inadequate completion of one or more of the embryonic processes outlined in Section 1.1.2. The early development of a particular tissue or organ system is arrested, delayed, or misdirected, resulting in persisting abnormalities of structure. Such *intrinsic* anomalies may be limited to a single anatomic region, involve an entire organ system, or produce a *malformation syndrome* affecting a number of different body systems.

Although defining an anomaly as a malformation does not imply any specific etiology, it does suggest that the error in development occurred early in gestation, either while tissue differentiation was taking place or during the organogenic period, when individual organ systems were developing. In the fetal period, the major phenomenon taking place is the growth of already differentiated systems, and true malformations arising during this time are quite rare.

1.2.2. Clinical Classification of Birth Defects

One way to approach the bewildering array of congenital defects is to consider their relationships to each other. An anomaly occurring alone may have considerably different meaning than the same anomaly occurring in conjunction with others. The subclassification outlined below helps sort out the different combinations in which abnormalities may occur.

1.2.2.1. Single-System Defects

Malformations that involve only a local region of a single organ system of the body make up the largest proportion of birth defects (Fig. 1.B). Such abnormalities include the commonest birth defects: cleft lip, club foot, pyloric stenosis, congenital hip dislocation, and congenital heart disease. Most of the disorders in this group are thought to be of multifactorial etiology, implying the cumulative effects of multiple genes of small effect and presumably an environmental "trigger" of unknown nature. These anomalies occur with increased frequency in some families and racial groups but do not follow the classic Mendelian patterns of distribution expected for disorders caused by major mutant genes. Instead, the more or less random distribution among family members suggests that they carry a statistically increased "load" of deleterious minor genes. None of the single-system defects, however, shows a high degree of concordance in identical twins, providing strong evidence for the influence of nongenetic factors in their causation.

Clinically (and presumably pathogenetically), these isolated defects appear to be identical with those that occur as part of a syndrome. This implies that there is a single common pathway leading to the same endpoint despite different initial etiologies.

1.2.2.2. Associations

Several clinical entities have now been described with physical features that are associated in a nonrandom fashion but in which the link among the various anomalies is not strong enough or consistent enough to justify definition as a syndrome. These conditions are presently called *associations* to emphasize the lack of uniformity in the clinical presentation from case to case. For example, the VACTERL association comprises abnormalities of the vertebrae, anal atresia, cardiac malformation, tracheoesophageal fistula, renal anomalies, and limb defects. Most children with this diagnosis, however, do not have all these anomalies but rather have varying assortments from this list.

This variability clearly presents problems for the diagnostician: How many features of the VACTERL association are necessary to permit the assumption of that diagnosis? Furthermore, associations have not been shown to have a genetic basis, nor have any teratogenic agents been identified. What cause can be postulated to explain the occurrence of such nonrandom but variable patterns of congenital abnormalities? Certainly, there remains a great deal to be learned about this type of congenital abnormality.

At this point, the primary value of the "association" designation is to prompt the search for hidden abnormalities that might fit the larger pattern. Thus, the presence of anal atresia in a newborn with feeding problems should lead to evaluation of the esophagus, spine, heart, and kidneys. The recurrence risk in these conditions is extremely small, based entirely on empiric data, and the prognosis depends almost entirely on the degree of severity and potential correctability of the individual structural lesions. Mental development often is normal, but statural growth may be somewhat poor in children with conditions in this category.

1.2.2.3. Sequences

There exist some patterns of multiple malformation that can be shown on developmental and embryologic grounds to be the result of a cascade of seemingly unrelated consequences, proceeding from one primary defect that itself is often a single-system malformation. During intrauterine life, this primary abnormality interferes with normal embryologic and fetal developmental processes, so that by the time of birth, the child is found to have what look like separate and distinct abnormalities that may involve widely separated body areas and different organ systems. For example, the primary abnormality in the Potter sequence is renal aplasia. The absence of urine production results in a markedly diminished volume of amniotic fluid during the last half of gestation. This, in turn, leads to intrauterine constraint, with deformities such as limb bowing and joint contractures as well as compressed "Potter facies." Oligohydramnios has one other deleterious effect: the absence of circulation of amniotic fluid into the bronchial tree apparently interferes with lung maturation. Therefore, newborns with the Potter sequence die of respiratory insufficiency rather than renal failure. The entire pattern of physical and functional consequences may be traced back to a single basic aberration of early development.

The importance of recognizing malformation sequences lies in their differentiation from other multiple-defect conditions whose implications for prognosis and recurrence risk may be quite different. The causes of most sequences are unknown, but some show features compatible with multifactorial inheritance, as might be expected by their derivation from a single underlying malformation.

1.2.2.4. Complexes

Another taxonomic category that has proven useful in dysmorphology is the developmental field complex. This term, popularized by Opitz, implies the existence of a noxious influence that acts on a particular geographic part of the developing embryo, resulting in abnormalities in adjacent structures that might be of quite disparate embryologic origin yet share a single locality at a particular point during development and thus share a similar fate when affected by the agent.

Many recognized complexes seem to be caused by vascular anomalies. Aberration of blood vessel formation in early embryogenesis can result in anomalous formation of structures normally served by those vessels: total absence of an artery, for example, may result in total absence of part or all of a developing limb; aberrant course of an embryonic artery may give rise to hypoplasia of the bone and muscle usually supplied, and so forth. In addition, vascular rupture can produce localized hemorrhage, which can damage adjacent tissues through direct pressure, through absence of nutrients and oxygen during a critical developmental stage, or possibly through biochemical reactions with blood products extravasated into embryonic tissues.

Examples of developmental field complexes include hemifacial microsomia (which has been produced in rodents and monkeys by inducing bleeding in the area of the face served by the stapedial artery), defects of the posterior axis ranging from sacral agenesis to sirenomelia, and possibly such conditions as the Poland anomaly and Moebius "syndrome."

1.2.2.5. Syndromes

As mentioned above, congenital abnormalities can occur singly or in combinations that may be more or less fixed. When a particular set of anomalies repeatedly occurs in a consistent pattern, the pattern is designated a *syndrome* (from the Greek "running together"). In the strictest sense, a syndrome is not a diagnosis but only a convenient label.

When the underlying cause of a syndrome is discovered, the shorthand designation should be abandoned in favor of a more definitive name; for example, Hurler syndrome becomes mucopolysaccharidosis, type I.

Birth defect syndromes usually are recognized after the report of a few individual cases that bear similarities to each other. As further cases are published, the syndrome is further defined by the confirmation (or refutation) of the original set of abnormalities, inclusion or exclusion of other anomalies, clarification of the prognosis and natural history of the disorder, and sometimes elucidation of its pathogenesis or etiology. In this way, the initial descriptions of the syndrome are refined and the limits of variability of its manifestations are explored.

Even after considerable refinement, however, diagnoses based on clinical observation show a great range of latitude, and thus there may be no "gold standard" against which a particular patient can be compared. No one congenital malformation is pathognomonic for a specific syndrome; furthermore, there is inherent variability in the manifestations of most dysmorphic disorders, both in type and in severity of the various structural abnormalities. The photographs in published reports provide good visual examples of some of the clinical features of a disorder, but they are usually chosen because of the severity or "classic appearance" of the feature illustrated. Written descriptions, especially those in the authoritative texts listed in References, are more helpful in expressing the spectrum of involvement in these conditions, but the terminology used is sometimes obscure. Syndrome diagnosis still relies heavily on the ability of the clinician to detect and correctly interpret physical and developmental findings and to recognize patterns in them.

The study of dysmorphic syndromes per se is important, since it can lead to a better understanding of the etiology and pathogenesis of birth defects. In addition, the recognition of a specific syndrome as the cause for a particular child's abnormalities permits much more accurate counseling for prognosis and recurrence risk and for direction of possible therapy. Unfortunately, several thousand malformation syndromes have been described, and more seem to be added daily. For this reason, there is little value in attempting to memorize the features of each disorder. Instead, the approach recommended in this book emphasizes recognition of individual clinical features which, combined with historical information and selected laboratory studies, can help determine the pattern of findings that may define a syndrome diagnosis. This process is outlined in the next chapter and is further explained in Chapter 5.

2

A Dysmorphologic Approach to the Child with Birth Defects

It has always been my habit to hide none of
my methods, either from my friend Watson or
from anyone who might take an intelligent
interest in them.
— "The Reigate Squires"

The process of dysmorphologic diagnosis employs the same tools used in all clinical diagnosis: the ability to obtain a meticulous history and perform a painstaking physical examination. The techniques differ only in focus from those used daily by every physician. A great deal of emphasis is placed on the family history and details of the pregnancy, while the physical examination is carried out with special attention to the relationships among structures and to some quite subtle physical clues. In addition, the dysmorphologist must be familiar with the basic principles of embryology and the wide range of normal physical variation.

A systematic approach makes the diagnostic process easier, more efficient, and more certain, but "system" does not imply "ritual." Every clinician develops his or her own style and sequence for physical examination and obtaining historical information. Likewise, each patient is different from every other, and any diagnostic scheme must be flexible enough to accommodate those differences without omitting important steps. Still, some common underlying principles can be defined to provide the framework for making a dysmorphologic diagnosis. The individual steps can be separated for purposes of discussion, but in practice they blend and overlap. Table 2.1 outlines these steps, which are discussed in detail below.

2.1. SUSPICION

Someone must bring the child with birth defects to the attention of the diagnostician. It is often important to know who first became suspicious that the child might not be entirely normal and what clues raised that concern. Perhaps it is not surprising that the majority of children seen in a dysmorphology clinic are first brought to the attention of a physician by the parents or a nurse in the newborn nursery. Parents are keen observers of their children and, of course, spend more time with them than does anyone else.

15

Table 2.1. Components of the Dysmorphologic Evaluation

Suspicion	Synthesis
Congenital abnormalities	"Pivotal" findings
Growth problems	Pattern recognition
Mental deficit	Comparison with known cases
	Personal experience
Analysis	Literature
History	
Pedigree	Confirmation
Family	Laboratory
Pregnancy	Clinical course
Birth	Birth of affected relatives
Health	
Growth	Intervention
Development	Treatment
Previous laboratory and X-ray studies	Counseling
Physical examination	Etiology
Anatomic regions	Prognosis
Organ systems	Recurrence risk
Measurements	
Photographs	Follow-up
Laboratory tests	Supportive counseling
X-ray studies	Testing of family members
Other	Surveillance for complications
Family investigations	Correction of diagnosis
Watchful waiting	Counseling for affected individual
	Complications
	Prognosis
	Reproductive options

2.1.1. Congenital Abnormalities

There seem to be three major categories of concern that bring children into the diagnostic process. The first is the presence of obvious major or multiple congenital abnormalities. Such children will have been seen by a pediatrician or other physician within hours of birth and usually will be referred for confirmation of that doctor's diagnostic impression, for identification of an unfamiliar pattern of abnormalities, or for help in deciding whether the outlook for survival justifies major surgical intervention or other heroic therapy.

At other times, a child simply "does not look right" to a physician or other health professional. There is often little that points to an obvious abnormality, but some physical features (most often the facial appearance) differ enough from those of other family members to raise concern.

2.1.2. Growth Problems

Growth deficit is another sign that may bring a child to the attention of the diagnostician. Small size at birth, disproportionate to gestational age, is frequently an important clue to prenatal dysmorphic processes, but more often, growth failure during the first months or years of life finally prompts referral to the dysmorphologist. In cases where growth is disproportionate, with, say, the trunk growing normally and the limbs growing slowly or the head increasing in size normally while the body and face lag behind, early referral is more likely, since parents and physicians become appropriately more concerned under these circumstances.

2.1.3. Mental Deficit

Finally, evidence of developmental delay or frank mental deficiency often prove to be the stimulus for diagnostic evaluation. In such cases, the parents and pediatrician may become more aware of minor congenital abnormalities or variants of normal, and these are seized upon as a possible "syndromic" explanation for the child's delay. Especially if such a referral takes place at an early age, there may be inappropriate concern over isolated or negligible birth defects, such as a single palmar crease on one hand.

Thus, a clear understanding of who is concerned and why provides the diagnostician a starting place for evaluation of the child. It is also important to learn at the outset what the parents have been told about their child's condition and what they expect from the diagnostic evaluation. Without this information, there is a risk of producing confusion or even alienating the parents or the referring professional.

2.2. ANALYSIS

Analysis entails breaking down something complex into its component parts. In dysmorphology, the "whole" is the diagnosis and the "parts" are the individual items of historical information and physical abnormality found in the specific patient (see Chapter 5). This is essentially a data-gathering stage, and it is vital not to jump to conclusions before all of the facts have been considered. Here, the importance of a systematic approach is paramount, since the number of pieces in the puzzle may be immense, and overlooking just a few of them may lead the examiner down an entirely erroneous path. Conversely, it is possible to gather so much information that the individual facts cannot be sorted out, and the forest is entirely obscured by the trees. A continuing exercise of judgment is required to recognize which information is likely to be useful, and this must be coupled with a willingness to go back to the source to gather further data if necessary.

Scrupulous record keeping is a necessity. Details of the history and physical examination should be recorded on the spot. A preprinted form such as the one shown in Appendix D is helpful both to keep the information in order and to prompt the examiner to include all pertinent facts.

2.2.1. History

A careful, thorough, and fully recorded history, complete with family pedigree, forms the foundation of the diagnostic process. The steps in obtaining such a history differ only in emphasis from those used in general pediatrics, but a complete review with some helpful special techniques is provided in Chapter 3.

If records are available from the referring source or from previous hospitalizations, copies should be made for inclusion in the patient's file. Birth records, growth charts, and the results of earlier laboratory and X-ray studies are particularly helpful; if possible, these should be obtained and reviewed before the scheduled visit.

2.2.2. Physical Examination

The heart of the dysmorphology evaluation lies in the detection or confirmation of major and minor structural anomalies, and therefore the physical examination is of enormous importance. Once again, the basic techniques of physical diagnosis are used, but the examination is fine tuned to promote detection of many subtle physical clues that might otherwise be overlooked. The most helpful approach is to conduct the examination by *anatomic region* and then to return to any suspicious *organ systems* as the occasion warrants. An example would be the observation of abnormal fingernails during examination of the hand, prompting specific attention to other ectodermal structures such as hair and teeth. Chapter 4 addresses the physical examination of each anatomic region, which should be of help in tailoring the diagnostician's approach to the specialized needs of the dysmorphologic evaluation.

Selected *measurements* of physical features can be extremely useful in confirming a clinical impression of abnormality. Standard tables and graphs of age norms for many such physical dimensions are available in several of the sources listed in References, and techniques of measurement are outlined in the discussion of individual anatomic regions in Chapter 4.

With the parents' permission, *photographs* can be taken of the patient, which often prove to be of great value. An instant photo can be placed in the chart as a memory aid for later review; more formal photographs of the face, hands, or other areas of interest are useful for comparison with illustrations of known syndrome diagnoses and for monitoring the patient's progress over time.

2.2.3. Laboratory Studies

First, a distinction should be made between tests required to make a diagnosis and those needed to guide therapy. A patient may have an acute or chronic illness that is entirely incidental to any dysmorphologic condition present. An inflamed throat usually must be cultured regardless of the child's underlying diagnosis, and the presence of a significant heart murmur demands a chest X-ray and electrocardiogram and perhaps more sophisticated tests to define the nature and severity of the heart lesion.

A large proportion of children seen in the dysmorphology clinic do not require any specialized laboratory or radiologic testing at all, but there are a few instances in which the diagnosis depends on (or cannot be confirmed without) appropriate studies.

A full chromosome *karyotype* usually is requested in one of two situations: for confirmation of the clinical impression of a known chromosomal syndrome, or in the case of an unrecognized pattern of multiple congenital anomalies. Abnormalities of three different organ systems, together with development delay and growth retardation, strongly suggest a chromosome aberration. About 15% of children with such a constellation of features are found to have abnormal karyotypes, often in the form of chromosomal deletions, translocations, or mosaicism. Most of these conditions are extremely rare, but if cases with similar karyotypes have been reported, their clinical course can provide valuable prognostic information. Occasionally, this testing may lead to discovery of a balanced chromosomal rearrangement carried by one of the parents, which can be of immense significance for reproductive counseling. Such carrier states are quite uncommon, however, and the value of chromosome studies must be weighed against their considerable cost.

Newer techniques of chromosome analysis have been developed to provide more precise information about chromosome structure. *Prometaphase banding* can reveal small deletions or translocations undetectable on routine banded karyotypes. The culture medium also can be manipulated during leukocyte incubation to increase *chromosome fragility,* permitting identification of clinically significant fragile sites.

A *buccal smear* stained for sex chromatin was used in the past for rapid determination of chromosomal sex and for initial screening for a girl with the Turner-Noonan phenotype or for a boy with stigmata suggesting multiple-XY syndrome. Because interpretation of this test is sometimes difficult, it has been supplanted almost entirely by more reliable lymphocyte karyotyping. When used, a buccal smear is helpful only when the diagnostic question concerns a numerical abnormality of the sex chromosomes; it has no value in detecting other chromosome aberrations.

Amino acid analysis, lysosomal enzyme studies, and other tests for inborn errors of metabolism should be reserved for cases in which a child shows physical features or a clinical course compatible with one of those diagnoses. They have no place as general screening tests for children with birth defects. For example, a newborn with polydactyly or abnormalities of the external ear is not a candidate for testing for metabolic disease, since such disorders are not known to produce these types of structural anomalies.

2.2.4. X-Ray and Special Studies

The value of radiography in dysmorphology also lies in its guided use. Radiographs are particularly helpful in evaluating children with short stature or bone abnormalities. The final diagnosis of a generalized skeletal dysplasia, for instance, often depends entirely on the radiologic appearance of the bones. When such a disorder is suspected, a *skeletal survey* should be done to evaluate bone structure in several areas of the body. Appropriate films might include anterior-posterior (AP) views of one arm and one leg, PA films of one hand and wrist, and AP and lateral views of the pelvis and spine. To these may be added AP and lateral skull radiographs, if indicated. In newborn babies and young infants, a single X-ray of the whole body on one film (a "babygram") often suffices to detect or rule out skeletal anomalies.

Estimation of *bone age* is another frequently used and valuable technique in the assessment of patients with growth discrepancies. This is done by comparing the apparent maturity of the patient's skeleton, as reflected in the sequential appearance of epiphyseal growth centers, with standards for chronological age. *Skull films* are a fundamental part of the evaluation for craniosynostosis, microcephaly, and other abnormalities involving the cranium, and specific X-ray examination of the limbs and other structures sometimes is of diagnostic value. As with the laboratory tests mentioned above, however, there is seldom justification for screening X-rays.

More specific and sophisticated radiologic studies may be required in special cases: *bone density measurements, estimation of the metacarpophalangeal ratios,* or *tomograms* of the facial bones are valuable in some instances.

A number of advanced noninvasive imaging techniques are becoming available, and many are being applied with great success to the diagnosis of birth defects. Among the most useful are the following:

- *CAT scans*—Especially valuable for intracranial fluid collections and calcifications.
- *Ultrasonography*—Used to evaluate hydrocephalus in the newborn and gross structure of the heart and kidneys.
- *Magnetic resonance imaging*—Provides exceptionally clear and detailed pictures of soft tissues.

Similarly, considerable progress is being made in new types of testing for neuromotor and sensory function.

- *Visual evoked response studies*—Useful for determining functional integrity of the retina and optic pathway.
- *Brainstem auditory evoked potential*—Permits testing of the hearing apparatus and auditory pathway even in children too young to respond to standard hearing tests.
- *Electromyography and nerve conduction studies*—Yield information concerning the integrity and functional capacity of the neuromotor unit.

Other new technologies will surely be developed to aid in confirmation of dysmorphologic diagnoses, but for the foreseeable future, their value will continue to be supportive to the clinical and deductive skills of the diagnostician.

2.2.5. Other Diagnostic Aids

In contrast with other areas of clinical medicine, dysmorphology occasionally uses one or two special diagnostic methods that may be helpful or even indispensable in achieving an accurate diagnosis. They are not always appropriate but sometimes provide the only means to clarify a diagnosis.

2.2.5.1. Family Investigations

Many inherited disorders share common features, and the final discrimination between two similar genetic conditions may depend on the detection of other affected family members. For example, both autosomal dominant and autosomal recessive forms of Robinow syndrome have been reported, and the two types are not easily distinguished clinically. In an isolated case, it would be impossible to offer accurate genetic counseling without the additional information provided by the occurrence of the same pattern of abnormalities in a relative.

At other times, it is necessary to examine close relatives of the patient to determine whether certain physical features may be occurring as isolated anomalies or variants within the family. The pedigree in Fig. 3.3 shows a family in which independent inheritance of a number of minor structural abnormalities created the erroneous impression of a birth defect "syndrome" in the proband.

Finally, family studies may be necessary to allow meaningful genetic counseling in instances of chromosome rearrangement in which one parent may be a balanced carrier or when an autosomal dominant condition is not fully penetrant. The family whose pedigree is shown in Fig. 3.2 carries such a gene, which was present in the father but had produced no effects in him. Only examination of the paternal grandparents allowed the determination that his risk for further affected offspring was 1 : 2 rather than the 1 : 40,000 figure that would have been quoted for a "new mutation."

2.2.5.2. Watchful Waiting

A second diagnostic procedure not often used in other disciplines simply involves waiting for further developments. This approach may seem negligent or callous, but in some instances it is both necessary and practical. The value of watchful waiting is based on two premises: development is by nature a sequential process, and some dysmorphic syndromes have a progressive course.

For example, a definitive diagnosis may not be possible for a 3-month-old girl who has hypotonia and a relatively small head circumference. With a full explanation to the parents, the diagnostician might choose to watch her progress for a period of several months. If her muscle tone gradually increases beyond normal to hypertonicity and her gross motor progress begins to lag behind her social skills, the most likely diagnosis may be prenatal brain damage. On the other hand, persistence of her hypotonia, with increasing appetite eventually leading to obesity, would strongly suggest the presence of Prader-Willi syndrome. The prognosis and therapeutic recommendations for the child, and counseling for the parents, would be quite different for these two conditions and would justify deferring the final diagnosis. Of course, the parents must be fully informed of the reason for postponing judgment concerning their child's condition and reassured that every effort will be made to attain an exact diagnosis as soon as possible. Furthermore, any specific therapy that is indicated should be provided as soon as its need becomes apparent. With these precautions, the "second look" may be the best and sometimes the only reasonable approach to a child with an unrecognized disorder.

2.3. SYNTHESIS AND CONFIRMATION

Ideally, the steps of synthesis and confirmation culminate the dysmorphologic evaluation with the achievement of a final diagnosis that incorporates and explains all pertinent facts obtained during the analysis phase. Clinical judgment, experience, and a knowledge of the literature in dysmorphology all play a part in this process, which is discussed in detail in Chapter 5.

2.4. INTERVENTION

The ultimate goal of all that has gone before is to help the patient and the family. Unfortunately, most birth defects are irreversible, some are untreatable, and a few are inevitably fatal. Nevertheless, the dysmorphologist can always provide some assistance, if not in the form of treatment, at least in emotional support and, often, relief of feelings of guilt or blame in the parents. When a specific diagnosis has been achieved, information about etiology, prognosis, and estimation of recurrence risk can be given. The scope of this book does not permit a thorough treatment of these issues, but several excellent texts with sections on genetic counseling are listed in References.

2.5. FOLLOW-UP

Clearly, the provision of an accurate diagnosis is only the first step in the long process of care for a child with congenital abnormalities, and the dysmorphologist may have a continuing role in working with the patient and the family. Sometimes the initial diagnosis is simply wrong or must be deferred (see Section 2.2.5.2), and reevaluation for diagnostic purposes may be necessary. At other times, the discovery of a genetic disease in the proband mandates examination of other family members who may be at risk. Further counseling for the patient, the parents, or other relatives may require follow-up visits. Finally, the dysmorphologist may be in the best position to maintain surveillance for the development of possible complications and may be the first to learn of new scientific developments of importance to his or her patients. For all of these reasons, it may be necessary to maintain contact with the patient and family for months or years after the initial diagnostic evaluation and to provide guidance for further testing or therapy in conjunction with the patient's primary physician.

The topic of continuing care for children with birth defects is enormously important but, once again, falls outside the scope of this book. Many texts and monographs that address various aspects of this subject are available, but there is at present no single source of specific information concerning the long-term care of individuals with a wide range of birth defect syndromes and genetic diseases.

3

Obtaining a Dysmorphologic History

It is a capital mistake to theorize before one
has data. Insensibly one begins to twist facts to
suit theories, instead of theories to suit facts.
—"A Scandal in Bohemia"

Every physician learns to take a thorough clinical history as the first step toward achieving a diagnosis. In dysmorphology, the same general rules of history taking apply, but the emphasis is somewhat different. This chapter discusses the rationale for these differences and reviews the process of obtaining diagnostically valuable data from the medical interview.

3.1. GENERAL PRINCIPLES

3.1.1. Interviewing Techniques

In dysmorphology, as in all of pediatrics, the medical history is obtained primarily from the parents (or other caretakers) of the affected child. Some older children or adult patients, however, can provide important details from their own recollection. When other relatives are present during the interview, they may also contribute useful information, especially concerning the health of the extended family. The best rule is to accept and record information from any source; it can be sifted and interpreted later.

Providing a detailed history is an unfamiliar and rather taxing exercise for many families, and every effort should be made to put the parents at ease and to make them as comfortable as possible. Needed are a private room or other quiet, secluded setting, comfortable chairs, plenty of time (at least 30 minutes), and a receptive atmosphere. Younger patients and siblings will soon become bored and restless during a long interview, and it often helps to provide a few playthings or, as a last resort, ask a family member to babysit a child in another room.

Listening is the prime responsibility in taking a history, but the hardest task is to listen actively: to allow people to tell their stories in their own words yet still obtain the needed information. Ideally, the questioner should only suggest topics and generally guide the interview. Some of the specific facts required for dysmorphologic diagnosis are rather obscure, however, and must be sought by asking direct questions. Questions also may be asked to clarify or amplify certain points, but interruptions should be kept to a minimum.

If the interview becomes a quiz session, the only answers obtained will be those to questions the interviewer thought to ask. On the other hand, a parent's undirected stream-of-consciousness monologue is likely to omit or gloss over pertinent facts. The middle ground is best.

It is usually necessary to take notes during the interview, but the examiner should try to maintain eye contact and must not let writing take priority over listening.

Try to refer to the patient by name as often as possible. Of course, terms such as "he," "she," or "the baby" can be used, but even the youngest infant is *never* an "it."

At the very beginning, the parents should be asked about their understanding of the child's problems and what they have been told by others. This information is important in two respects: first, it helps the examiner avoid confusing or even alienating the parents by flatly contradicting their assumptions; second, it allows a rough estimate of the family's level of medical sophistication, to guide later discussion and explanation. The goal is to achieve the best possible basis for common understanding between physician and family. This is especially vital in regard to technical terms or colloquialisms that might come up during the interview. Unless everyone has the same idea about the meaning of words such as *echocardiogram* or *brain damage,* miscommunication is sure to result.

The historical interview has one other important but often unstated function: developing trust. While the examiner learns about the patient and the family, the parents are getting to know the examiner. In this unconscious "sizing up" process, the parents make judgments concerning the interviewer's knowledge, patience, and compassion. (Someone once said, "No one cares how much you know until they know how much you care.") If a sense of trust and mutual respect is generated in the first few minutes of the interview, the groundwork is laid for a working partnership to address the child's problems.

3.1.2. Obstacles to Obtaining a Dysmorphologic History

Some of the impediments to gathering an adequate dysmorphology history are obvious but common: too little time for the interview or an impatient attitude, the use of medical jargon by the examiner, a distracting setting (only the most cursory history can be obtained at the patient's bedside), or questioning that is too directed. All of these factors are, or should be subject to correction by the interviewer.

Subtler and harder to deal with are the emotional obstacles that are often raised after the birth of a "defective" child. By definition, dysmorphic abnormalities are evidence that something has gone wrong, and this inevitably produces feelings of anger, shame, guilt, and denial in the parents. These emotions can interfere with their ability to recall and communicate important facts. Sometimes the interviewer also may have to deal with his or her own feelings of discouragement or even revulsion over the child's condition and an accompanying reluctance to "bother" the parents. The detailed questioning involved in obtaining a medical history may strike some parents (and, indeed, some examiners) as painful or intrusive. Nevertheless, the ultimate goal of providing an explanation for the anomalies both justifies and necessitates a thorough investigation of the history, and every effort must be put forth to make the process as productive and painless as possible.

Much depends on the attitude and approach of the interviewer and on the development of a sense of trust and mutual concern. The parents may be expecting to hear more bad news or to be blamed for the child's problems. They may also be worried that they will not know the answer to some critical question or that some hidden fault will be found in the family tree. All of these concerns can be put to rest if the interviewer provides consistent support for the parents and makes clear that the purpose of the interview is simply to gather information, not to make judgments. The examiner is enlisting the parents' assistance in solving a mystery; they are expert witnesses, not defendants.

Rarely, emotional conflicts sparked by the birth of a dysmorphic child may separate family members into two opposing camps. Often, one parent blames the other for the child's problems, or the extended family blames both parents, or the grandparents deny that the child has any abnormalities whatever. Under such circumstances, gathering an adequate history may be very difficult, since important information may be withheld or distorted. When family dynamics of this kind are found or suspected, the interviewer must make a special effort to remain accepting and nonjudgmental. Taking sides is always counterproductive. The emphasis should be firmly fixed on obtaining the needed information in an objective fashion, for the benefit of the patient.

Specific questions about causation often arise early in the interview, and sometimes they can be addressed immediately. ("I can understand the concern that your automobile accident had something to do with Sean's problems. As a matter of fact, the cleft lip had already occurred well before that time.") As a rule, however, it is best to reserve such explanations for the end of the evaluation, when all available facts are at hand. Even the most anxious parents usually understand that some questions cannot be answered intelligently until the evaluation is completed. They simply should be reassured that there will be plenty of time then for a complete discussion of their concerns.

When it is necessary to obtain information from the parents of a critically ill newborn infant, a special approach is called for. The parents will be shocked and bewildered by their baby's unexpected problems, and the examiner must be especially gentle, considerate, and supportive. In such cases, the interview should be kept as brief as possible or divided into several short sessions, if necessary, so that the parents can spend more time with the baby. It is often helpful to reverse the usual order of events and examine the child first. This approach permits the physician to provide the parents at least some information about their baby, and this may allow the parents to direct their attention more fully to the necessary questions that follow.

3.1.3. Sequence of Obtaining the History

Within the limits imposed by the admonition to listen first, there are advantages in following a systematic approach to obtaining the history so as not to miss anything of significance but avoid prolonging the interview unnecessarily. On occasion, of course, it may be necessary to change the sequence or return to an earlier topic for clarification or further information. Beginning with the family history provides an opportunity for the examiner to indicate interest in the people involved and not just in the child's abnormalities. This approach also seems to give the parents a comfortable and usually neutral starting place for the history-taking process. The sequence of topics then follows naturally along the lines described in the next section. The best way to end the historical portion of the evaluation is simply to indicate to the parents that it is now time to examine the child.

3.2. CONTENTS OF THE DYSMORPHOLOGIC HISTORY

This section outlines the general subject matter of a dysmorphologic history. Under each subheading are listed several questions as examples of ways to elicit pertinent information. Of course, these categories and questions are meant to be neither rigid nor exhaustive, and the history taker will immediately tailor them to his or her own style and the needs of the moment. However, the items listed have proven to be important in most instances, and some approximation of this data base should be obtained for every patient.

3.2.1. Outside Records

A great deal of valuable historical data can be obtained from existing medical records and the results of earlier evaluations. Obtaining such information is especially important with respect to matters about which the parents cannot be expected to have detailed information, such as results of prenatal diagnostic testing, medical birth history, growth and development milestones, and laboratory and X-ray results. Whenever possible, such records should be obtained for review before the time of the first contact with the family. In any event, they should be studied before a final diagnosis is put forth or definitive counseling is offered. Review of outside records will at the least prevent redundant testing and occasionally will provide information that materially aids in defining the diagnosis.

3.2.2. Family History

The most practical method of recording a family history is by constructing a *pedigree*. This is simply a schematic diagram of the family, providing a graphic depiction of the relationships among family members and a brief summary of any conditions that might be of genetic significance. The main virtues of a pedigree are its easy interpretation and compact format; its major drawback is the confusion that may be caused by the use of obscure symbols. Several systems of pedigree recording have been devised, using a variety of icons and charting protocols. The symbols shown in Fig. 3.1 have gained widespread acceptance in the United States. Whatever system is chosen, it should be used consistently, with clear labeling and a legend to explain the symbols used, even at the rough-draft stage (Fig. 3.2). A pedigree to be included in a formal evaluation report or publication can be "cleaned up" and redrawn using a simple plastic template. This not only improves its appearance, but also makes the information easier to interpret.

Any family members with abnormalities similar to those seen in the patient should be examined if possible. Most such anomalies will be found to be familial *normal variants* and thus can be excluded from consideration. Some autosomal dominant conditions, however, can show a great deal of variability between one affected individual and another, and mild cases may remain asymptomatic and undiagnosed. This *variable expressivity* has significant implications for genetic counseling. In Waardenburg syndrome, for example, a parent may show only telecanthus and early graying of the hair, while her offspring may have the complete pattern: telecanthus, sky-blue irides, deafness, and a white forelock. In such a case, the partial involvement of other family members may provide important clues both to the underlying diagnosis and to its mode of transmission, and recurrence risk assessment can be tailored accordingly. Occasionally, individuals who carry a mutant dominant gene show no abnormal features, but may have offspring in whom the gene pro-

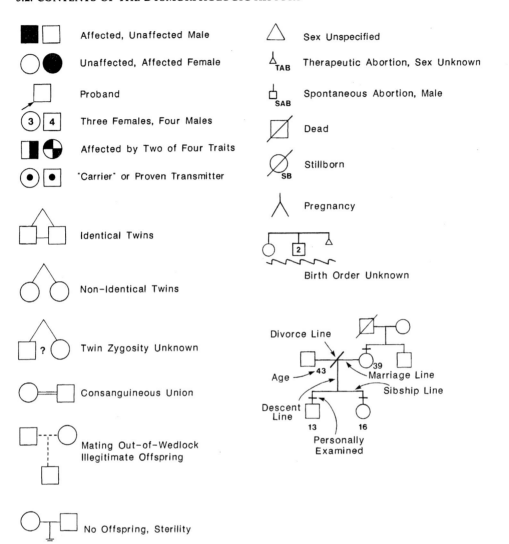

Figure 3.1. Standard pedigree symbols.

duces its characteristic effects. Pedigrees of such families are said to show **failure of penetrance** with the genetic disorder seeming to "skip" one or more generations (Fig. 3.3).

Sometimes, the presence of various features of the patient's phenotype in several relatives may point to the independent inheritance of the different anomalies or minor variants, often from both sides of the family. In such cases, the coincidental clustering of unrelated abnormalities usually is peculiar to one particular family rather than forming a syndrome as such (Fig. 3.2).

In obtaining a family history, it is important to ask about relatives with other abnormalities in addition to those displayed by the patient. In rare instances, these may represent malformations or diseases of genetic origin that bear directly upon the patient's problems. More commonly, it will be possible to reassure the parents about the incidental nature of such abnormalities, especially in distantly related family members.

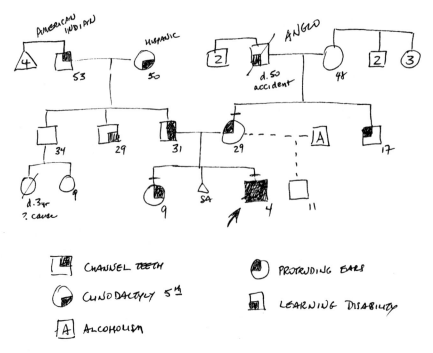

Figure 3.2. Rough-draft pedigree showing coincidental occurrence of multiple minor anomalies in a family.

Consanguinity implies that two people can trace their genetic lineage back to a common ancestor; i.e., they are blood relatives. The discovery of consanguinity between parents is of primary importance for conditions with an autosomal recessive genetic cause. The concern is that both parents may have inherited a single copy of the same mutant autosomal recessive gene. If each then contributes the mutant gene to their child, the "double dose" will cause a genetic disease. Clues to possible consanguinity include forebears with the same surname on both sides of the family, origin of the families in the same limited geographic area, or, occasionally, membership in a religious or ethnic group

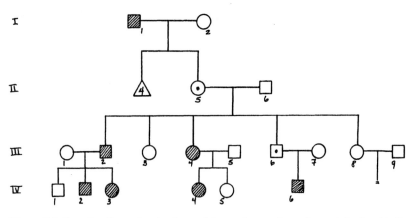

Figure 3.3. Formal pedigree showing incomplete penetrance of an autosomal dominant trait.

whose small size or established customs promotes some degree of inbreeding. Often, the most productive way to search for such risk of consanguinity is simply to ask the parents, "Is there any chance that the two of you are related to each other?" Alternatively, the question might be phrased, "Were there any people in your two families, even generations back, who had the same last name or came from the same town?"

Finally, it is important to include in the record an indication of the ethnic origins of the families. Inbreeding aside, some genetic conditions are much more prevalent in certain ethnic groups, and such information may provide a valuable clue to the diagnosis of these disorders.

3.2.3. Parental History

In addition to the general family history, specific information about the parents themselves should be sought. The points to be covered are listed below.

1. Age at conception of the propositus. Several chromosomal abnormalities are more frequent in the offspring of mothers over the age of 35, and new mutations for some autosomal dominant conditions are much more frequent in children born to older fathers. Furthermore, there is a small but significant increase in the risk for low birth weight, chromosomal abnormalities, and some other birth defects in children born to very young mothers.

2. Occupation of both parents. Although there is as yet no conclusive proof linking birth defects with particular occupations, information should be obtained about exposures to such suspected teratogens as ionizing radiation and certain organic chemicals and pesticides.

3. General health status. Inquiry should be made about the presence of any chronic disease in either parent and about any treatment being received, especially radiation therapy or drugs given to the mother during the pregnancy in question.

4. Outcome of previous pregnancies. A history of repeated spontaneous abortions or stillbirths may indicate an occult chromosomal or genetic cause. Impaired fertility may also be a clue to such conditions. Information about living children will have been obtained as part of the family history, but if any pregnancies have been lost or any children have died at an early age, further inquiry is in order. Special attention should be paid to any congenital anomalies found in abortuses or stillborns and to the age and cause of death in older children. When available, autopsy reports and other records can be of great value.

3.2.4. Pregnancy History

Every effort should be made to obtain complete information about the gestation leading to the birth of the affected child. After the birth of a baby with congenital abnormalities, parental recall may be slanted toward remembering events that they feel might have been responsible for the problems. Sometimes this selective memory obscures facts that may not have seemed important but bear more relation to the actual etiology of the abnormality. Therefore, it is best to use a consistent and systematic approach to obtaining this part of the history. It is also helpful to ask at each step how the occurrences during the pregnancy in question compared with those in any previous pregnancies. This portion of the history can conveniently be divided into two sections: maternal factors and fetal factors.

3.2.4.1. Maternal Factors

1. Nutrition. Did the mother engage in any fad diets or other alterations in her usual eating patterns? Were prenatal vitamins taken? Did prolonged morning sickness interfere with food intake?

2. Weight gain. Did the mother achieve a weight gain appropriate for the length of gestation? Was there any period of excessive or deficient gain?

3. Gestational timing. Was this a full-term pregnancy? Was the estimated date of confinement based on menstrual timing, estimated uterine size, or specific testing (fetal ultrasound or amniotic fluid analysis)?

4. Teratogenic exposure. Were any drugs taken during the pregnancy? (Note should be made of any prescribed or illicit drug use, with an estimate of the gestational timing and duration of exposure.) Did the mother drink alcohol during the pregnancy? (Try to obtain an estimate of the amount and frequency of alcohol use.) Did she smoke cigarettes? Were there any exposures to toxic substances, chemicals, or radiation? Was she in contact with children or others with apparent viral diseases?

5. Complications. Did the mother suffer any illness during this pregnancy? Was there any evidence of infection or unexplained high fever? Did vaginal bleeding or leakage of amniotic fluid occur? Was there premature rupture of the fetal membranes or early onset of labor? Was amniocentesis or chorionic villus sampling performed because of advanced maternal age or for any other reason?

3.2.4.2. Fetal Factors

1. Growth. Did the baby seem to grow consistently throughout gestation, or was there concern about too slow or too rapid growth?

2. Fetal movement. When did the mother first feel the baby moving? Was the movement vigorous? Was there any point at which activity stopped or became unusually strong? Were the baby's movements always felt in just one part of the abdomen?

3.2.5. Birth History

Events surrounding the birth of the child may be critical, especially if there is a functional abnormality of the nervous system. Mental and motor deficits or visual and hearing defects may form part of a syndrome diagnosis, or they may be caused by hypoxemia, bleeding, or trauma during the birth process. Therefore, answers to questions such as the following are necessary.

1. Antepartum status. Was there any change in the baby's condition just before birth? Did fetal movement increase or decrease drastically? Was any special monitoring done? If so, did it show an abnormality or prompt a change in plans for the delivery?

2. Length of labor. How long was the labor? Were any drugs given to stimulate labor?

3. Mode of delivery. Did the baby come out head first? (If not, what was the presenting part?) If a cesarean section was done, what were the indications? Was there anything unusual about the delivery (prolapsed cord, placenta previa, placental abruption, multiple birth, etc.)? Was there any abnormality of the afterbirth or the umbilical cord?

4. Baby's condition at birth. Did the baby breathe and cry right away? Did his color seem normal? (If not, describe.) Did he seem to move normally?

5. Measurements. How much did the baby weigh at birth? Length? Head size?

6. Abnormalities. Did the nurses or doctors mention any physical abnormalities that the baby showed right at birth? Did the baby need extra oxygen or any special treatment immediately after birth?

3.2.6. Neonatal Status

Next, data about the child's progress during the first few weeks of life are gathered. Nursery records can be helpful, but most parents are quite well informed about this period of their baby's life. It is during this time that occult structural anomalies such as congenital heart disease may begin to produce problems, and the first signs of neurological damage may become evident.

1. Feeding. Were there any unusual problems in feeding? Did the baby have a good, strong suck? Was there an unusual amount of vomiting? Did he seem relaxed and content during and after feeding? Did he seem to get sweaty or turn blue while eating?

2. Weight gain. After the first 2 weeks, did she seem to gain weight steadily? Did she grow about as fast as expected?

3. Development. Did the baby move his arms and legs vigorously? Would he look at faces for a few moments? Did he seem to respond normally to loud sounds and bright light? What was his personality like? Placid, fussy, always hungry, always sleepy?

4. Complications. Were there any infections or other illnesses in the first few weeks of life? Did she have more (or longer-lasting) jaundice than expected? Were there any problems such as seizures, floppiness, breath-holding spells, or fever during this period? Did there seem to be any trouble with her urination or bowel movements?

3.2.7. Subsequent History

Finally, information is obtained about the child's course since infancy, along the lines of a standard pediatric history but again with a few special emphases.

1. General health. Is the child usually healthy? Have there been any unusual or prolonged illnesses? Does he suffer from repeated infections? Have there ever been any seizures? Has he been hospitalized for anything?

2. Growth. Has she been growing about normally in weight? How about height? Does she seem to be growing at about the same rate as her brothers and sisters? Has there ever been a time when she just seemed to stop growing for a while? Has she begun having periods yet? Are they regular?

3. Developmental progress. How does he seem to be doing in learning things? Do you remember how old he was when he first rolled over? Crawled? Pulled up on the furniture? When did he take his first steps? How old was he when he said his first word? How about putting two words together? Does he go to school now? What grade is he in? Does he need any special help in school? In what areas? How are his grades?

4. Behavior. Would you say your daughter is a quiet girl or a busy girl? Can she sit with a toy or watch television for 10 minutes or so? Does she have a lot of temper tantrums? Does she like to play with other kids, or is she a loner? Imagine for a moment that you don't know her: How old would you say she is?

5. *Special testing or therapy.* Has he ever had any special tests for intelligence (speech, vision, hearing)? Have any medical tests been done beyond the routine ones? Any X-rays, special blood tests, or anything that had to be done in the hospital? Has he had any operations? Does he see anyone for speech (physical, occupational) therapy or counseling?

6. *Wrap-up.* Is there anything else important that we haven't talked about?

3.3. A WORD OF ENCOURAGEMENT

On paper, the process of eliciting a dysmorphologic history seems terribly complicated, inordinately time consuming, and basically boring. Take heart; it need be none of these things. Obviously, not every question has to be asked about every child. A great deal of information will be provided spontaneously by the parents if they are given the chance to do so. Furthermore, the whole procedure becomes much more interesting and meaningful when it takes place in the context of a real patient. The time and effort invested in gathering a comprehensive history are richly rewarded by the rapport established with the family, not to mention the value of obtaining the information base essential for diagnosis and counseling.

4

The Physical Examination in Dysmorphology

The world is full of obvious things which
nobody by any chance ever observes.
—The Hound of the Baskervilles

Although the value of the medical history is immense, the physical examination forms the cornerstone of dysmorphologic diagnosis. Children with multiple birth defect syndromes may display a bewildering array of individual abnormalities that seem to defy analysis or even description. It is necessary first to detect and then to identify all of the various anomalies before they can be assembled into some meaningful diagnostic pattern. Furthermore, the terminology used to describe these structural defects may be obscure and unfamiliar, which hampers the search for related information in the literature.

The following chapter is intended to introduce the clinician to a broad sampling of congenital anomalies, both major and minor. Techniques for their detection are described, and their significance in dysmorphologic diagnosis is outlined. The most common or preferred terminology for each physical variant or abnormality is printed in boldface, while italics are used for normal anatomic features as well as secondary definitions and synonyms. (These typefaces are used only at the first occurrence of each term.)

The chapter is organized by anatomic zones, arranged roughly in the order of the usual physical examination. In each section, a brief discussion of the embryology of the region is followed by a description of its normal anatomy and clinical landmarks. Methods for examining each zone, including any specialized techniques and measurements which may prove useful, are then addressed.

Discussion of structural abnormalities in each section begins with *minor variants* that are often found in normal individuals but may have diagnostic significance in some instances. These are further subdivided into two groups: *spectrum variants,* which show a continuous range of variability, and *minor anomalies,* which are discrete and functionally insignificant malformations that also may vary in severity but represent real departures from normal anatomic development.

The effects of mechanical stress on developing structures as they apply to each anatomical zone are discussed in the subsections on *deformations* and *disruptions.* Although tissue *dysplasias* commonly affect a similar tissue type throughout the body, their manifestations may be more prominent and thus easier to detect in some regions than others. For this reason, a separate entry on this topic is included in each section. Finally, true *malformations*, intrinsic structural anomalies, are considered in detail.

This arrangement by anatomic zones is intended to help clinicians in their examinations of patients by consolidating all information on a particular body region in an easily accessible form.

4.1. SKULL

Abnormal skull conformation may result from intrinsic aberrations of cranial bone growth, deforming extrinsic forces, or abnormalities in the shape of the underlying brain. In early life, the calvarium grows in response to brain growth. The base of the skull and the facial skeleton (except the mandible) develop from cartilaginous models, and their growth is largely independent from that of the brain and calvarium.

In utero and for the first several weeks of life, the skull plates and their intervening sutures are remarkably pliable and can suffer considerable temporary deformation without permanent harm. This ensures continued protection of the brain during passage of the head through the birth canal. However, this malleability can also result in a variety of deformations in response to more prolonged or severe extrinsic mechanical forces.

4.1.1. Embryology and Development

The *neurocranium,* which surrounds and protects the brain, consists of two parts: the *calvarium* or (cranial vault) and the *skull base*. The calvarium is made up of convex plates of membranous bone that grow outward from symmetrically placed growth centers in the parietal, frontal, and occipital regions. These plates continue to enlarge by bone deposition at the periphery, narrowing the intervening space to form linear skull *sutures* between adjacent plates. These widen into the *fontanels* occupying the space between the rounded corners at the junction of three or more plates (Fig. 4.1.1).

The skull base is formed by the basilar part of the occipital bone, the ethmoid, sphenoid, and segments of the temporal bones. Unlike the calvarial plates, these structures grow from cartilaginous models (endochondral bone), and thus their size and shape can be affected by genetic conditions such as the chondrodystrophies that cause disordered growth of cartilage.

4.1.2. Anatomy and Landmarks

In early infancy, the cranium is somewhat more box shaped than in later life, largely because of the *parietal* and *frontal prominences* that mark the topological centers of the major cranial growth plates. The intervening sutures and fontanels provide useful landmarks for skull configuration (Fig. 4.1.1). The *metopic suture* is usually closed in the full-term neonate, but the *sagittal, coronal,* and *lambdoid sutures* are usually palpable. The *anterior fontanel* has the shape of a parallelogram, while the *posterior fontanel* may be triangular, depressed, or completely closed at the time of birth. The *mastoid fontanels* lie

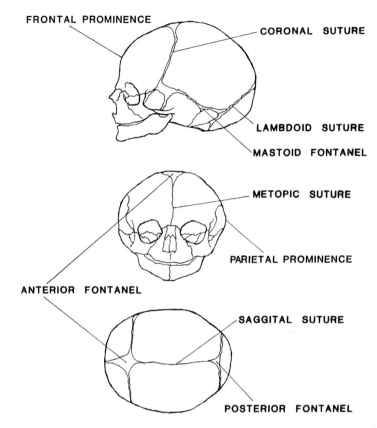

Figure 4.1.1. Skull configuration in the newborn, showing fontanels, sutures, and anatomic landmarks.

just behind the ears and are normally closed at birth, although a depression may be palpated over the site. The *brow ridges* are not well demarcated at this age, nor is the midline *occipital prominence* or *inion.*

With completion of the most rapid period of extrauterine brain growth at about 2 years, the calvarium assumes the typical ovoid shape, and the usual bony prominences of the adult skull begin to appear. Useful clinical landmarks include the *nasion,* inion, *vertex,* and the *mastoid processes* (Fig. 4.1.2).

4.1.3. Examination Techniques

Inspection of the skull for general conformation and symmetry should be done from directly overhead as well as from the front and side to permit detection of even minor degrees of asymmetry. At this stage, special attention should be paid to the contours of the frontal and occipital zones and to the overall impression of proportions of the cranium to the facial features.

Palpation is especially important in young infants, when the patency and relationships of the sutures and fontanels can be ascertained. In newborns with large heads,

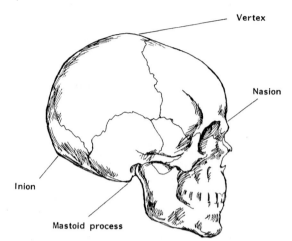

Figure 4.1.2. Mature skull showing bony landmarks.

bulging or increased resistance to compression over the fontanels should be assessed, and the width of the sutures should also be estimated. If a ridge is palpable along a suture line, it is important to try to determine whether it has the "clifflike" configuration of simple overlapping of the skull plates or the symmetrical "mountainlike" pattern associated with premature sutural fusion (Fig. 4.1.3A,B). The ridging produced by sutural overlap also extends much farther along the suture than that of *craniosynostosis,* which is often palpable over just 1 cm or less.

When one palpates the head of a newborn, gentle pressure should be applied with the fingertips, as when testing fruit for ripeness. A yielding, "ping-pong ball" consistency in a local area of the calvarium indicates the presence of *craniotabes,* a thinning of the skull vault usually caused by extrinsic pressure. Once this finding has been elicited, further

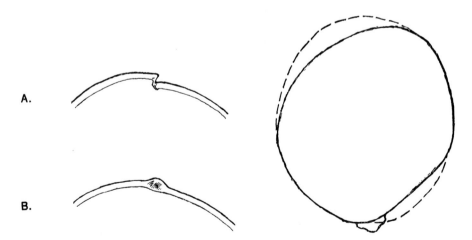

Figure 4.1.3. Localized skull abnormalities. (A) Cross section of overlapping sutures. (B) Cross section of zone of craniosynostosis. (C) Plagiocephaly seen from above. The dashed line indicates normal skull contours.

demonstrations should be avoided because it is possible to rupture small blood vessels on the surface of the brain by vigorous or repeated compressions.

Percussion of the skull can be a useful technique to determine whether sutural fusion has taken place. If the sutures are still open, gentle percussion or drumming of the fingers of one hand on the skull will produce a vibratory "cracked-pot" resonance detectable by the fingers of the other hand, resting lightly on the other side of the skull (MacEwen's sign).

In rare instances, auscultation of the skull is worthwhile, primarily to detect the bruit of an intracranial vascular abnormality.

The most important measurement of the skull is that of the *occipitofrontal circumference*. This is done with a flexible measuring tape, preferably one of metal or fiberglass, passing over the most prominent parts of the forehead and occiput. Care must be taken not to include an ear, a braid, or a barrette under the tape, which should be pulled just tightly enough to indent the skin of the forehead. Three measurements are taken by this method, with repositioning of the tape each time, and the largest value is recorded to the nearest millimeter.

In infants, the anterior fontanel can be measured in the usual AP and lateral axes, but this is sometimes difficult or misleading if the fontanels are wide. In such instances, measurement should be done along a diagonal axis, and values should be compared with published norms. A variety of other measurements of the skull have been used by structural anthropologists, but most of these have little relevance to the clinical examination.

4.1.4. Minor Variants

4.1.4.1. Spectrum Variants

The **general shape** of the skull varies somewhat among racial groups, ranging from the tall, boxlike cranium seen in the Nordic races to that of the American Indian, which tends to be wider than it is long. Of course, a spectrum of normal variation in skull configuration may be seen among individuals in any racial group. Regardless of the ratio of length to width, the normal values for head circumference still fall in the same range.

Very mild degrees of skull **asymmetry** can sometimes be seen in normal individuals, but more marked asymmetry may be caused by intrauterine deformation or unilateral craniosynostosis (see below).

At birth, **fontanel size** is quite variable. In the normal term newborn, the anterior fontanel may range from 1 to 5 cm in diagonal measurement, whereas the posterior fontanel may be from as much as 1 cm across to completely closed. However, the mastoid fontanels are never normally open after about gestational week 34, and their patency strongly suggests the presence of raised intracranial pressure. A **third fontanel** often appears as a widening of the sagittal suture near the junction of its middle and posterior thirds. This represents slightly slowed growth of the constituent plates of the parietal bones and can be distinguished easily from the posterior fontanel by its location and round or oval outline. Because bone growth is unusually slow in the area of the third fontanel, its size or patency may not reflect brain growth as do the other fontanels. For example, an easily palpable third fontanel may be present in neonates with severe microcephaly whose anterior and posterior fontanels are completely closed.

The presence of **wide sutures** may be a sign of increased intracranial pressure or of abnormally slow membranous bone growth. Either of these effects may be transient, and in newborns, separation of the calvarial plates by 2–5 mm has no more significance than the normal variability in size of the anterior fontanel. If the sutures remain wide beyond the first postnatal month, however, a pathological cause may be present.

4.1.4.2. Minor Anomalies

Because of the largely passive nature of skull development, only a small number of intrinsic minor anomalies has been described. Among these are **parietal foramina,** rounded defects that lie close to the center of the parietal bones at the site of the parietal emissary veins. Ranging in size from 1 mm to 3–4 cm, these anomalies are usually bilateral and sometimes appear as multiple bone defects. Even large parietal foramina are usually not symptomatic, but they may cause concern in infancy because of bulging (and sometimes pulsation) of the overlying scalp. By 3 years of age, the defects may still be palpable but have usually reached their final size and are no longer pulsatile.

Another example of minor intrinsic abnormality of the bones of the skull is *localized hyperostosis.* The two most common forms are **frontal bossing** and **parietal bossing.** In both, there is a symmetric buildup of bone forming a low dome that resembles the boss on a shield. In the case of parietal bossing, these mounds form over the greatest convexity of the parietal bones; in the case of frontal bossing, the prominences are seen over the forehead on either side of the midline, almost vertically above the orbits. Frontal bossing should be differentiated from simple **prominence of the forehead,** in which the entire brow bulges forward but no distinct bony mounds are seen. Parietal bossing is often seen with *trigonocephaly* (see below).

The appearance of an unusually **short** or **tall forehead** simply is judged by the vertical distance between the brow ridge and the top of the head. Considerable racial and familial variation exists in this measurement, which may be further emphasized or obscured by a high or low anterior hairline (see Section 4.16). A **sloping forehead** also may appear short; however, a severe backslant usually signifies hypoplasia of the frontal lobes and is commonly associated with marked microcephaly.

4.1.5. Abnormalities

4.1.5.1. Deformations

The most common abnormalities of the skull are deformational in nature. A number of these conditions have their origin in the perinatal period, when strong but transient mechanical forces are applied to the fetal head. Most babies born from a vertex presentation show some degree of **molding** of the skull (Fig. 4.1.4A). The presenting portion of the head is usually the most prominent, reflecting the pressures applied by the bones and soft tissues of the maternal pelvis as the baby passed through the birth canal. If the head was retroflexed in utero, the skull will have a teardrop shape, with a prominent **occipital shelf** (Fig. 4.1.4B). Such babies frequently display a "position of comfort" in which the neck is held in extreme hyperextension.

Molding is usually accompanied by **overriding sutures:** the pressures exerted in the

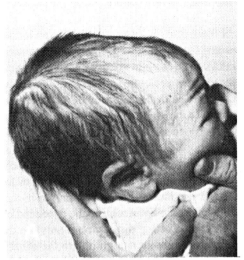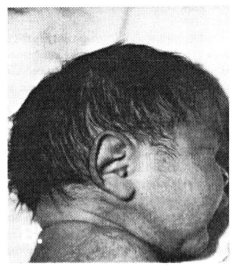

Figure 4.1.4. Skull molding in the neonate. (A) Elongated cranium with prominent occiput. (B) Breech head with prominent brow and occipital shelf.

birth canal force one skull plate up over its neighbor as far as is permitted by the connective tissue in the suture (Fig. 4.1.3A). This may be sufficient to create an impression of closed fontanels until the overlapping spontaneously corrects itself and may also make measurements of head circumference spuriously low. Overriding occurs most frequently in the sagittal suture, with the coronal and lambdoid sutures less often affected. Overlapping at the metopic suture is extremely rare, and ridging in this zone should suggest craniosynostosis (see below) until proven otherwise.

When the fetal head is engaged in the pelvis for a prolonged period before birth, deforming pressures may be directed along a diagonal axis. This can distort the skull in such a way that the transverse section resembles a parallelogram instead of a rectangle (Fig. 4.1.3C). Flattening over diagonally opposite corners of the head (e.g., left frontal and right parietooccipital zones) is called *asynclitism of the skull* or **plagiocephaly.** In severe instances, asymmetry of the facial features and even disturbance of the visual axis of the eye on the affected side may be seen (see Section 4.2).

Despite the striking appearance produced by these deformations in the newborn, they are well-recognized and transient abnormalities that usually correct themselves in the first few weeks or months of life, since the deforming forces are no longer active. In occasional cases of severe plagiocephaly, however, restoration of normal cranial contours is very slow, and if little or no improvement is seen by the age of 4–6 months, intervention may be necessary.

The size of the skull is almost entirely dependent on the volume of its contents. The growth of the brain causes the calvarium to enlarge in a passive fashion, as if it were a rubber bathing cap. When we measure head circumference, we are really obtaining a rough estimate of brain size, and thus the conditions termed **microcephaly** and **mac-**

rocephaly might better be called *micrencephaly* and *macrencephaly,* signifying small or large brain.

During normal development, as the rate of brain growth slows, the skull is no longer under expansive stress, and the sutures narrow and eventually close. In a similar manner, bony fusion between two neighboring skull plates can be brought about by any mechanical force that allows their edges to remain in contact for a prolonged time. Thus, in severe microcephaly, the cessation of brain growth, coupled with normal growth of the cranial plates, produces **premature craniostenosis** of all sutures. In such cases, it should be noted that the small brain causes a small skull, not vice versa. Early sutural fusion does not "lock in" the brain so that it ceases to grow.

A different situation prevails when brain growth is normal but a bony bridge spans the gap between two cranial plates. In such a case, skull growth is impeded only in the direction PERPENDICULAR to the fused suture, and the brain, growing wherever it can, distorts the calvarium in characteristic ways. Such **craniosynostosis** can be produced by at least three mechanisms. The rarest are genetic causes acting directly (and only) on the integrity of the sutures themselves. Somewhat more common as a group are the genetic disorders such as Crouzon syndrome, which cause aberrant bone growth at the skull base. This leads to early fusion of the basilar sutures, with frequent involvement of the sutures of the cranial vault as well. Most common of all is premature fusion brought about by intrauterine constraint, where compression holds together the edges of opposing cranial plates, allowing premature fusion to take place.

Certain abnormal skull configurations are typical of premature craniosynostosis of specific sutures (Fig. 4.1.5). In **scaphocephaly** (*dolichocephaly*), the sagittal suture is involved, and the head assumes an elongated configuration in the AP axis. Bilateral coronal synostosis results in **brachycephaly,** broadening the skull with reduction of its AP diameter. Unilateral coronal fusion leads to plagiocephaly and also can produce progressive facial asymmetry (see Section 4.2). **Trigonocephaly** is a triangular head shape with a prowlike forehead, produced by stenosis of the metopic suture. **Turricephaly** is the tower-shaped skull caused by early fusion of the lambdoid, coronal, and metopic sutures in combination.

When multiple sutures are fused, bizarre distortions of the cranial vault can be seen. For example, several genetic syndromes show disordered bone growth and early fusion of sutures at the skull base, producing a characteristic facial appearance and *acrocephaly* of the skull (Fig. 4.1.6A). In the anomaly referred to as **Kleeblattschadel** or *cloverleaf skull* (Fig. 4.1.6B), all of the cranial sutures are prematurely fused and the brain is forced to grow through the anterior and temporal fontanels, which imparts a grossly abnormal appearance to the skull. In multiple-suture synostosis, prompt surgical intervention may prevent or ameliorate serious neurologic complications. Large portions of cranial bone, sometimes almost the entire cranium, are removed, and new bone regenerates from the dura within a period of weeks, often with intact sutures and fontanels.

4.1.5.2. Disruptions

Destruction of skull tissue may be seen in the *amniotic band* complex, in which the placenta sometimes adheres to the scalp or the bands themselves are stretched tight across the face and head (see Appendix C).

A much milder skull disruption, craniotabes, can be caused by localized direct pressure on the head during late intrauterine life. The source of such pressure may be a maternal uterine fibroid, the knee of a twin, or some other firm object impinging on the skull. Both tables of the calvarium are thinned in a zone ranging from about 3 to over 10 cm in diameter. The skull in this region is quite yielding and flexible to palpation (see Section 4.1.3), but the overlying scalp is usually intact.

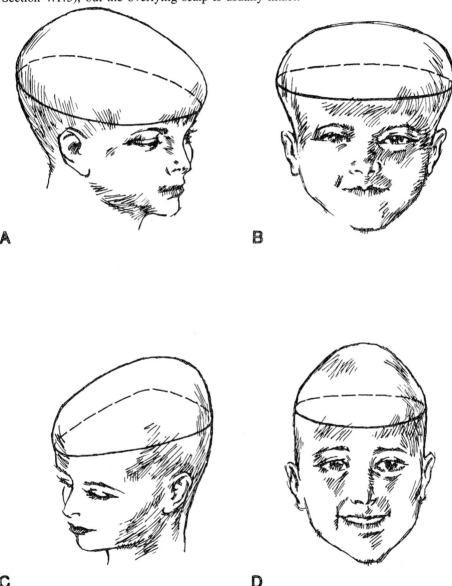

Figure 4.1.5. Characteristic skull shapes in craniosynostosis. (A) Scaphocephaly with sagittal suture fusion. (B) Brachycephaly from bilateral stenosis of the coronal sutures. (C) Trigonocephaly in premature closure of the metopic suture. (D) Turricephaly with coronal and lambdoid suture fusion.

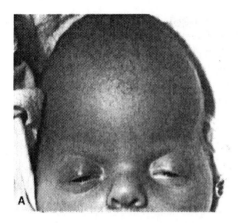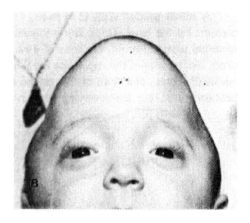

Figure 4.1.6. Effects of multiple-suture craniosynostosis on face and skull configuration. (A) Premature fusion of basilar skull sutures in Apert syndrome. Note bulging forehead, depressed nasal bridge, and downslanted palpebral fissures. (B) Synostosis of all cranial sutures. The brain is growing upward through the region of the anterior fontanel and laterally through the temporal fontanels (Kleeblattschadel).

4.1.5.3. Dysplasias

The bones of the skull may be involved in a number of generalized skeletal dysplasias, all of which are manifested by one of two clinical features: bony overgrowth or delayed closure of the fontanels. Excessive growth of the cranial bones is a relatively slow process and may be localized, producing signs such as parietal or frontal bossing. More widespread hyperplasia, with thickening of the entire skull, may cause gradual stenosis of neural canals, leading to deafness or blindness.

Slowed growth of the calvarial plates results in broad cranial sutures and large fontanels that may take years to fully close. Often, *wormian bones* form in the spaces between the skull plates and may be palpable as "islands" within the open fontanels. The cranium often assumes a bulbous shape, reminiscent of a lightbulb, and this together with the wide sutures often raises a suspicion of increased intracranial pressure, but other signs of central nervous system pathology are absent.

4.1.5.4. Malformations

Primary malformations of the skull are limited to those associated with incomplete neural tube closure. Isolated midline defects of cranial bone define the sites and size of *meningoceles* and *encephaloceles*. Total absence of the neurocranium is seen in *anencephaly*, in which the remaining disorganized rudiments of brain lie exposed to the exterior, unprotected by dura, skull, or scalp.

4.1.6. Summary

The bony calvarium is essentially a passive structure, and most of its congenital anomalies are deformations produced by extrinsic mechanical forces.

4.2. FACE—GENERAL

All of us spend a great deal of time observing the faces of people around us, but we often find it difficult to describe those characteristics which define a family resemblance or allow us to recognize a friend in a roomful of strangers. This is because myriad subtle differences in facial structures blend together to create an overall "gestalt" that we can identify without conscious effort. The contributions of individual facial features will be addressed in later sections; here we will examine the face as a whole, considering factors of proportion and overall configuration.

The physiognomists of the 19th century tried to link personality traits and behavior with particular facial characteristics, defining a "spiritual face," a "criminal face," and so on. Today these beliefs seem quaint, yet there are still some who would suggest that there are characteristic facies associated with mental deficiency or behavioral disorders. In fact, the variety of human faces seems almost endless, and neither mental ability, personality, nor social status defines the overall facial appearance.

4.2.1. Embryology and Development

The face is embryologically quite complex, made up of contributions from the neural crest, branchial arches, and mesodermal tissues. In general terms, the face is built up from paired lateral structures of branchial arch origin that fuse at the midline. These are sheathed by neural crest cells that migrate from their original positions over the first six to seven somites, coursing both laterally around the sides of the face and centrally over the forehead and down as far as the philtrum (Fig. 4.2.1).

Differential growth of the components of the facial skeleton lead to subtle differences in the size and relationship among the facial features, providing the wide variety of distinctive family and individual appearances that we take for granted.

4.2.2. Anatomy and Landmarks

In this section, only a few facial landmarks are necessary: in full frontal view, the brow ridges, *zygomatic arches,* and the *midfacial zone,* along with the facial proportions in length and width (Fig. 4.2.2); from the lateral aspect, the *external auditory meatus* and the *facial plane,* defined by the most prominent points of the brow ridges and the lower maxilla (Fig. 4.3.3A). The proportions of the face change with age. The forehead of the newborn baby occupies nearly half the height of the face, reflecting the large cranial

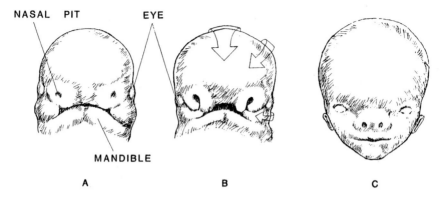

Figure 4.2.1. Early facial development. (A) Frontal view of embryonic face at about 4.5 weeks of gestation. The stomodeum is well defined. (B) Frontal view of 5 weeks of gestation. Mesenchymal tissue from the prechordal plate is migrating down over the frontal process, while neural crest cells are moving into the region laterally, above and below the eye. The median and lateral nasal processes are beginning to coalesce with the maxillary process. (C) Face of a 10-week fetus.

volume necessary to accommodate the rapidly growing brain. Throughout childhood, growth of the midface, maxilla, and mandible outstrips that of the upper face; by adult life, the brow accounts for just one-third of the height of the facial profile. Furthermore, the facial features become more sharply sculptured with increasing age, and both of these phenomena must be taken into consideration when judging *facial maturity*.

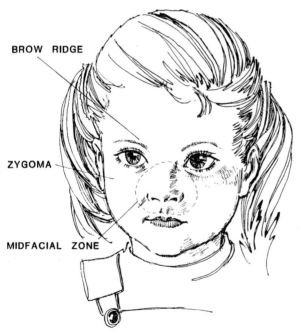

Figure 4.2.2. Face showing clinical landmarks.

4.2.3. Examination Techniques

Inspection is really the only mode of examination applicable to the overall evaluation of facial structure and proportion. It is important, however, to distinguish between a general gestalt of abnormal facial appearance and specific abnormalities of individual facial features. Terms such as "syndrome facies" or "funny-looking face" are not helpful, and an effort must be made to define the unusual appearance as clearly as possible to aid later considerations of possible diagnoses.

The face should be inspected from several directions during the course of the exam, since some relationships among the various facial features can be better appreciated from a particular viewpoint. For example, the impression of a prominent forehead in the full-face view can best be confirmed by observation from the side, and facial asymmetry is often appreciated better when the patient's head is tilted far back so that the examiner has a tangential view of the face from below.

Attention should also be directed toward abnormalities of *facial expression* during the examination (see Section 4.21). Older patients should be asked to smile, close their eyes tightly, and wrinkle their brows; infants are observed at rest and while crying.

4.2.4. Minor Variants

Normal variation in the general appearance of the face is almost impossible to define because the spectrum is so broad. For purposes of dysmorphologic diagnosis, perhaps the most important consideration is whether the patient's face resembles that of other members of the family. (This gives a whole new meaning to the phrase "relative facial abnormality.") Hence, when a patient has an unusual general facial appearance, it is vital to examine other family members, especially the parents. Conversely, a striking underlying family characteristic may obscure the typical facies of a specific syndrome diagnosis, as when the inheritance of a broad, flat face is accompanied by myopathic disease that normally would produce a marked facial narrowing, the combination resulting in a face of essentially "average" proportions.

A **broad face** is characteristic of some American Indian and Oriental groups and some black families, whereas some racial groups from the Mediterranean and Near East tend to have a **narrow face.**

A **pinched face** refers to an appearance of small facial features clustered close together. This certainly can be a familial trait, but when very severe it may suggest a diagnosis such as Hallermann-Streiff syndrome (Fig. 4.2.3A). Similarly, some normal individuals have faces that look older than their chronological age, often because of diminished subcutaneous fat, which reveals the contours of the facial skeleton. Carried to the extreme, such an appearance blends into the **prematurely aged** face seen in the progeria syndromes (Fig. 4.2.3B).

4.2.5. Abnormalities

4.2.5.1. Deformations

Facial asymmetry is the most common consequence of deforming forces acting on otherwise normal structures of the face. This may be caused by prolonged direct pressure

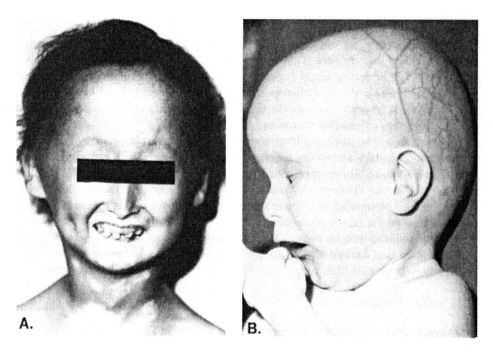

Figure 4.2.3. Generalized slow growth of facial features. (A) Small, pinched facies in Hallerman–Streiff syndrome. (B) Appearance of premature aging with slow facial growth in progeria syndrome.

in utero, where it usually will be associated with plagiocephaly (see Section 4.1) and can be expected to resolve gradually over the first 6–9 months of life. In contrast, asymmetry as a secondary result of premature fusion of the lower portion of one coronal suture will tend to worsen with time. This may become severe enough to offset the visual axis of one eye, leading to *amblyopia* (Fig. 4.2.4A). Failing this, the child may unconsciously tilt his head in order to keep the eyes in the same horizontal plane, and a muscular *torticollis* may develop. Rarely, a compensatory *scoliosis* can appear, completing the cascade of dysmorphic features derived from a single early developmental anomaly.

Prolonged intrauterine compression of the entire face, as when oligohydramnios permits the face to be pressed against the uterine wall, leads to **Potter facies.** Frequent findings in these circumstances include a flattened nose, vertical creases below the eyes, and large, floppy ears (Fig. 4.2.5A).

The muscles that attach to the facial skeleton help to mold its contours. When their activity is absent, intrinsic bone growth is unmodified, and an elongated, narrow **myopathic face** is the result (Fig. 4.2.5B). A somewhat similar facial configuration has been described in children with severe allergic rhinitis who are habitual mouth breathers. These **allergic facies** probably are produced by much the same mechanism of muscle imbalance, but in this case originating in the open-mouthed breathing position.

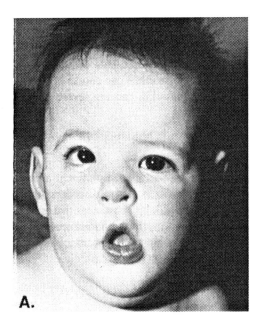
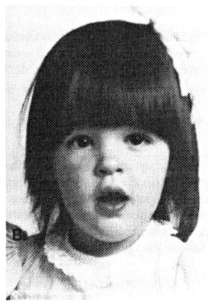

Figure 4.2.4. Facial deformation. (A) Facial asymmetry from premature synostosis of sphenotemporal suture at right cranial base. Note flattening of right cheek and temporal zone and upward deviation of right eye caused by distortion of the orbit. (B) The same child 18 months after corrective surgery, showing restitution of facial contours.

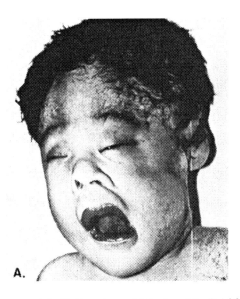
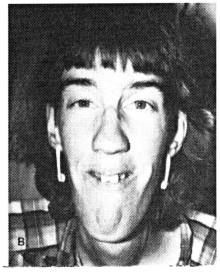

Figure 4.2.5. (A) Flattening and distortion of the facial features caused by prenatal constraint. (Photo courtesy of Dr. John Graham, Los Angeles, Calif., and Dr. Will Cochran, Boston, Mass. Reprinted by permission of Grune & Stratton, Inc., from Seminars in Perinatology, **7** (4):270–273.) (B) Narrow, elongated face seen in neuropathic disorders.

4.2.5.2. Disruptions

The **facial clefting** that results from swallowed amniotic bands often does not follow the normal planes of fusion of the embryonic face and thus represents destruction of previously normal tissue by extrinsic mechanical force. These clefts can course in almost any direction but often lead diagonally upward through the orbit, causing severe disruption of the eye (see Appendix C).

4.2.5.3. Dysplasias

A few dysplastic diseases affect the general facial appearance. Prominent among these are the storage diseases that produce **coarse facial features.** These disorders are all marked by the retention of large amounts of insoluble intracellular substances that gradually distend the skin and soft tissues of the face, forming a firm, thickened intracutaneous layer. This progressive coarsening eventually leads to a "pugilistic" appearance in such disorders as mucopolysaccharidosis type 1 (Hurler syndrome) (Fig. 4.2.6).

4.2.5.4. Malformations

In a number of conditions in which skeletal maturation is compromised, the patient retains a disproportionately **immature facial appearance** in relation to age. This is particularly striking in patients with panhypopituitarism or isolated growth hormone deficiency, and hormone administration, if begun in childhood, leads to a restoration of more normal facial proportions.

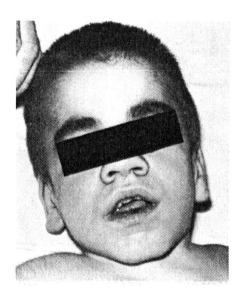

Figure 4.2.6. Generalized facial dysplasia. Coarse facial features in Hurler syndrome (mucopolysaccharidosis type 1).

Triangular facies is often the result of a disparity between the growth of the cranium, paced by normal brain growth, and the growth of the facial skeleton, whose bones may share in an intrinsic growth deficiency. Most chondrodystrophies do not affect the face in this way, but a few conditions, such as Silver syndrome, typically show such a pattern.

A **hypoplastic midface** is caused by inadequate growth of the central maxilla. In its extreme forms, this gives the face a "dished-in" appearance, and the mandible may seem prognathic in contrast. The nose also may be short or have a low bridge (see Section 4.6). In **lateral facial hypoplasia,** the malar eminence and zygoma are flattened, making the midface seem more prominent and producing a downward slant of the palpebral fissures (see Section 4.4).

4.2.6. Summary

The overall gestalt of facial appearance may be of considerable importance in dysmorphologic diagnosis, but due allowance must be made for the wide spectrum of normal variability and especially for family resemblance.

4.3. EARS

The external ear is a relatively simple structure but one with complex antecedents and a wide variety of normal and abnormal structural variations. Abnormalities of auricular configuration are mentioned as part of more than 100 syndrome diagnoses. Unfortunately, in most such conditions, ear anomalies are nonspecific, and their value in diagnosis is usually supportive rather than primary.

4.3.1. Embryology and Development

The external ear is formed from the six hillocks of His, which originate from zones of the first and second branchial arches surrounding the first branchial cleft. At about weeks 6–7 of gestation, these mounds of tissue begin to grow and coalesce while migrating laterally and upward from their original embryonic position near the midline below the mandible. The greater portion of the pinna is of second-arch origin, while the tragus and antitragus and the anterior wall of the auditory canal derive from the first branchial arch (Fig. 4.3.1). The auricle grows in response to both intrinsic and external stimuli and is one of the few body structures that continues to grow throughout life.

4.3.2. Anatomy and Landmarks

The cartilaginous framework of the pinna molds its surface into a convoluted pattern that has several consistent features (Fig. 4.3.2). The *helix* forms the outer border of the upper and posterior two-thirds of the pinna. The *helical root* begins at the upper insertion of the ear into the skin of the lateral head and swings down and back to blend with the floor of the *concha*. The *tragus* shields the entrance of the *external auditory canal* into the concha and is balanced by the *antitragus* lying just above the *lobe*. The sharp ridge of the

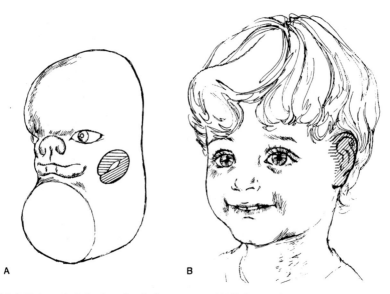

Figure 4.3.1. Embryonic derivation of auricular structures. (A) Embryo at 6 weeks, with schematic depiction of ear primordia. Horizontal shading indicates contribution of first branchial arch tissues; diagonal shading shows tissues of second branchial arch origin. (B) Fully formed ear, showing first-arch derivatives limited to tragus and helical insertion. The major portion of the pinna originates from tissues of the second branchial arch.

anthelix curves upward parallel to the posterior rim of the helix before branching into a prominent, almost horizontal *lower crus,* which ends under the helical root, and a rounded *upper crus,* which extends diagonally upward to support the upper curve of the helix.

4.3.3. Examination Techniques

4.3.3.1. Ear Placement

Ear position is best judged in relation to other landmarks of the head and face rather than by absolute measurements. A convenient technique is to view the face from the side,

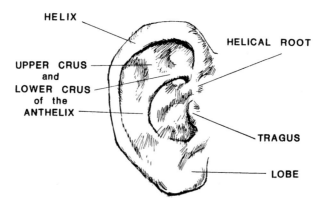

Figure 4.3.2. Normal anatomy and landmarks of the auricle.

visualizing a vertical plane touching the brow ridges above each eye and the most prominent point of the maxilla below the nose. A line perpendicular to this facial plane, passing
backward from the lateral canthus of the eye, normally should cut the insertion of the
auricle on the side of the head (Fig. 4.3.3A). Care must be taken in instances where
micrognathia or a receding or bulging forehead create the impression of a tilted facial
plane. Failure of complete migration of the ear anlage leads to **low-set ears,** whose
position can lie anywhere between the original midline location and a point just slightly
caudal to the normal site. Low-set ears are often posteriorly rotated as well, since the
process of migration and maturation of the embryonic tissues of the pinna involves a 90°
forward rotation of the auricle to its final position. The long axis of the pinna usually
makes an angle of approximately 15° with the vertical axis of the head (Fig. 4.3.4A). An
angle of more than about 20° should be recorded as **posterior rotation of the ear.**

In some cases, an optical illusion of low ear placement can be created by an unusually large cranial vault or by a small external ear. This effect is often seen in premature
infants with a skull flattened from side to side or in older children with hydrocephalus.

Angulation of the auricle away from the head can be seen from a position directly in
front of or behind the patient but is best judged by looking down from above the top of the
head. The ear normally makes an angle of about 15° with the side of the head (Fig.
4.3.4B).

4.3.3.2. Ear Size

Ear length is easily measured by using a transparent plastic ruler placed along the
longest axis of the pinna. Graphs of auricular size by age are found in several of the
sources given in References, allowing validation of clinical impressions of ear size. A

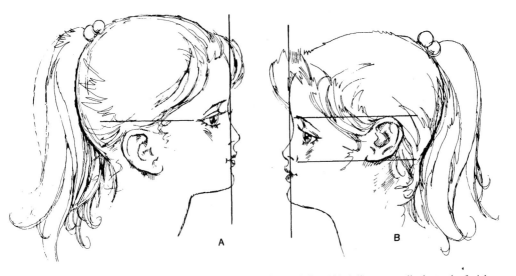

Figure 4.3.3. Methods for clinical assessment of ear position and size. (A) A line perpendicular to the facial
plane, passing backward at the level of the outer canthus of the eye, should intersect the root of the helix where it
joins the skin of the lateral scalp. This ear is low set and posteriorly rotated. (B) The upper and lower limits of the
pinna normally lie at the level of the eyebrow and the base of the alae nasi, respectively.

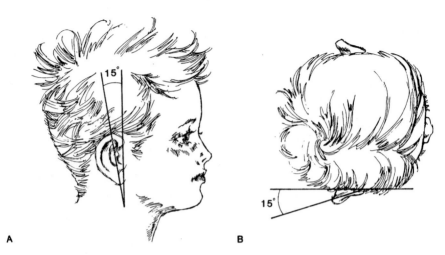

Figure 4.3.4. Angulation of the auricle. (A) The longest diameter of the ear usually is tilted back about 15° from the vertical plane of the head. (B) Similarly, the pinna protrudes at about a 15° angle from the side of the head in the horizontal plane.

quick estimate of the relation of the size of the ear to that of the other facial features can be obtained by using "artists' criteria." Imaginary lines perpendicular to the facial plane are drawn back from the lateral tip of the eyebrow and the junction of the alae nasi with the upper lip. These lines should bracket the entire pinna (Fig. 4.3.3B).

4.3.4. Minor Variants

A fairly wide range of structural variants of the auricle have been described; when found in isolation, they have no significance for hearing loss or other functional or structural problems. Many of these normal variants are familial, usually following a dominant inheritance pattern, and thus can serve as genetic markers. For this reason, examination of parents or other family members can often clarify the significance of minor deviations from the average in ear structure.

Preauricular pits and preauricular tags (Fig. 4.3.5) occur in about 0.5–1% of individuals, with wide variance in frequency among different racial groups. They are believed to represent remnants of early embryonic branchial cleft or arch structures.

Variations in the form of the helix are relatively common. An **overturned helix** often may be seen as a temporary deformation in the ear of newborn babies but sometimes is severe enough to persist as a permanent minor anomaly (Fig. 4.3.6A). The term **Mozart ear** refers to the attentuation and backward sweep of the upper helix said to have been present in the composer and his family (Fig. 4.3.6B). An accentuation of the usual slight irregularity of cartilage at the junction between the upper and posterior curve of the helix forms the **Darwinian tubercle** (Fig. 4.3.6C). Some irregularity of the curve of the helix may be seen, and sometimes this is severe enough to produce a truly **indented upper helix** (Fig. 4.3.6D).

The size and site of attachment of the ear lobes seems to be heritable: **unattached**

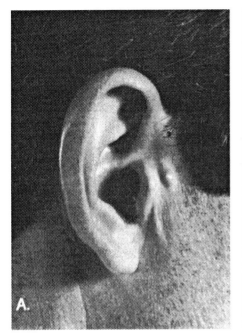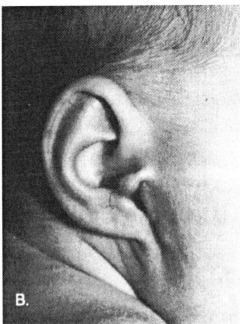

Figure 4.3.5. Preauricular pits and tags. (A) A small, blind skin pit at the insertion of the helix. Also present is a typical moundlike skin tag anterior to the tragus. (B) A larger, pedunculated preauricular tag. An associated cleft is seen between the tragus and the lobe of the ear.

lobes (Fig. 4.3.6E) are thought to be dominant to **attached lobes** (Fig. 4.3.6F), whereas **absent lobes** are distinct from both and inherited through a different autosomal dominant gene (Fig. 4.3.6D). **Creased earlobes** (Fig. 4.3.6G) are a feature of some rare syndromes, whereas **cleft** or **perforated ear lobes** (Fig. 4.3.6H) probably result from lack of complete fusion between the two most medial embryonic hillocks.

A very rare but quite striking developmental anomaly is **cryptotia,** in which the upper curve of the helix seems to be tucked up under a fold of normal skin on the lateral scalp (Fig. 4.3.7A). This condition does not appear to be familial and is not associated with hearing loss or any consistent abnormalities in other body systems.

4.3.5. Abnormalities

4.3.5.1. Deformations

Ear cartilage is both pliable and exposed and thus quite susceptible to deformation from extrinsic pressure. This may take the form of simple **distortion of the pinna,** as when the shoulder impinges on the ear during late intrauterine life (Fig. 4.3.8A). This type of deformation rapidly disappears after removal of the deforming force (Fig. 4.3.8B).

Pressure that tends to flatten the ear against the head produces overgrowth of the ear. This seems to be partly the result of "ironing out" the contours of the auricle and partly an

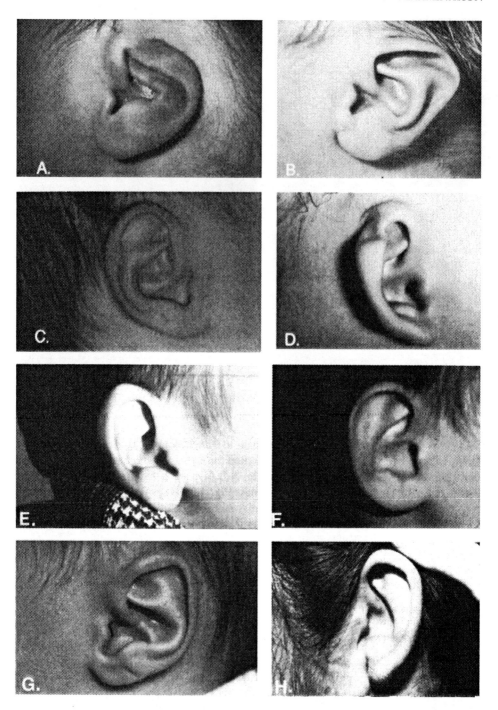

Figure 4.3.6. Structural variants of the pinna. (A) Overturned helix, creating the appearance of a triangular, posteriorly rotated auricle. (B) Mozart ear. (C) Darwinian tubercle of the helix. Note attached lobe. (D) Indentation of helical cartilage. (E) Large, detached earlobe. (F) Small earlobe. (G) Creased earlobe. (H) Congenitally cleft earlobe.

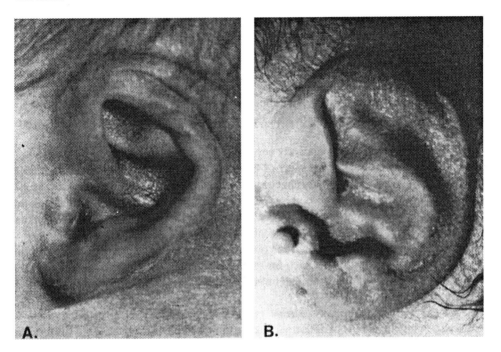

Figure 4.3.7. Anomalous appearance of structurally intact auricles. (A) Cryptotia, with upper helix tucked under a skin fold on the lateral scalp. (B) Large, flattened ear associated with oligohydramnios and intrauterine constraint.

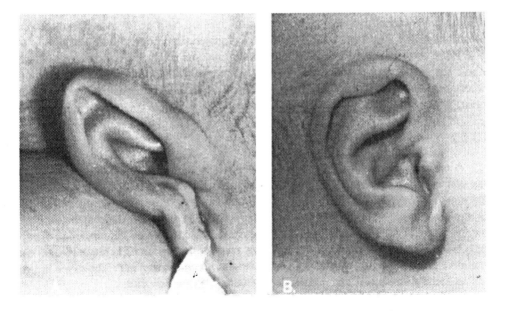

Figure 4.3.8. Deformed pinna. (A) Appearance of auricle at birth. Elevation of the shoulder and a laterally tipped head in utero combined to crumple the pinna upward and forward. (B) Normal auricular shape at 6 months.

actual increase in the growth rate of the auricular cartilage. The cartilage tends to be thinner and softer than normal, lending a floppy, feltlike consistency to the pinna (Fig. 4.3.7B). Bilateral **large, flattened ears** are often caused by prolonged intrauterine compression as a result of *oligohydramnios*. Associated abnormalities often include Potter facies, limitation of joint movement, and lung hypoplasia. Any of these indications of prolonged oligohydramnios should prompt an immediate evaluation of the genitourinary system, since renal agenesis or hypoplasia is the most common occult cause of this pattern of clinical features.

Asymmetric ear size is relatively common in the newborn and is most often caused by unequal pressures on the two sides of the head during the last months of intrauterine life. Factors involved in such asymmetric pressure include uterine abnormalities (e.g., scarring, fibroids, or a bicornuate uterus), multiple pregnancy, or torticollis, in which the baby's ear is pressed firmly against a shoulder or the inner wall of the uterus. Postnatal compression from torticollis, neuromuscular disease, or even consistent propping of a baby with one side of the head down can produce asymmetry of the ears on the same basis through the first year of life. A search for such mechanical factors should be undertaken if the architecture of the pinna is normal but the length differs by more than 3 mm between the two sides.

An ear with an essentially normal cartilaginous skeleton but a distorted shape is usually showing the effects of abnormal muscle pull. The pinna is anchored to the head by the posterior and superior auricular muscles, which insert on the upper and posterior aspects of the cup of cartilage that forms the concha. These muscles serve both to hold the ear close to the side of the head and to stabilize its cartilaginous skeleton. Weakness or absence of the auricular muscles results in various deformities of the auricle. When the superior muscle band is absent, a **lop ear** results; if only the posterior slip is missing, a **protruding ear** is seen; and if both are gone, a **cup ear** is found (Fig. 4.3.9). Some children with generalized severe hypotonia or dystonia will show these characteristic distortions of the auricle as a local indication of generalized poor muscle function.

There are, however, a few intrinsic malformations of auricular cartilage that can mimic the shape of a distorted ear. Careful inspection should allow discrimination between these two possibilities, since in a distorted ear the cartilaginous landmarks remain intact, although altered in their spatial relationships.

4.3.5.2. Disruptions

A normally developing auricle may be injured or partly destroyed by mechanical or vascular events involving the lateral facial zone. **Upward** or **forward displacement of the ear** is extremely rare and is seen primarily in conditions involving considerable disruption of tissue on the side of the face (Fig. 4.3.10). In all such instances, the ear canal is either absent or "left behind" in its normal position but markedly diminished in diameter. Direct injury to the pinna at any age may result in formation of hematomas that can distort or destroy neighboring cartilage, leading to a **cauliflower ear.** The pinna is firm and irregularly thickened and sometimes contains calcium deposits.

4.3.5.3. Dysplasias

In one skeletal disorder, diastrophic dysplasia, fluid-filled cysts commonly form in the ear cartilage during infancy. Their later resolution leads to distortion and thickening of

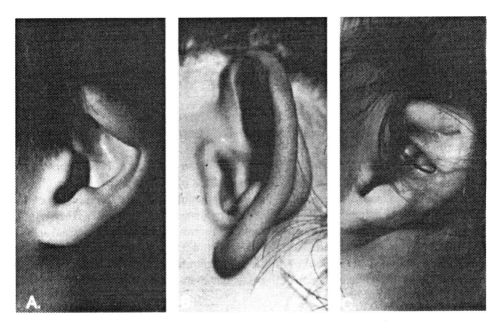

Figure 4.3.9. Distortion of the pinna from weakness of auricular muscles. (A) Lop ear. (B) Protruding or bat ear. (C) Cup ear.

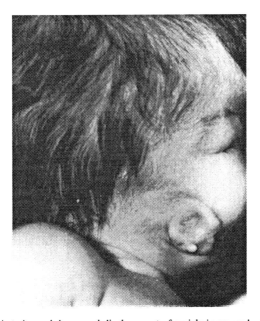

Figure 4.3.10. Anterior and downward displacement of auricle in severe hemifacial microsomia.

the pinna similar to the cauliflower ear described above (see Fig. 4.3.13F). The tissues of the auricle also may be diffusely thickened by the intracellular deposits found in the storage diseases.

4.3.5.4. Malformations

Intrinsic structural abnormalities of the auricle involve aberrant development of the cartilaginous skeleton of the ear. Such abnormalities may be seen in isolation or as part of many syndrome diagnoses.

Inadequate neural crest and/or mesenchymal tissue in the proximal portions of the first and second branchial arches results in hypoplasia of the pinna or **microtia** ("small ear"), the most common isolated intrinsic malformation of the auricle. The severity of this abnormality ranges in an unbroken spectrum from a small but structurally fairly normal ear through "rolled" remnants of cartilage and skin surrounding a narrow external auditory canal to total absence of auricular structures (Fig. 4.3.11). As might be expected, the most common functional problem associated with microtia is hearing loss, based on both atresia of the canal and involvement of the ossicular chain in the developmental anomalies of the first and second branchial arches.

When microtia is unilateral (the right side is more commonly involved), moderate to severe hearing loss in the contralateral, normally formed ear still occurs very frequently, and hearing should be carefully assessed bilaterally. A subtle form of microtia is **absence of the superior crus of the anthelix** (Fig. 4.3.12). This minor malformation is easy to miss but is associated with at least a 15% incidence of ipsilateral hearing loss.

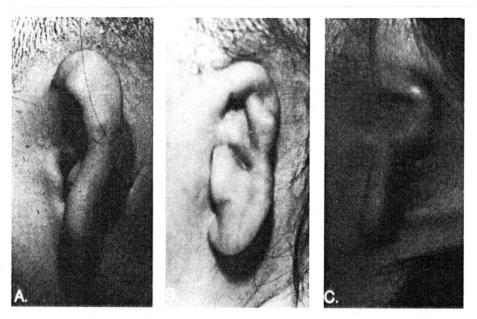

Figure 4.3.11. Spectrum of microtia. (A) Grade I—small, distorted pinna with intact external auditory canal. (B) Grade II—smaller auricle with disorganized cartilage and slitlike blind external canal. (C) Grade III—"rolled" remnant of auricular cartilage with complete absence of auditory meatus.

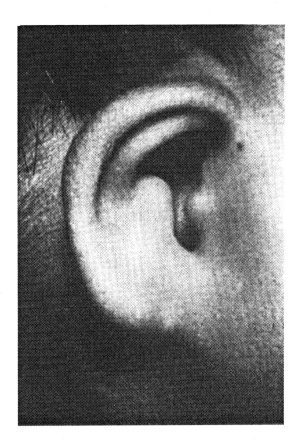

Figure 4.3.12. Absence of the superior crus of the anthelix. The upper portion of the auricle is foreshortened such that the upper curve of the helix lies immediately above the lower crus of the anthelix. Note also the small preauricular pit.

Varying degrees of microtia usually are seen in syndromes involving developmental anomalies of the branchial arches, such as Treacher Collins syndrome and hemifacial microsomia.

A large number of other dysmorphic syndromes include ear abnormalities as a feature, but in most instances these are facultative rather than required parts of the syndrome and thus are only of marginal help in making a dysmorphologic diagnosis. Examples shown in Fig. 4.3.13A–C include the attenuated, sometimes **pointed ears** seen in Trisomy 18, the **crumpled ears** of Beale syndrome, and the **small, square ears** found in children with Down syndrome. **Triangular ears** (Fig. 4.3.13D) are a common feature of children with Turner or Noonan syndrome, probably based on the massive cervical edema present during midgestation that places unusual tractive forces on the developing auricular tissues. In fetal alcohol syndrome, overdevelopment of the root of the helix produces a **railroad track** configuration (Fig. 4.3.13E); in Beckwith syndrome, a diagonally creased earlobe is frequently seen (Fig. 4.3.6G).

Contrary to widespread belief based on a few published reports, a general association between malformation of the ear and kidney abnormalities has not been substantiated. The branchiootorenal syndrome is one of the few disorders in which a relatively constant relationship between auricular and genitourinary abnormalities is seen.

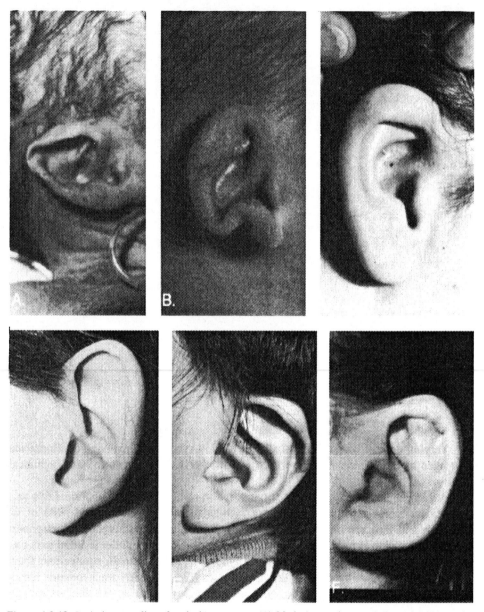

Figure 4.3.13. Intrinsic anomalies of auricular structure. (A) Marked posterior angulation, pixielike ear in trisomy 18. (B) Small, crumpled pinna in Beale syndrome. (C) Small, thickened, squared-off auricle in Down syndrome. (D) Elongated, triangular configuration of external ear in Turner syndrome. (E) Prominent helical root (railroad track ear) in fetal alcohol syndrome. (F) Irregularly thickened, cauliflower ear in diastrophic dysplasia.

4.3.6. Summary

True malformations of the pinna, especially those which are not familial, should prompt a search for hearing loss. Unusually large or asymmetric ears often indicate mechanical compression and, when seen in the newborn period, may provide an early clue to renal agenesis or other causes of oligohydramnios. Abnormal placement of the pinna suggests arrest of migration, which may be associated with other abnormalities of branchial arch development, while distortion of the auricle suggests inadequate structure or function of the periauricular muscles.

4.4. PERIOCULAR REGION

The structure that surround, support, and protect the optic globe contribute a great deal to the overall appearance of the face. Whereas the size and shape of the eyeball itself is relatively consistent from person to person, the periocular structures show a wide range of normal and abnormal forms, some of which provide valuable clues for dysmorphologic diagnosis.

4.4.1. Embryology and Development

The optic globe develops from an early outpouching on the lateral aspect of the forebrain (see Section 4.5.1), and as it grows and differentiates, it induces the formation of the periocular structures. The bony *orbit* is derived from extensions of the anterior plate mesoderm, with contributions from neural crest tissue as well as the maxillary process of the first branchial arch. The *eyelids* form as folds of surface ectoderm, with a central core of mesenchyme above and below the eye. They grow toward each other and finally fuse at about week 10 of gestation. This fusion persists until about 26 weeks, after the bulbar and palpebral conjunctivae have formed, when they open again. The *nasolacrimal duct* begins as a solid cord of ectoderm that detaches from the surface and sinks into the underlying mesoderm. It later canalizes; the lower end opens into the nasal cavity, and the upper end expands to form the *lacrimal sac*.

In addition to its role in the induction of these periocular structures, the eye also has a suppressive effect on hair growth in a large circular area surrounding the orbit. Only the eyebrows and lashes normally form in this area, but some newborns have darkly pigmented hair extending from the anterolateral scalp hairline down to the lateral brow (see Section 4.16).

4.4.2. Anatomy and Landmarks

Viewed from the front, the free edges of the upper and lower eyelids can be seen to have different degrees of curvature. The upper lid is more acutely arched than the lower, since it must follow the contour of the cornea (Fig. 4.4.1). The margin of the upper lid lies just above the pupil when the gaze is directed straight ahead, and when the eye looks upward or downward, the lid follows to retain about the same position relative to the iris. In forward gaze, the border of the lower lid normally rests just at the lower margin of the iris.

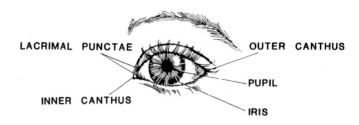

LACRIMAL PUNCTAE   OUTER CANTHUS

                                             —PUPIL

INNER CANTHUS

                                             —IRIS

Figure 4.4.1. Superficial anatomy and landmarks of the eye and periocular region.

The space between the upper and lower lids is the *palpebral fissure*. The *inner canthus* and *outer canthus* are the points where the upper and lower lids meet. The angle of the outer canthus is more acute than that of the inner. Just lateral to the inner canthus on the margins of the lids are the *lacrimal punctae,* the openings of the lacrimal ducts, each atop a small papilla. The *eyelashes* are arranged in two staggered rows along the lid margin. Those of the upper lid are long and curved upward, while the shorter lower lashes curve less.

The *eyebrows* arch along the edge of the superior orbital margin, beginning at a point vertically above the inner canthus and thinning out as they pass beyond the outer canthus. The base of each eyebrow hair seems to be aimed at a point just above and medial to the inner canthus.

4.4.3. Examination Techniques

Inspection and measurement are the techniques applicable to examination of the structures surrounding the eye. Attention should be paid to the spacing of the orbits and the configuration of the lids, brows, and lashes.

For centuries, artists have used various landmarks and rules of thumb to give the faces in their paintings a lifelike and normal quality. Some of these techniques are valuable for dysmorphology. For example, a quick estimate of eye spacing can be obtained by the approximation used by portrait artists: "an eye and an eye and an eye." In other words, the distance between the inner corners of the two eyes normally is about the same as the distance between the inner and outer canthi of one eye (Fig. 4.4.2).

The impressions gained by simple inspection may be verified by specific measurements between landmarks in the ocular zone. Orbital spacing is determined clinically by measuring the distance between the centers of the pupils with the eyes in forward gaze (*interpupillary distance*). A more precise measurement can be obtained from frontal radiographs of the face, measuring between the inner orbital margins (*interorbital distance*). The *inner canthal distance, outer canthal distance,* and *palpebral fissure length* are measured between the ocular canthi as shown in Fig. 4.4.3, but this can be done accurately only when the patient's eyes are fully open. Tables of normal values for all of these measurements are available in standard texts.

In the frontal view, an imaginary line drawn through the inner and outer corners of one eye should cut the same structures on the other side. If the outer canthus falls more than 2 mm above or below this line, *upslanted* or *downslanted palpebral fissures* are present (Fig. 4.4.4). Care should be exercised, however, in making such a judgment,

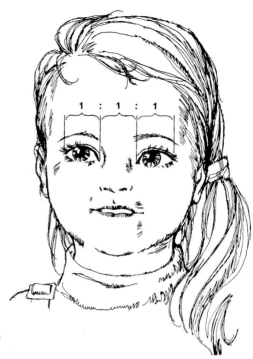

Figure 4.4.2. Normal spacing of the orbits: "an eye and an eye and an eye."

especially in evaluating photographs. A small forward or backward tilt of the head may create a false impression of the plane of the intercanthal line (Fig. 4.4.5).

Normally, no sclera can be seen directly above the iris in any direction of gaze, but when the eyes are protuberant or when there is *retraction of the upper lid,* the sclera becomes visible, producing a "startled" appearance. Lid retraction with consistent downward gaze leads to the familiar "sunset sign." In contrast, *ptosis* or *drooping of the eyelid* narrows the palpebral fissure. A mild degree of ptosis can be detected by comparing, in the two eyes, the distance between the upper lid margin and the secondary fold of skin that

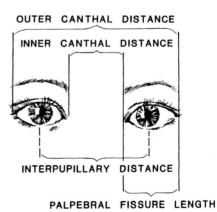

Figure 4.4.3. Terminology for measurements in the periocular zone.

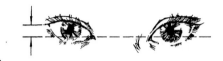

A

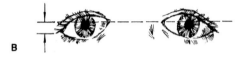

B

Figure 4.4.4. Palpebral fissure slant. (A) Upslanting palpebral fissures. The outer canthi lie above the line joining the inner canthi. (B) Downslanting palpebral fissures.

commonly traverses the lid 3 or 4 mm above the lashes (Fig. 4.4.6A). Bilateral ptosis commonly results in a backward tilt of the head as the child attempts to peer out from beneath the drooping lids (Fig. 4.4.6B).

A lateral view of the face provides an impression of the depth to which the globes are set in the orbits and is especially helpful if the eyes seem *deep set* or *protuberant*. The lashes should also be inspected from the side, since the angle of curvature they make in exiting from the lid margin may be a clue to neuromuscular disease (See Section 4.5.1).

4.4.4. Minor Variants

4.4.4.1. Spectrum Variants

There is considerable variability in normal individuals and families in the configuration of the ocular zone. Mild *hypertelorism,* reflected in a slightly increased interpupillary distance, such as seen in Jacqueline Kennedy Onassis, is fairly common, and so are minor degrees of *hypotelorism.*

Most newborn babies have a relatively low nasal bridge, and the "excess" skin over the area often forms an **inner epicanthic fold.** This crescent-shaped fold originates in the skin below the eye and sweeps upward to blend with the upper lid, covering the inner

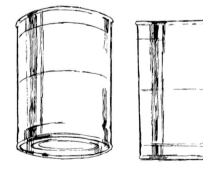
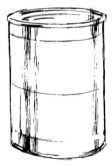

Figure 4.4.5. Effect of head tilt on the apparent slant of palpebral fissures. A horizontal line drawn around a cylinder will appear to curve downward at the ends if the top of the cylinder is tipped away from the examiner and upward when the top is tilted forward.

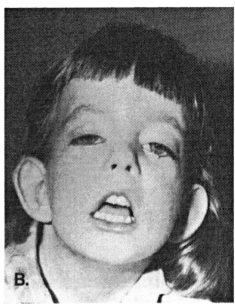

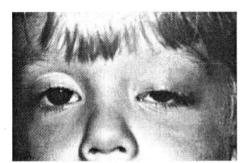

Figure 4.4.6. Ptosis of the eyelids. (A) Unilateral ptosis with eyelid margin covering iris: high risk for disuse amblyopia. (Photo courtesy of Dr. Frank Durso, Albuquerque, N.M.) (B) Bilateral ptosis in a child with generalized muscular weakness. Note the protruding ears and the backward tilt of the head needed to permit vision from beneath the drooping lids.

canthus (Fig. 4.4.7A). During continuing development of the facial skeleton in the first year of life, the growing nasal bridge gradually tents up the skin between the eyes, and the fold disappears. Persistence of an infantile epicanthic fold past 18 months of life is unusual and generally indicates slow midfacial growth. In members of Asian races and certain American Indian groups, a somewhat different **Oriental epicanthic fold** is normally present. This fold begins at the lower lid margin and swings upward over the medial portion of the upper lid (Fig. 4.4.7B). This is commonly associated with redundant skin over the upper lid, bringing the secondary skin fold down close to the lid margin. Both types of epicanthic folds can create a false impression of ocular hypertelorism because of the apparent increase in breadth of the interocular zone.

Mildly upslanted palpebral fissures can be seen as a familial feature, often associated with slight *midfacial hypoplasia.* Similarly, downslanting palpebral fissures may occur in individuals with mild *malar hypoplasia*. Here, one can imagine that the slant of the eye fissures results from too little support at the lateral margins, allowing a "droop" of the outer portion of the orbit.

The term **almond-shaped eyes** refers to the appearance of the palpebral fissures when the curvatures of the upper and lower lids are almost equal (Fig. 4.4.8). Generally this is caused by an unusually shallow arc of the upper lid and again can be seen as a normal feature in some Oriental and American Indian individuals, but it may also serve as a clue to a very mild degree of microphthalmia.

Individuals with dark, abundant facial hair often have luxurious eyebrows that approach each other in the midline. If the brows are actually fused, the term **synophrys** is

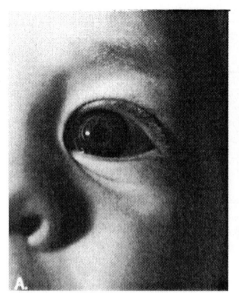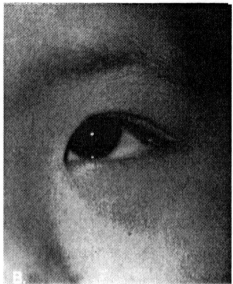

Figure 4.4.7. Epicanthic folds. (A) Classic inner epicanthic fold obscuring the inner portions of both lids and the inner canthus. (B) Oriental epicanthic fold joining the lower lid at the inner canthus. Note the associated redundancy of skin on the upper lid.

used to describe the resulting single band of eyebrow that traverses the glabella (Fig. 4.4.9). In a similar fashion, racial and familial tendencies influence the growth of the eyelashes; lightly pigmented, short, or **sparse lashes** may be a normal feature in some children, whereas dark-colored, tangled, or **luxurious lashes** are found in others. Interestingly, eyelashes in children of both sexes seem to attain their greatest length and density between the ages of six months and five years (see Section 4.16).

4.4.4.2. Minor Anomalies

Ptosis of the eyelid implies that the levator palpebral muscle is weak, allowing the lid to sag downward, partly covering the pupil. Unilateral ptosis may be familial but is often of traumatic origin, whereas bilateral ptosis is suggestive of a generalized neuromuscular abnormality (Fig. 4.4.6B).

A tendency of the lid margin to roll inward, allowing the lashes to make contact with the cornea, is called **entropion.** This may be a temporary condition, but if not corrected promptly, it can lead to corneal abrasion and eventual scarring.

The tear ducts normally open within a few days to a few weeks after birth. In early infancy, excessive tearing from one eye may be the first indication of **lacrimal duct stenosis** or **atresia.** The blockage of tear drainage usually occurs distal to lacrimal sac, which can become first distended and, soon after, infected. A cystic mass can be found below the inner canthus, and often tears (or pus) can be expressed from the lacrimal puncta by gentle pressure over this zone.

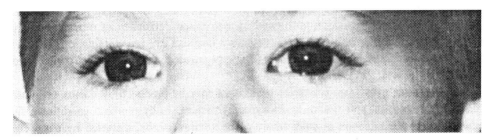

Figure 4.4.8. Almond-shaped palpebral fissures in Prader-Willi syndrome. The upper and lower lids have nearly equal curvatures.

4.4.5. Abnormalities

4.4.5.1. Deformations

There are only a few examples of true deformation of structures of the ocular zone. **Asymmetry of the orbits,** whether the result of direct deforming pressure or the disconjugate growth of orbital structures secondary to *premature synostosis,* can distort the optic axis and lead to *strabismus* and amblyopia (see Section 4.2).

The usual gentle upward curve of the eyelashes may be lost when there is inadequate tone in the levator palpebrae muscle. Thus, **straight** or **drooping lashes** may be found on ptotic eyelids and may serve as a subtle indication of generalized muscle hypotonia in such disorders as Prader-Willi syndrome or the congenital muscular atrophies (see Section 4.16).

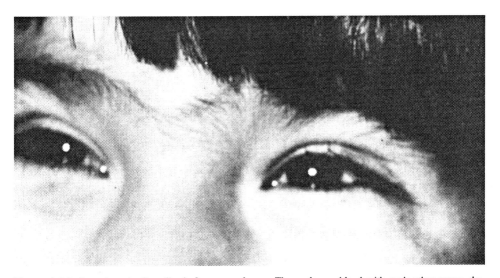

Figure 4.4.9. Synophrys in Cornelia de Lange syndrome. The eyebrows blend with each other across the midline.

The optic globes are supported within the orbits by a cuplike pad of fat and connective tissue. When this cushion is thinned by nutritional deficiency or other cause, the eyeball recedes further into the orbit, creating a deep-set eye (*enophthalmia*). The skin around the eye sinks and often becomes hyperpigmented, producing an "owlish" appearance (Fig. 4.4.10A).

Protruding eyes (*exophthalmia*) sometimes may be produced by edema or hyperplasia of intraorbital soft tissue, as in hyperthyroidism. In dysmorphic conditions, the cause of this phenomenon is more likely to be *shallow orbits,* distorted by basal craniosynostosis, as in the Crouzon or Apert syndromes (Fig. 4.4.10B).

4.4.5.2. Disruptions

The orbital zone may be involved in disruption by amniotic bands that cut across the tissues of the upper face (see Appendix C). Beyond this rare occurrence, there are no characteristic disruptive lesions of the ocular zone.

4.4.5.3. Dysplasias

Individual tissues around the eye may share in the generalized effects of some dysplastic diseases. The skin of the lids may become thickened in the *mucopolysaccharidoses* and other storage disorders, while hyperostosis of the brow ridges can distort the upper orbits in a few rare bone dysplasias. In general, however, there are no dysplastic changes that are peculiar to the periocular region.

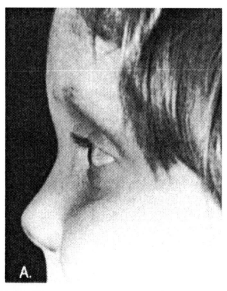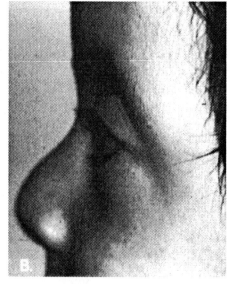

Figure 4.4.10. Orbital depth. (A) Deep-set eyes. Note the distance between the convexity of the cornea and the facial plane in this straight lateral photograph. (B) Shallow orbits with protruding eyes (compare with panel A).

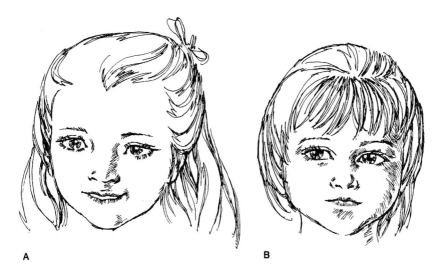

Figure 4.4.11. Horizontal spacing of the orbits. (A) Ocular hypertelorism. The nasal bridge is relatively wide. (B) Ocular hypotelorism.

4.4.5.4. Malformations

Moderate or severe **ocular hypertelorism,** with a measured distance between the pupils (or the bony orbits) more than three standard deviations above the mean, is seen as part of a number of syndrome diagnoses and may be associated with strabismus and amblyopia if the orbital separation is sufficient to prevent binocular fusion (Fig. 4.4.11A).

Conversely, a diminished distance between the eyes is known as **ocular hypotelorism** and may be an indication of abnormal development of the olfactory and frontal lobes of the brain (Fig. 4.4.11B). In the extreme, the two eyes actually fuse into one structure during early development because of the absence of adequate intervening tissues. This is **cyclopia,** which is invariably associated with major abnormalities of brain conformation and absence of the olfactory tracts (Fig. 4.4.12).

There are several other developmental abnormalities that can produce the illusion of hypertelorism. An appearance somewhat similar to that produced by epicanthic folds is found with **telecanthus,** in which the inner canthi are displaced laterally even though the globes (and the orbits) are normally situated (Fig. 4.4.13). In contrast to true hypertelorism, telecanthus is marked by the reduction or absence of visible sclera medial to the iris and by lateral displacement of the lacrimal punctae. Both telecanthus and epicanthic folds can also produce a mistaken impression of strabismus because the pupils seem to lie eccentrically in the palpebral fissure.

Clefts of the eyelids can occur as the termination of a facial cleft extending into the orbit (see Fig. 4.7.6) but also can appear as local defects in Treacher Collins syndrome (lower lid) and Goldenhar syndrome (upper lid) (Fig. 4.4.14). When clefting affects the lower lid, it most commonly occurs at the junction between the medial two-thirds and lateral third. The mildest detectable degree of these localized clefts is the absence of lashes over a space of a few millimeters along the lid.

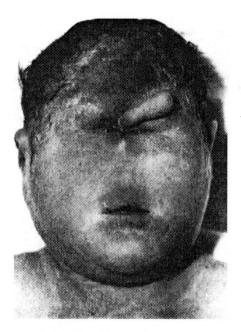

Figure 4.4.12. Cyclopia, with a single wide orbit, partially fused optic globes, a midline proboscis, and microstomia.

Ectropion is a condition in which the lower lid is patulous and droops well below its usual position against the globe at the lower limbus of the iris. This may be the cause of chronic conjunctivitis (Fig. 4.4.15).

The term **blepharophimosis** refers to a restriction of the space between the upper and lower lids when the sizes of the orbit and globe are normal. The palpebral fissures are reduced in both height and width by associated telecanthus and ptosis (Fig. 4.4.16A). A

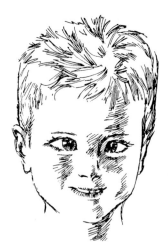

Figure 4.4.13. Telecanthus. Note the absence of visible sclera medial to the iris.

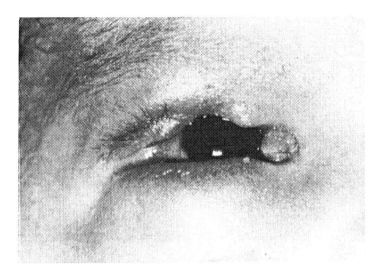

Figure 4.4.14. Cleft upper lid in Goldenhar syndrome.

quite similar appearance is created by **short palpebral fissures** such as are seen in fetal alcohol syndrome (Fig. 4.4.16B). In this case, however, the vertical measurement between the lids may be close to normal, and both the outer and inner canthi are displaced toward the midline of the eye. Autopsy in a few affected individuals has suggested that a mild degree of microphthalmia may be the basis for this abnormality of lid development.

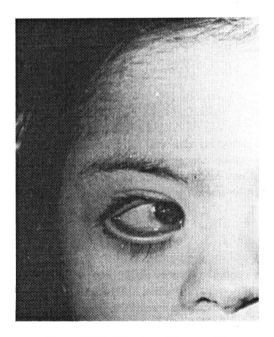

Figure 4.4.15. Ectropion of the lower lid.

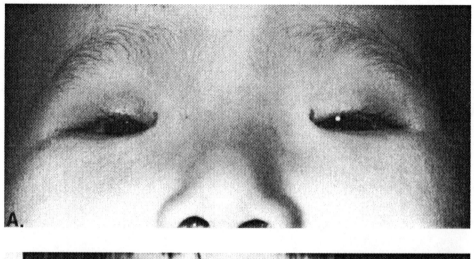

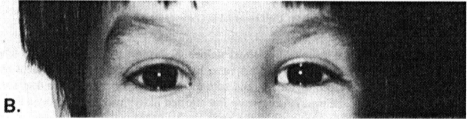

Figure 4.4.16. Shortened palpebral fissures. (A) Short and narrow palpebral fissures with telecanthus in familial blepharophimosis syndrome. (B) Mild shortening of palpebral fissures in fetal alcohol syndrome.

4.4.6. Summary

Structures in the periocular zone can provide clues to a number of syndrome diagnoses as well as information concerning early eye development. An illusion of hypertelorism or strabismus may be produced by several distinct abnormalities in this region, and care must be taken to determine the real cause of such an appearance.

4.5. EYES

The eye is the most complex sensory organ, and its development spans a considerable portion of intrauterine life. Very distinctive ophthalmologic anomalies are found in many dysmorphic syndromes, and therefore careful examination of the eye is of immense value in the diagnosis of children with multiple malformations.

4.5.1. Embryology and Development

The eye originates as an outward bulge on the lateral wall of the forebrain at the beginning of week 4 of gestation, forming the hollow *optic vesicle* (Fig. 4.5.1A). When its outer surface comes into contact with the overlying ectoderm, both layers promptly begin to invaginate, in a manner similar to pushing in one side of a tennis ball, forming the double-walled *optic cup*. This process is not entirely symmetric, so that the inferior rim of the optic cup becomes deeply indented, producing the *choroid fissure*. Meanwhile, the invaginated portion of surface ectoderm pinches off to become the *lens placode,* taking its place just inside the optic cup as the choroid fissure begins to fuse (Fig. 4.5.1B).

By week 7, the proximal portion of the choroid fissure has closed, and the pigment cells of neural crest origin have migrated into the outer layer of the optic cup, while the inner layer is beginning to differentiate into rod and cone cells. The definitive *lens* is now forming, and the mesenchyme surrounding the optic cup is beginning to condense into the fibrous *sclera* and the pigmented *choroid* layers (Fig. 4.5.2A). Within the mesoderm at the anterior pole of the eye, the *pupillary muscles* appear, soon to be incorporated within the *iris,* which extends inward from the edges of the optic cup anterior to the lens. All around the base of the inner surface of the iris, the *ciliary muscles* develop; these are joined to the perimeter of the lens by the *suspensory ligaments.*

At about intrauterine week 15, the major structures of the eye are complete (Fig. 4.5.2B). Fusion of mesenchymal connective tissue with surface ectoderm at the anterior

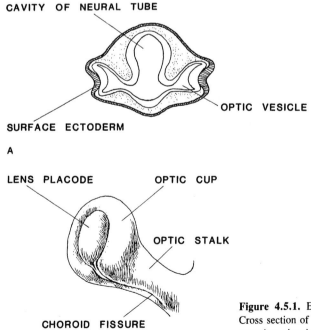

Figure 4.5.1. Early embryogenesis of the eye. (A) Cross section of the neural tube at about 4.5 weeks of gestation, showing early invagination of the optic vesicles. (B) The optic cup at about 5.5 weeks.

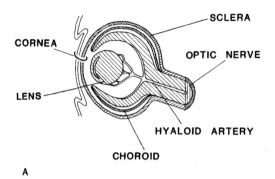

CORNEA

SCLERA

OPTIC NERVE

LENS

HYALOID ARTERY

CHOROID

A

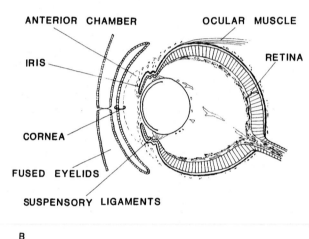

ANTERIOR CHAMBER

OCULAR MUSCLE

IRIS

RETINA

CORNEA

FUSED EYELIDS

SUSPENSORY LIGAMENTS

B

Figure 4.5.2. Later stages of eye development. (A) Sagittal section of the optic globe at about 6 weeks of gestation, showing the lens primordium and neural tissues destined to become the retina. [After Moore (1982).] (B) Section of the eye at 15 weeks, showing fused lids, formation of the anterior chamber, and degeneration of the hyaloid artery. [After Langman (1969).]

pole has given rise to the *cornea,* which has become separated from the lens and iris by a fluid-filled space, the *anterior chamber.* The *iridopupillary membrane,* which earlier formed a temporary barrier between the anterior chamber and the lens and iris, normally will have completely disappeared by this time, and the *ocular muscles* will have condensed out of the remaining mesenchymal tissue surrounding the eyeball. The pigmented and neural layers of the *retina* are now defined, and axons of retinal nerve cells can be seen converging on the *optic nerve* leading to the brain.

4.5.2. Anatomy and Landmarks

The outer circumference of the cornea at its junction with the sclera lies immediately over the outer border of the iris (Fig. 4.4.1). The *pupil* is centered in the iris, and the lens, in turn, is concentric with the pupil. These structures define the *optic axis* of the eye, which terminates on the retina at the *macula,* lateral to the optic nerve.

4.5.3. Examination Techniques

Simple inspection of the eye provides information about the color of the sclera and iris, the clarity of the cornea and lens, and the configuration of the pupil. In older

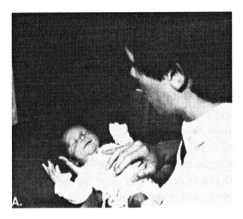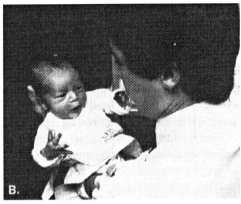

Figure 4.5.3. Eye-opening maneuver for young infants. (A) Baby is cradled in the supine position. (B) When raised abruptly to vertical position, baby opens eyes.

children, inspection may be accomplished easily with the use of a penlight, but in infants, and especially in newborns, some special maneuvers are valuable.

Attempts to open the eyes of a newborn by brute force are doomed to failure, since the baby's reflexive resistance combines with periorbital edema, slippery skin, and eversion of the upper lid to defeat the examiner. A better technique consists of cradling the baby face up with the head cupped in one hand and the back supported by the forearm (Fig. 4.5.3A). The infant is then swung upward quickly to a vertical position (Fig. 4.5.3B); this motion will usually cause spontaneous eye opening, although the maneuver may need to be repeated a few times for a sleepy baby.

Next, with the baby supported upright and en face, the examiner swings his body in a quarter circle from right to left and then back again (Fig. 4.5.4). This movement produces

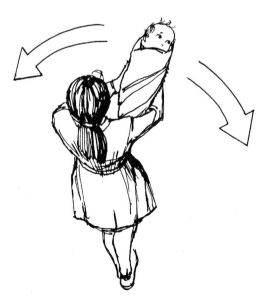

Figure 4.5.4. Technique for testing lateral eye movements in infants. Swinging the baby in an arc to the left and right causes the eyes and head to deviate in the same direction.

lateral deviation of the infant's eyes in the same direction as the rotation, permitting evaluation of the ocular movement in the horizontal plane and also providing a good view of the sclerae.

Testing *extraocular movements* in older children and adults only requires their following a moving light or the examiner's wiggling fingers into all four quadrants of the visual field. Sometimes it is necessary to steady the child's chin with the free hand to prevent her turning her head to follow the moving object. If strabismus is suspected, the diagnostic techniques outlined in Appendix A may be useful.

Inspection of the sclera can reveal variations from its usual translucent white color as well as the presence of abnormalities such as pterygia and lipomas. The iris is examined for overall structure, color, and the shape and placement of the pupil as well as for pupillary light responses. As with other paired structures, the two eyes are compared for each of these features.

With a high-diopter positive lens setting ($+8$ to $+12$), the direct ophthalmoscope is helpful in examining the anterior chamber, iris, and lens. Directing the light beam (and the line of vision) somewhat obliquely at these anterior structures provides a good view and is more comfortable for the patient. Mild degrees of *corneal clouding* and small or diffuse *cataracts* may sometimes be detected in this fashion, but more commonly they will be suspected when there is difficulty focusing the ophthalmoscope on the retina. More severe opacification of the lens is usually seen first as an alteration in the *red reflex:* a central "shadow" may be seen, and the retinal light reflex may appear unusually bright and pale or may be virtually absent in such cases.

When *dislocation of the lens* is suspected, the examiner should observe the iris through the ophthalmoscope while percussing the lateral skull gently with the heel of the hand. This maneuver may produce a to-and-fro motion, like a curtain swaying in a breeze, in that portion of the iris which is not supported posteriorly by the lens (*iridodonesis*).

Adequate funduscopic examination is often impossible in small children without the use of midriatics; but at the minimum, a retinal reflex should be sought in each eye, and at least a glimpse of the retina itself should be obtained.

If there is a marked clouding of the cornea or enlargement of the globe that might suggest *glaucoma,* palpation of the eye is in order. This is accomplished by gently pressing on the closed lid lateral to the cornea with one finger while palpating with a finger of the opposite hand to get an estimate of the firmness of the globe. The examiner's eye should be tested similarly to provide a comparison with normal. This admittedly is a subjective and inexact test, but it may lend support to a suspicion of increased intraocular pressure, which would justify immediate ophthalmological referral.

The most pertinent measurement of the eye itself is the corneal diameter, which is normally about 10 mm. Since the eye has attained most of its eventual size by the time of birth, this dimension remains remarkably stable throughout life.

4.5.4. Minor Variants

4.5.4.1. Spectrum Variants

Small **refractive errors** and mild degrees of **astigmatism** are common in the general population and are noteworthy only if severe, progressive, or familial. In particular, moderate to severe **myopia** is a feature of several dysmorphic syndromes.

In infants, the scleral envelope normally is rather thin, and the underlying darkly pigmented choroid layer sometimes imparts a bluish tinge to the bulbar sclera. This normal **blue sclera** of infancy disappears by 1 year of age as denser connective tissue is gradually laid down in the outer layers of the eyeball. Hypopigmentation of the choroid layer may permit scleral vessels to be seen in a ghostly pattern behind the normal retinal vasculature (**tigroid retina**).

At birth, many babies have a dark, hazy blue iris color, and the definitive **pigmentation** of the iris develops gradually during the first 6–10 months of postnatal life. Normal eye color varies over a continuous gradation from pale blue to almost black and usually reflects the eye color of both parents. As with all polygenic physical features, however, some individuals may inherit a gene mix that produces a phenotype unlike that of either parent, and it is entirely possible for a brown-eyed couple to have a blue-eyed child.

Although the pupil is usually centered in the iris, a mild degree of eccentricity is relatively common; a more severe degree, designated **corectopia,** is seen in Fig. 4.5.5A. Some slight irregularity of the inner margin of the iris is not unusual, but a pupil in the shape of a teardrop suggests the presence of **synechiae,** while an elliptical pupil should spur the search for an associated **coloboma** of the retina (see below).

4.5.4.2. Minor Anomalies

Minor structural anomalies of the eye that can be detected by simple examination include small colobomas of the iris, which may range from an elliptical pupil to a defect reaching the outer edge of the iris (usually in the inferonasal quadrant) (Fig. 4.5.5B). When the defect extends into the retina, vision may be affected and the anomaly can no longer be classified as minor.

Pigmentary abnormalities of the iris are quite frequent and usually benign, most often representing somatic mutation in one primordial pigment-producing cell. When the entire iris of one eye is of a distinctly different color than the other, the term used is **heterochromia iridis** (Fig. 4.5.6A). A wedge-shaped segment of anomalous eye color is properly called **heterochromia iridum** (Fig. 4.5.6B). **Brushfield spots** are small, slightly

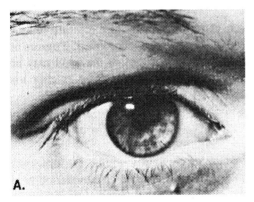
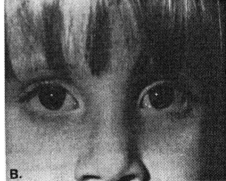

Figure 4.5.5. Anomalies of the pupil. (A) Corectopia, with the pupil placed off center in the iris. (B) Iris colobomas, producing an elliptical or keyhole-shaped pupil.

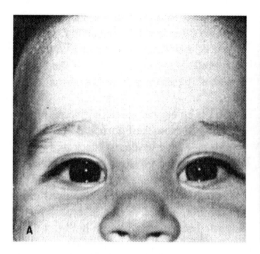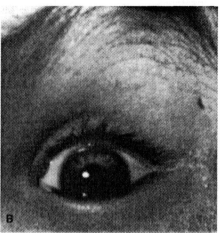

Figure 4.5.6. Pigmentary anomalies of the iris. (A) Heterochromia iridis. Note the very subtle difference between the two eyes in the shading of the iris. The right iris was medium brown, the left gray-blue. (B) Heterochromia iridum. The upper third of the iris was pale blue, in contrast to the dark brown color of the remainder.

elevated zones of depigmented iris that form an irregular ring about one-third of the way in from the limbus of the iris (Fig. 4.5.7). Seen in some normal individuals, they have no functional significance but may be a clue to the diagnosis of Down syndrome, in which they are associated with peripheral iris hypoplasia.

A **pterygium** is a small, raised fibrous growth, triangular in shape, with its apex near the limbus of the cornea and its base on the sclera of the lateral globe. This benign tumor may produce problems if it continues to enlarge and extends onto the cornea.

4.5.5. Abnormalities

4.5.5.1. Deformations

Deformations of optic structures based on extrinsic mechanical forces are few. A shallow orbit may lead to protuberant eyes, but the eye itself is not deformed. **Tumors** of the eye or orbit may compress or distend the globe. Irregularities of the pupil may be caused by **synechiae**, strands of scarlike connective tissue adherent to the anterior iris and, often, to the internal surface of the cornea.

4.5.5.2. Disruptions

The dysmorphic signs produced by destruction of previously normal eye structures before birth range the gamut from **retinitis pigmentosa** as a result of intrauterine viral infections to mechanical disruption of the optic globe by amniotic bands (see Appendix C). Malignant tumors, especially **retinoblastoma**, may invade adjacent structures or

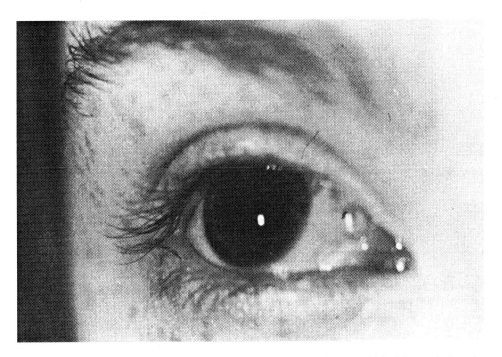

Figure 4.5.7. Brushfield spots. These pale dots are arranged in an arc about one-third of the way in from the outer margin of the iris.

destroy ocular tissues by direct pressure, but most are discovered before reaching this stage, usually by detection of a **white pupil**.

Prenatal glaucoma can create intraocular pressures high enough to destroy sensitive tissues of the eye. Actual distension of the globe with enlargement of the cornea characterizes **buphthalmos** ("ox eye"), which may progress rapidly after birth to result in permanent blindness (Fig. 4.5.8).

4.5.5.3. Dysplasias

Several types of metabolic abnormality and generalized tissue dysplasia affect the developing eye. Cataract may occur after insult to the lens at virtually any point after week 4 of gestation (including postnatal life), but the phase of development of the lens will influence the size and shape of the opacity. For example, a *central* or **nuclear cataract** would result from abnormalities occurring before gestational week 6 whereas a *lamellar* or **zonular cataract** would be more likely after the secondary lens fibers have begun to proliferate at 8–0 weeks (Fig. 4.5.9A). Subsequently, injury to the lens leaves its mark on progressively more superficial layers, although damage and opacity eventually may extend widely within the lens. In many metabolic disorders, the fetus is protected in utero by placental clearance of deleterious substances (as in Lowe syndrome) or lack of exposure to exogenous agents (as in galactosemia). Thus, as a rule, such disorders are marked by cataract formation that begins weeks to months after birth.

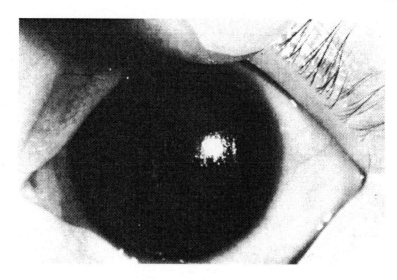

Figure 4.5.8. Congenital glaucoma (buphthalmos). The anterior chamber is enlarged and tense, and the cornea is cloudy. (Photo courtesy of Dr. Frank Durso, Albuquerque, N.M.)

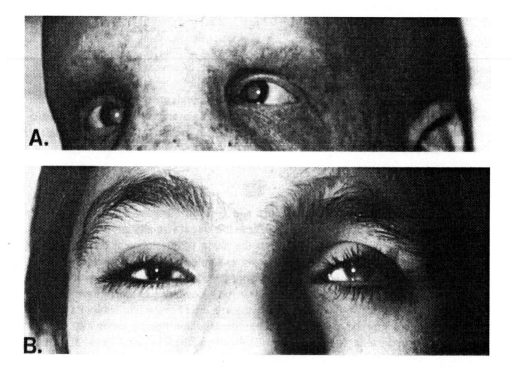

Figure 4.5.9. Opacities of the optic media. (A) Dense nuclear cataract in Rothmund poikiloderma syndrome. (B) Corneal clouding bilaterally, with moderate microphthalmia on the right.

Corneal opacities usually develop during postnatal life in the mucopolysac-charidoses and some other metabolic disorders. A slit-lamp examination may be necessary to detect the fine dustlike corneal densities in their earliest stages. Widespread involvement of other body systems usually will be evident in these diseases by the time corneal clouding becomes clinically obvious (Fig. 4.5.9B).

Inadequate melanin production as seen in several types of oculocutaneous **albinism** should be detectable after about gestational week 25. The usual presentation is that of a baby with very pale to bone-white hair and photophobia. When light is shined into the eyes, it is reflected brightly through both the pupil and the stroma of the iris itself as a very pink "red reflex." Fine horizontal *nystagmus* is a frequent accompanying feature.

In neurofibromatosis, **Lisch nodules** appear as pigmented, heaped-up zones of various sizes on the surface of the iris. Unlike Brushfield spots, they are unevenly distributed and may be found anywhere on the iris. While they have no functional significance, these lesions become more numerous in mid to late childhood and may be diagnostically helpful.

4.5.5.4. Malformations

The eye is susceptible to a variety of errors in morphogenesis because of its complex structure and the intricate processes involved in the formation of its component parts. These malformations can be roughly categorized by the phase of eye development during which they occur (Fig. 4.5.10).

Phase I: Organogenesis—conception through week 5. **Anophthalmos**, or complete absence of the eye, results if the optic vesicle fails to form. Because the developing vesicle and optic cup induce the formation of the orbital and other periocular structures, this extremely rare abnormality results in total absence of these structures as well (Fig. 4.5.11A). Much more frequent (although still rare) is **microphthalmos**, in which a slightly small to vestigial eyeball is accompanied by variable hypoplasia of the eyelids, lacrimal apparatus, and orbit. Formation of a microphthalmic eye may take place at any point over a long span of embryonic and early fetal development, probably involving a number of different pathogenic mechanisms. As a general rule, if there is any evidence of periocular structures (lids, lashes, lacrimal glands, or a palpable orbit), some vestige of an optic globe will be found, but it may be demonstrable only by histologic sections. Mild degrees of microphthalmos may show no abnormalities of eye structure apart from small size and may be detected only by careful measurement or formal ophthalmologic evaluation (Figs. 4.5.10B and 4.5.11B).

When there has been inadequate early development of the forebrain, the optic vesicles may fuse with each other in the midline, producing *synophthalmos* or cyclopia (Fig. 4.4.12). Usually some degree of pairing of optic structures is preserved, although a single large median orbit is the rule.

Failure of complete closure of the choroid fissure in the embryonic optic cup leads to **ocular coloboma**, a failure of tissue formation that may involve structures from the optic nerve forward through the retina to the iris and *ciliary body,* in varying combinations and degrees of severity. The line of closure of the primitive fissure is along the inferior and medial side of the optic cup, and therefore the defects are found along this same line after birth: *iris colobomas* are usually seen at the 7 o'clock position in the left eye and at the 5

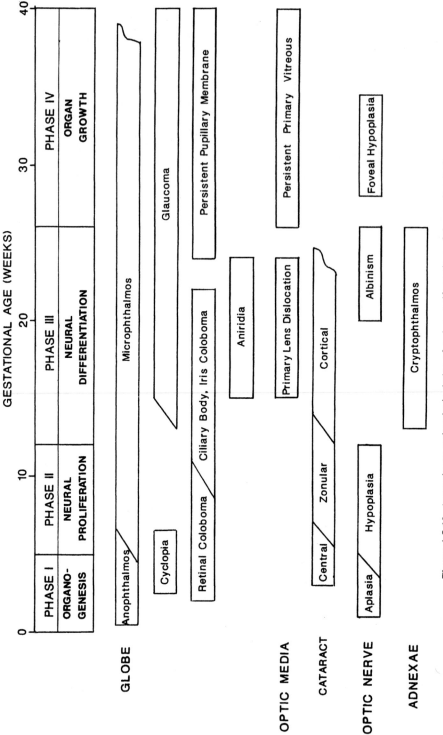

Figure 4.5.10. Approximate embryologic timing of various malformations of the eye (see text).

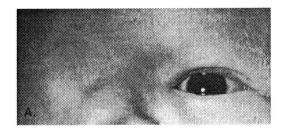

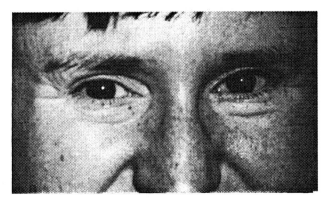

Figure 4.5.11. Generalized hypoplasia of the eye. (A) Complete anophthalmia, with no palpable globe or orbit. In this child, the entire right face was undeveloped, suggesting a vascular basis for the maldevelopment. (B) Very mild microphthalmia of the right eye. Note the slightly wider expanse of the right upper lid.

o'clock position on the right (Fig. 4.5.5B). Very rarely, colobomas are found in other zones of the eye, but the origin of these defects is not clear. If a retinal lesion is extensive or the optic nerve is involved, segmental blindness will be present.

Phase II: Week 6–12. At the beginning of phase II, rapid proliferation of the nerve cells lining the optic cup occurs, and their axons begin to converge on the optic stalk, where they pass out along the *hyaloid artery* to form the optic nerve. If nerve cell proliferation is impeded, **hypoplasia of the optic nerve** results, and the nerve head will appear small and white on funduscopic examination. Amblyopia, nystagmus, and poor visual acuity are frequently associated.

Also during this phase, the *primary vitreous* secreted during month 1 of development is being surrounded and replaced by the avascular *secondary vitreous*. **Persistence of hyperplastic primary vitreous** may result in mild microphthalmia and a dense, hazy zone behind the lens that produces *leukocoria,* a bright yellow-white light reflex. Usually unilateral, this condition may be complicated by glaucoma or *retinal detachment.*

Phase III: Week 13–26. Phase III of ocular development is marked by differentiation of the definitive retinal cells and by formation of the iris and ciliary body. **Aniridia** is a total or partial failure of iris development, producing the appearance of a very large, immobile pupil (Fig. 4.5.12A). It may be seen in isolation or, more commonly, associated with nystagmus, ptosis, glaucoma or *blindness.* Wilms tumor is strongly linked with aniridia in children with an interstitial deletion of chromosome 11.

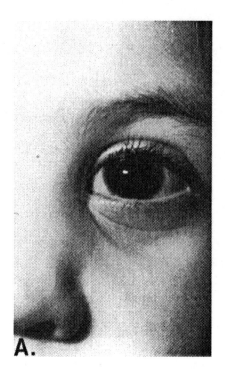 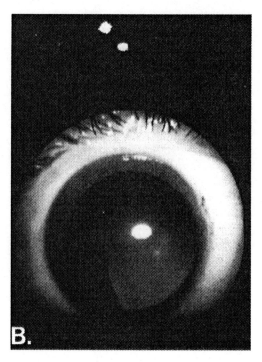

Figure 4.5.12. Deficits of mesenchymal elements in the anterior eye. (A) Aniridia. A fringe of iris is present just inside the limbus. (B) Dislocated lens. The lens has drifted laterally (note its curved edge seen through the dilated pupil) because of deficient suspensory fibers in the zonule. (Photo courtesy of Dr. Frank Durso, Albuquerque, N.M.)

The *suspensory ligaments* are elaborated by the ciliary body and attach to the periphery of the lens during this stage of development. In some disorders of connective tissue, these fibers are weak or unusually stretchable, and this eventually may allow **dislocation of the lens**. In Marfan syndrome, this usually takes place in late childhood, if at all, and results in strabismus and diminished visual acuity. The edge of the dislocated lens often can be seen coursing across the pupil, and iridodonesis sometimes can be elicited (Fig. 4.5.12B).

Abnormalities in development of the structures at the circumference of the anterior chamber during this period may impede normal fluid drainage, leading to congenital glaucoma (Fig. 4.5.8). One mechanism by which this can occur is through *persistence of the pupillary membrane* lying between the iris and the anterior chamber. Strands of mesodermal tissue connecting the iris and the posterior surface of the cornea may partially occlude the canal of Schlemm, interfering with the flow of aqueous humor.

The eyelids normally fuse over the developing eye by week 10 of intrauterine life and open again by about week 26 (see Section 4.4.1). When the lids fail to open, **cryptophthalmos** results. The eye is completely covered with skin and remains underdeveloped and sightless.

Phase IV: Week 27 to birth. During phase IV, the formation of ocular structures is largely complete, light perception is present, and simple growth is accompanied by programmed atrophy of some the embryonic vessels and by completion of the pigmentation of the posterior layer of the iris. Some degree of central control of *ocular movements* is being attained, and at least intermittent conjugate gaze is present. At this stage, the eye is quite susceptible to the adverse effects of high oxygen concentrations, which can produce **retrolental fibroplasia.** This, in turn, can lead to retinal detachment and degeneration, with permanent blindness.

Late in gestation or during the first months of life, mixed-tissue tumors may develop on the sclera in children with Goldenhar syndrome. These **epibulbar dermoids** are rounded, raised white masses appearing lateral to the cornea (Fig. 4.5.1). They may overlap the limbus and must be distinguished from benign pterygia which tend to be flatter and more pink.

4.5.6. Summary

As the most accessible structure derived from the neural tube, the eye provides valuable information about early developmental aberrations of the central nervous system. Furthermore, a knowledge of the sequential stages of optic development may provide insight into the gestational timing of dysmorphic processes. Prompt recognition of some eye anomalies may permit treatment that will avert permanent blindness.

4.6. NOSE

Situated as it is in the center of the face, the nose contributes a great deal to the overall gestalt of facial appearance. It shares in the complex embryonic development of the midface, and its abnormalities are hallmarks of a number of dysmorphic syndromes.

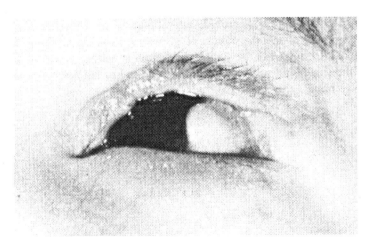

Figure 4.5.13. Epibulbar dermoid. The rounded, glistening white mass can be seen encroaching on the corneal border in the eye of this child with Goldenhar syndrome.

4.6.1. Embryology and Development

The embryogenesis of the nose is remarkably complex, considering the relatively simple structure that is eventually produced. During week 5 of gestation, paired mesodermal swellings between the *first branchial cleft* and the *frontal prominence* undergo considerable differential growth to form the horseshoe-shaped *nasal ridges* surrounding the *nasal pits* (Fig. 4.2.1A). As the maxillary segment of the first arch grows medially, it is separated from the lateral nasal ridge by the deep *nasolacrimal groove,* in which develops the nasolacrimal duct (Fig. 4.2.1B). The lateral part of the nasal ridges form the *alae nasi,* while the medial portions approach each other, eventually to fuse into the *columella.* Meanwhile, cells originating in the prechordal plate have started their long migration down over the midforehead to form the frontal skull, the dorsum of the nose, the *nasal septum,* and the base of the *philtral groove,* completing their journey with the production of the small projection at the center of the upper lip (Fig. 4.2.1C).

As with the external ear, the nose continues to grow throughout life, although quite slowly after the second decade.

4.6.2. Anatomy and Landmarks

The nose is a three-dimensional object. It grows in length from *nasion* to tip, in width from side to side, and away from the facial plane in height. Final nasal shape depends on the size and relationship between the paired *nasal bones,* the *alar cartilages,* and the median *upper nasal cartilage,* which is continuous with the septum. The *nasal bridge* is that portion of the nose lying between the orbits—approximately the upper half of the nose. The alae nasi arch out in either direction from the *nasal tip* to form the outer margin of the nostril or *naris.* The medial borders of the nares form the margins of the columella, which covers the outer end of the nasal septum (Fig. 4.6.1).

4.6.3. Examination Techniques

Visual inspection of the nose provides an estimate of its size relative to other facial structures, its symmetry, and the effects of growth in three dimensions. Whereas the height of the nasal bridge can be judged best from the side, a frontal view permits evaluation of the length and width of the entire nose and of the columella as well as the form of the alae nasi.

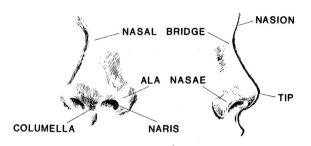

Figure 4.6.1. Superficial anatomy and landmarks of the nose.

One way of estimating the length of the nose is by observing the distance between the base of the columella and the *vermilion border* of the upper lip. The length of the face between the brow line and the mouth is determined primarily by the development of the maxilla. Only two structures, the nose and the *philtrum,* occupy this zone of the central face, so a change in the length of one will usually be accompanied by a compensatory change in the length of the other. Thus, a long nose often results in a short philtrum, and vice versa (Fig. 4.6.2).

In newborns, it is important to ascertain the adequacy of nasal air flow, since babies at this age are obligate nose breathers. The easiest test is simply pressing one nostril closed with a fingertip while the baby is sucking a pacifier or bottle. Distress or gasping during this maneuver suggests that the other nasal passage is fully or partially occluded. Confirmation can be obtained by attempting to pass a small catheter or feeding tube through each nostril into the oropharynx.

Since telecanthus or a *low nasal bridge* may create the impression of a *broad nasal bridge,* it is best to complete the examination with palpation of the nasal bridge to determine the size and shape of the bone underlying the soft tissue in this region.

4.6.4. Minor Variants

4.6.4.1. Spectrum Variants

There is a wide normal range of nasal size and general shape, with strong elements of heritability. Here again, comparison of the characteristics in the patient with those of the parents is valuable.

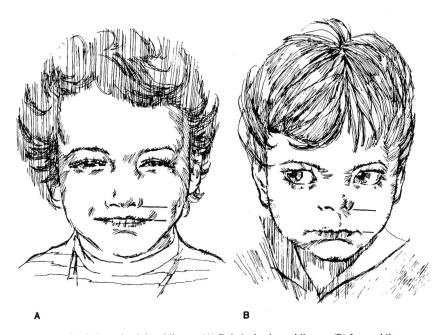

A   **B**

Figure 4.6.2. Length of the philtrum. (A) Relatively short philtrum. (B) Long philtrum.

A low nasal bridge is the rule for infants under the age of 1 year, since the nasal bones and cartilages are incompletely formed at birth and continue to grow throughout childhood. For the same reason, the infant's nose usually appears shorter in relation to facial length than does that of the adult. In later life, a persisting low nasal bridge (*saddle nose*) may signify slow maturation of the facial skeleton (Fig. 4.6.3). On the other hand, a high, arched nasal bridge leads to the appearance of a **beaked nose**, which may be seen in syndrome diagnoses featuring premature synostosis at the base of the skull, such as Crouzon syndrome and acrocephalosyndactyly.

Nasal length varies within fairly wide limits, ranging from a simple "pug" nose to an overhanging nasal tip. When the dorsum of the nose is very short, the nasal tip is essentially pulled upward, resulting in **anteverted nares** (Fig. 4.6.4). Similarly, **nasal width** shows considerable variation by family and racial group.

4.6.4.2. Minor Anomalies

A **short columella** pulls down the nasal tip and distorts the nares, producing a flattened appearance (Fig. 4.6.5A). A **bulbous nose** with a rounded, overhanging tip may be a familial variant, but is also seen in such conditions as trichorhinophalangeal syndrome (Fig. 4.6.5B). **Hypoplasia of the alae nasi** gives a narrow, pinched appearance that again is sometimes called a beaked nose (Fig. 4.6.5C). If the breadth of the dorsum of the nose does not widen normally from base to tip, a somewhat tubular contour results. When combined with a mild degree of alar hypoplasia, such a **cylindrical nose** is a frequent feature of Waardenburg syndrome (Fig. 4.6.5D). A **broad nasal bridge** implies palpable widening of the nasal bones and is seen in some normal individuals with mild hypertelorism.

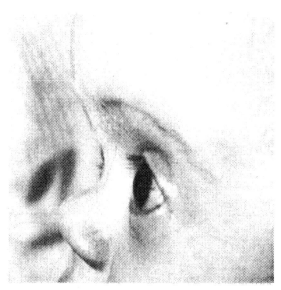

Figure 4.6.3. Low nasal bridge.

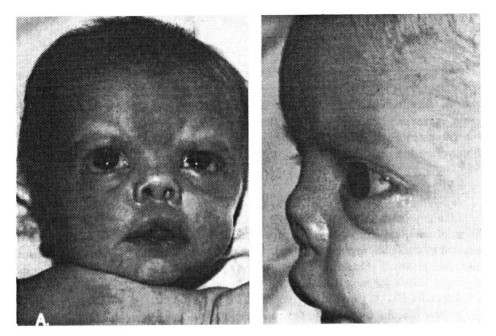

Figure 4.6.4. Short nose. (A) Frontal view, showing anteverted nares and tented upper lip in Robinow syndrome. (B) Lateral view of the same child. Note foreshortening of the dorsum of the nose and the tilted plane of nostril openings.

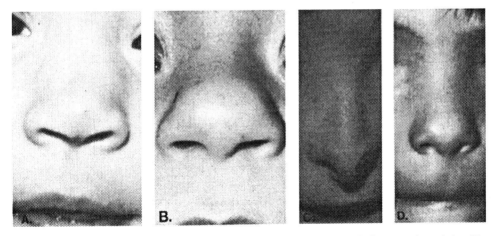

Figure 4.6.5. Minor variants of nasal configuration. (A) Short columella with downturned nasal tip. (B) Bulbous nasal tip. (C) Columella and nasal tip extending beyond hypoplastic alae nasi. Note the short philtrum. (D) Broad, high nasal bridge producing a "tubular" appearance of the nose.

4.6.5. Abnormalities

4.6.5.1. Deformations

Not infrequently, the nose is distorted by intrauterine constraint and babies at birth are found to have the nasal tip pushed to one side, asymmetric nares, and a **deviated nasal septum**. This last deformity can often be corrected with relative ease in the newborn period, preventing breathing difficulties and obviating the need for later surgical intervention. More severe degrees of deformation are often seen with Potter facies caused by oligohydramnios (Fig. 4.6.6).

4.6.5.2. Disruptions

Like any other superficial structure of the body, the nose may be damaged by the effects of amniotic bands. Because of a tendency for these bands to be swallowed or aspirated by the fetus, severe orofacial clefting may occur which does not follow the usual embryonic planes of closure. These defects may pass upward through the alae nasi or cut diagonally across the nose but never will be found to have an exact midline orientation (see Appendix C).

In later life, direct trauma to the nose may cause damage or destruction of the nasal cartilages, resulting in a flattened, asymmetric, or *pugilistic nose*.

4.6.5.3. Dysplasias

Nasal structures may be coarsened by soft tissue deposition of storage materials in disorders such as the mucopolysaccharidoses and oligosaccharidoses (Fig. 4.2.6A).

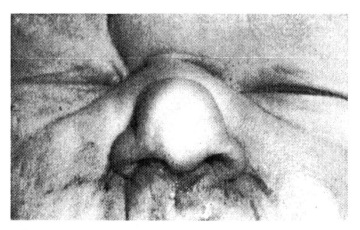

Figure 4.6.6. Nasal deformation and facial skin creases resulting from compression in the oligohydramnios sequence.

4.6.5.4. *Malformations*

The embryologic formation and subsequent migration of the mesenchymal cells of the prechordal plate seem to depend on the normal development of the underlying forebrain. When this anterior portion of the neural tube fails to form properly, a number of sequelae arise: the frontal eminence remains small, and the deficiency of neural and mesenchymal tissue in the midline permits the optic cups on the two sides to arise much closer to each other than is normal, sometimes partially fusing in the midline. In such cases, there is a severe deficiency of the primordial tissues that usually form the nose, and cellular migration is impeded by the aberrant midfacial development. There is a spectrum of severity of this holoprosencephaly sequence and a corresponding spectrum of abnormal nasal development: in cyclopia, the nasal structures are represented by a tubular **proboscis** emerging above the fused eyes (Fig. 4.4.12); a bulky nose with a midline **single nostril** might accompany marked hypotelorism in cebocephaly, while the mildest degree of arhinencephaly might be found with only a low nasal bridge.

The opposite type of anomaly occurs when too much tissue develops in (or migrates into) the upper midfacial zone, causing various degrees of **frontonasal dysplasia**. The mechanism for this malformation seems to be either an absolute excess of cells from the prechordal plate or an interference with their downward migration, causing them to "pile up" at some intermediate location. The nasal bridge is extremely broad, and extreme hypertelorism is always present (Fig. 4.6.7A). In severe cases, the nostrils may be separated by several centimeters, and there is often a midline deficiency of the upper lip (Fig. 4.6.7B). In other instances, the frontonasal mesoderm seems to have been halted midway in its migration, and the deficit of tissue distal to the roadblock causes a bifid or dimpled nasal tip, variable hypoplasia of the distal nasal septum and columella, and a short, tented upper lip without a philtrum (Fig. 4.6.7C).

A seemingly much more minor nasal abnormality but one that may have implications for severe occult abnormalities is the existence of a median **nasal pit** (Fig. 4.6.8). As is the case with similar lesions anywhere on the midline of the head or back, such a defect may mark the end of a tract that connects directly with the central nervous system. Danger signs include hairs implanted in the pit, fluid emerging from its depths, or any underlying bony defect or cystic mass. Of similar significance is a bulging over the nasal bridge, appearing when a baby cries (Fig. 4.6.9). This indicates the presence of an **anterior cephalocele** and demands neurosurgical investigation because of the possibility of extension into the nasopharynx.

One other serious nasal malformation is often missed in examinations of the newborn. Total or partial obstruction of the posterior opening of the nasal passage is known as **choanal atresia** or **stenosis** and results from persistence or incomplete perforation of the **oronasal membrane** (see Section 4.8). This condition should be suspected if an infant seems to have respiratory difficulty only when feeding or prefers to breathe through the mouth. Inability to pass a small catheter or feeding tube through the nose into the oropharynx should prompt immediate consultation with an ear-nose-throat specialist and radiographic confirmation.

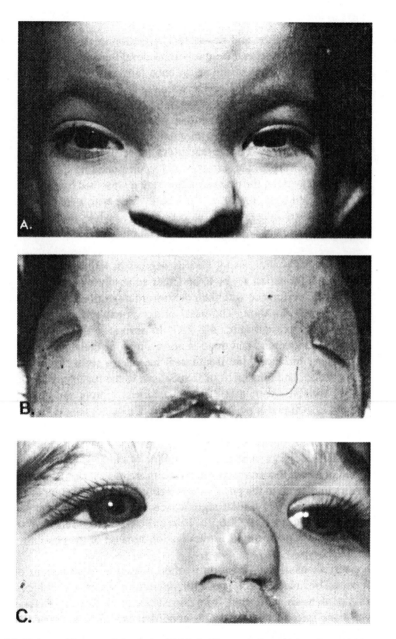

Figure 4.6.7. Variants of frontonasal dysplasia. (A) Marked hypertelorism with broad nasal bridge and repaired bilateral cleft lip. (B) Extreme ocular hypertelorism with widely separated alae nasi and aberrant formation of philtrum and upper lip. (Photo courtesy of Dr. Herb Koffler, Albuquerque, N.M.) (C) Hypertelorism, telecanthus, and wide nasal bridge but deficient nasal tip, columella, and alae nasi. Note extremely short philtrum and tented upper lip.

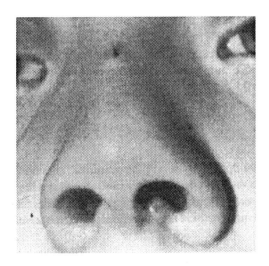

Figure 4.6.8. Midline pit on the nasal bridge. Note hairs emerging from the depths of the pit.

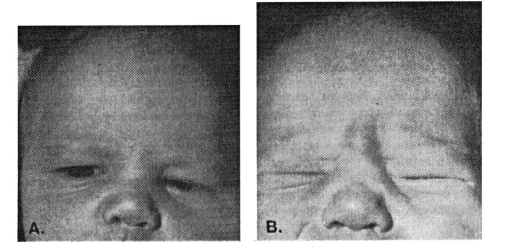

Figure 4.6.9. Anterior encephalocele. (A) Baby at rest. (B) Bulging over occult encephalocele when baby cries.

4.6.6. Summary

Because of its developmental history and relationships to surrounding structures, the configuration of the nose may provide valuable information about embryogenic events occurring between weeks 5 and 10 of gestation.

4.7. PERIORAL REGION

In humans, the mouth not only serves the primitive functions of eating and breathing but also is used for two distinctly human activities: speech and the display of subtle facial expressions. For this reason, even minor structural anomalies in this region may have cosmetic or functional implications disproportionate to their severity.

4.7.1. Embryology and Development

The skeletal structures surrounding the oral cavity originate from the maxillary and mandibular portions of the *first branchial arch,* with a small contribution from the *prechordal plate mesoderm.* The musculature and soft tissues derive from regional mesenchyme, with some contribution from neural crest cells (see Sections 4.2 and 4.6).

The *mandible* is composed of both membranous and endochondral bone (Meckel's cartilage) of first-arch origin. Midline fusion of the *mandibular prominences* occurs at about the time of closure of the anterior neural tube (4–4.5 weeks), while union of the bilateral *maxillary prominences* with the median *premaxilla* is not complete until 7–8 weeks. The premaxilla contributes the cartilage that will form the small *primary palate* as well as the midportion of the upper *alveolar arch,* bearing the central and lateral incisor teeth (see Section 4.8). The *prolabium* overlies the premaxilla and contributes the soft tissue structures forming the bottom of the philtral groove and the midportion of the upper *vermilion.* This is thought to be the furthest extension of neural crest cells that have migrated down the midline from the prechordal plate.

4.7.2. Anatomy and Landmarks

The philtrum lies between the base of the nose and the vermilion (*carmine margin*) of the upper lip and bears a central shallow philtral groove, bordered by low ridges. The lower end of this depression indents the vermilion to form a "cupid's bow." The upper and lower lips meet at the *oral commissures* or *angles of the mouth,* which themselves usually lie vertically below the pupils of the eyes. The *nasolabial folds* curve down from the alae nasi, demarcating the *cheeks* from the lips. In the midline, the *mentum* of the mandible marks the central point of the chin, while the *body* of the mandible extends backward to form a variably obtuse angle with the mandibular *ramus* (Fig. 4.7.1).

4.7.3. Examination Techniques

Most of the perioral zone can be evaluated by inspection alone. In the frontal view, the size and symmetry of the mouth, lips, and nasolabial folds can be ascertained. The

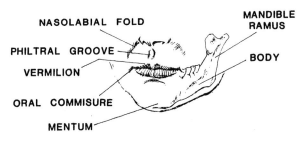

Figure 4.7.1. Anatomy and landmarks of the perioral region.

length and configuration of the upper lip and philtrum should be noted, as well as the contour of the chin and cheeks. If *micrognathia* is suspected, the lips should be spread apart with the mouth closed, allowing examination of the alignment of the upper and lower teeth (or, in infants, the *alveolar margins*). The relative size of the mandible is easiest to judge from the lateral aspect, and the cheeks and angle of the mandible should also be inspected from this point of view.

Palpation of the mandible is sometimes valuable, and special attention should be paid to the mentum and mandibular angle.

4.7.4. Minor Variants

4.7.4.1. Spectrum Variants

As in most other facial features, there is a wide latitude of variability in the perioral structures. A mildly large or small mouth (**relative macrostomia** or **microstomia**) and lower jaw (**prognathia** or **retrognathia**) and **thick** or **thin lips** may appear as family characteristics. Similarly, the length of the philtrum varies in roughly inverse proportion to the length of the nose (see Section 4.6.3); therefore, a **long philtrum** may indicate a short nose, while a **short philtrum** has the opposite connotation (Fig. 4.6.2). **Downturned corners of the mouth** sometimes reflects relative overgrowth in the width of the upper lip and, when combined with a short philtrum and thick lower lip, produces an appearance sometimes called **carp mouth** (Fig. 4.7.2A).

4.7.4.2. Minor Anomalies

Absence of the lateral ridges of the philtrum produces a **flat** or **smooth philtrum**, which may be associated with a long upper lip and loss of the usual cupid's bow configuration of the carmine margin (**rainbow vermilion**). Moreover, in such instances the upper vermilion is often turned under, producing the appearance of a **narrow carmine margin** (Fig. 4.7.2B).

Small, blind **angular lip pits** may occur at the corners of the mouth. No fistulas or underlying abnormalities are associated with this minor anomaly.

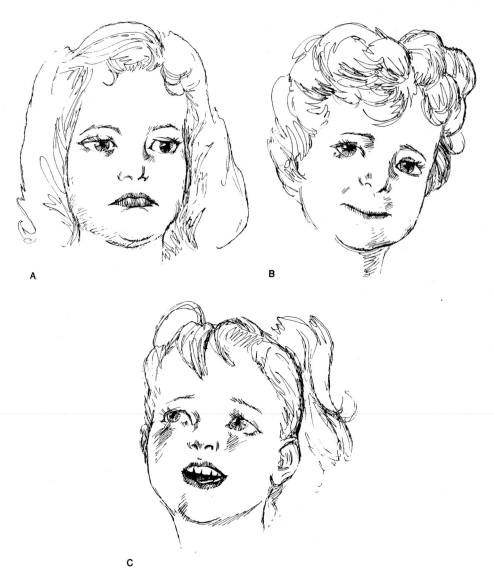

Figure 4.7.2. Minor variants of perioral configuration. (A) Full lower lip with depressed angles of the mouth (carp mouth). (B) Long, smooth philtrum. Note narrow vermilion lacking a cupid's bow. (C) Mandibular asymmetry with asynclitism of the dental arches.

4.7.5. Abnormalities

4.7.5.1. Deformations

The most common deformational abnormalities of the lower face involve the mandible. Intrauterine constraint that puts pressure on the developing jaw may produce mild to moderate micrognathia. This is especially frequent in babies born from a face presentation or a breech position with extended head. After birth, a "receding chin" may be evident, and the baby may be most comfortable lying on her side with her neck hyperextended. If the lips are parted while the jaws are held together, the lower alveolar margin may be found to lie several millimeters behind the upper.

If intrauterine pressure has been asymmetric, **unilateral mandibular hypoplasia** may be seen. Usually, the head has been tipped laterally for a long period, with one side of the jaw pressed against the shoulder, clavicle, or uterine wall. Asymmetry of the jaw often will be obvious, but again, examination of the alveolar margins can assist in diagnosing milder degrees of involvement: the upper and lower alveoli will not meet squarely but will show a gap on the unaffected side (Fig. 4.7.2C).

In both unilateral and bilateral deformation, the intrinsic growth potential of the mandible is unimpaired, and once the baby has been born and the abnormal pressure relieved, catch-up growth is rapid. The jaw will grow faster than the remainder of the facial skeleton, and normal facial contours are usually attained within the first year of life.

A more subtle deformation may be found in individuals of any age who have diminished or absent function of the facial muscles. A **flattened nasolabial fold** may be present on the affected side in cases of unilateral facial nerve palsy or may be bilateral in generalized neuromuscular disease (Fig. 4.7.3A).

In some rare disorders, aberrant muscle pull is apparently responsible for the production of abnormal **chin creases**. These usually are seen as horizontal or H-shaped creases just above the mentum and may become more evident with increasing age in childhood.

4.7.5.2. Disruptions

Severe and widespread damage to structures in the perioral region can be produced by amniotic bands. The fetus is thought to inhale or swallow the free end of a strand, which becomes adherent to tissues of the pharynx or esophagus. With one end anchored in the pharynx and the other still attached to the placenta, these strands can slice through the fragile fetal tissues in virtually any plane, producing major facial clefts that do not correspond to normal lines of embryonic fusion (see Appendix C).

4.7.5.3. Dysplasias

The lips and soft tissues around the mouth are thickened by deposition of intracellular substances in the storage diseases (Fig. 4.2.6A), and large or **prominent lips** are seen in a number of other conditions, including Williams syndrome and hypohydrotic ectodermal dysplasia. Even more striking localized enlargement may be caused by dysplasia or blockage of lymphatic drainage in facial **lymphangioma** (Fig. 4.7.3B).

The vermilion of the lips is a tissue transitional between skin and mucous membrane and sometimes can be involved with hamartomatous lesions caused by dysplastic disorders. **Angiofibromas** can be seen on the lips as raised, red to yellow papules or plaques in conditions such as Goltz syndrome.

Generalized overgrowth of the mandible (**macrognathia**) is a cardinal feature of hyperpituitarism, often caused by a pituitary tumor, but also can be seen as a part of some dysmorphic conditions such as Sotos syndrome (Fig. 4.7.4).

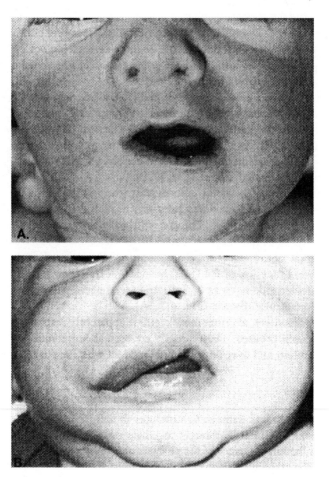

Figure 4.7.3. Deformation of perioral structures. (A) Lower facial asymmetry caused by right-sided seventh-nerve palsy. (B) Enlargement and distortion of upper lip secondary to lymphangioma.

4.7.5.4. Malformations

The most common major anomaly affecting the perioral region is **cleft lip**. This malformation represents a failure of normal tissue proliferation and fusion in the region of the embryonic furrow where the median and lateral nasal processes meet the maxillary process. The resulting defect may be partial or complete, unilateral or bilateral (Fig. 4.8.9A and B). The line of clefting is paramedian and follows the ridge at either side of the philtrum (Fig. 4.7.5A). The mildest form results in an intact lip with only a linear scarlike lesion running along the margin of the philtrum; the most severe type penetrates the alveolus and interferes with normal palatal closure, resulting in an associated **cleft palate**.

In complete bilateral cleft lip, a midline nubbin of tissue is seen attached to the columella of the nose (Fig. 4.7.5B). This represents the remnants of the intermaxillary

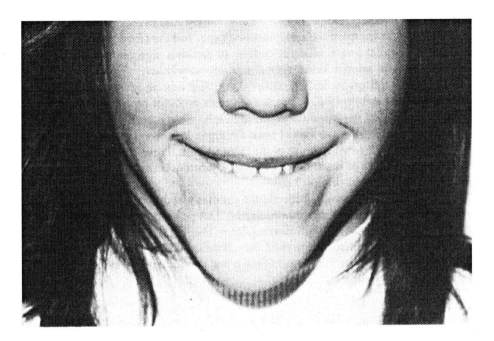

Figure 4.7.4. Macrognathia in Sotos syndrome.

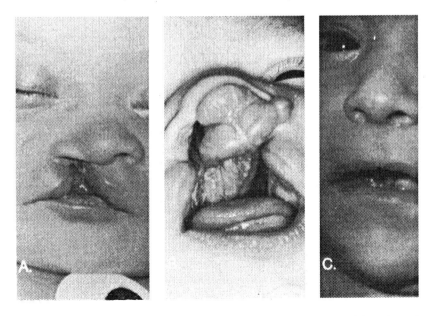

Figure 4.7.5. Cleft lip. (A) Unilateral incomplete cleft. The alveolar ridge is intact. (B) Bilateral complete cleft lip and palate. Note midline tissue mass incorporating premaxilla and prolabium. (C) Small midline cleft of vermilion. Note poorly modeled philtrum.

segment, the unpaired median structure that normally would have formed the floor of the philtral groove, the center of the upper alveolar ridge, and the primary palate. *Absence* of this rudimentary tissue in a bilateral cleft is an ominous sign pointing to major maldevelopment of the anterior brain, typically *holoprosencephaly*.

A **median cleft** of the lip is extremely rare and may be associated with a broad, dimpled, or cleft nasal tip (Fig. 4.7.5C). Such cases probably represent the mildest form of *median facial cleft syndrome* (frontonasal dysplasia) (see Section 4.6.5.4).

Oblique facial clefts can extend from the upper lip upward to the inner canthus of the eye, following the general course of the lacrimal duct. These rare malformations seem to result from a deficit of tissue along the line of juncture between the maxillary process and the lateral nasal fold (Fig. 4.7.6).

Failure of complete fusion between the maxillary and mandibular segments of the first branchial arch results in **true macrostomia**. This defect may be unilateral or bilateral and is frequently associated with hearing loss. The angle of the mouth is displaced laterally and upward, extending beyond the vermilion borders of the lips (Fig. 4.7.6). Cutaneous pits and tags may be found along a line connecting the oral commissure with the external auditory canal.

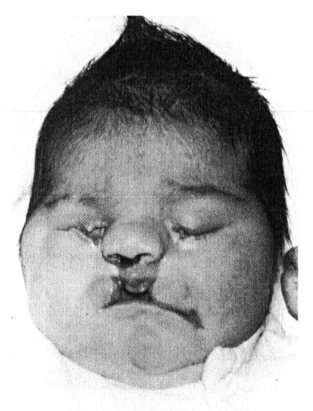

Figure 4.7.6. Bilateral oblique facial clefts extending to the lower lids. Also note macrostomia on the left.

Moderate to severe degrees of micrognathia may result from lack of intrinsic mandibular growth in a number of congenital disorders. In this malformed type of small jaw, there is little or no catch-up growth during early childhood (Fig. 4.7.7). When the hypoplasia is extreme, the oral cavity is too small to contain the tongue, giving rise to the Pierre Robin complex (see Section 4.8.5.4).

Lower lip pits are seen as part of a few rare syndromes. They are usually bilateral, situated on the vermilion to either side of the midline, and may have underlying fistulas that exude a mucoid substance.

4.7.6. Summary

The perioral zone is susceptible to abnormalities of all types and of varying degrees of severity. Fortunately, some of the most common anomalies either resolve spontaneously or can be surgically corrected. The more clinically severe anomalies often occur in isolation and are less likely to be pertinent for dysmorphologic diagnosis than are the milder ones.

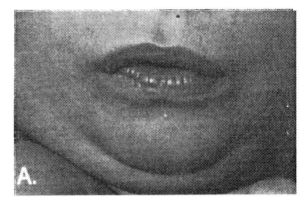

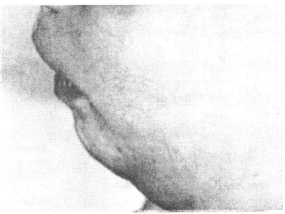

Figure 4.7.7. Micrognathia. (A) Frontal view. Note "double chin" appearance. (B) Lateral view.

4.8. ORAL CAVITY

The structures of the mouth are derived from all three embryonic tissue layers and thus can display a wide variety of developmental abnormalities, some of which are particularly useful in suggesting or helping confirm a dysmorphic syndrome diagnosis. Unfortunately, the oral cavity is one part of the face for which our instinctive concepts of "normal" are not well developed, and special attention must be directed to this part of the examination so as not to miss subtle but important abnormalities.

4.8.1. Embryology and Development

The oral cavity originates as the *stomodeum,* a deep depression lying between the frontonasal prominence and the mandibular portion of the first branchial arch (Fig. 4.2.1A). Initially, the stomodeum is separated from the *foregut* or *primitive pharynx* by the *oropharyngeal membrane,* but at about 3.5 weeks of gestation this structure breaks down, allowing free communication between the digestive tract and the amniotic cavity. A few days later, the anterior two-thirds of the tongue begins to form on the floor of the pharynx from one midline and two lateral swellings. As the tongue grows upward into the pharynx, a lateral projection of the pharyngeal wall appears at either side to form the *palatal shelves,* while the nasal septum descends from above (Fig. 4.8.1A).

Continued differential growth of the palatal shelves causes them to swing up into a horizontal plane above the tongue, and at about 7.5 weeks they begin to fuse with the triangular *primary palate* anteriorly. By 9 weeks, the free edges of the shelves have met each other and the nasal septum in the midline, and fusion proceeds anteriorly and posteriorly, forming the *secondary palate* (Fig. 4.8.1B). The roof of the mouth is completely closed by week 12 and soon begins to ossify as the *hard palate,* which separates

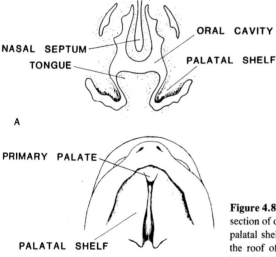

NASAL SEPTUM

TONGUE

ORAL CAVITY

PALATAL SHELF

A

PRIMARY PALATE

PALATAL SHELF

B

Figure 4.8.1. Embryogenesis of the palate. (A) Coronal section of oral cavity at 6.5 weeks of gestation, showing palatal shelves still in vertical orientation. (B) View of the roof of the mouth from below at 7.5 weeks, just before fusion of the palatal shelves to form the secondary palate. [After Langman (1969).]

the oral cavity from the nasopharynx. That portion of the roof of the mouth extending backward beyond the posterior edge of the nasal septum remains unsupported by bone and is called the *soft palate*. The *uvula* is the rearmost extension of the palate and the last part to fuse.

The *teeth* first appear at about gestational week 6 as buds of ectoderm extending down into the mesenchyme of the early mandible and maxilla. A mesodermal core becomes the *dentin* and pulp of the tooth, while the surrounding ectoderm gives rise to the dental *enamel*. The teeth are formed well before birth but continue to grow and differentiate beyond the time of dental eruption. Each incisor tooth develops from three closely adjacent growth centers that normally fuse together completely before eruption but may leave an irregular "picket fence" appearance of the incisal edges in young children.

4.8.2. Anatomy and Landmarks

The *labial mucosa* on the inner surfaces of the lips is continuous laterally with the *buccal mucosa* that lines the inner surface of the cheeks. A raised fold of mucosa extends from the central base of the upper *alveolar ridge* onto the interior of the upper lip, forming the *labial frenulum*. A similar but smaller frenulum is found in the midline of the lower lip. The teeth surmount the alveolar ridges (*gums*), forming the upper and lower *dental arches*. The *primary* or *deciduous dentition* consists of *upper* and *lower central incisors, lateral incisors, canines,* and *first* and *second molars*. These are eventually replaced by the *secondary* or *permanent dentition,* which includes new copies of all of the primary teeth plus the *first* and *second premolars* and the *third molars* (wisdom teeth). An appreciation for the usual pattern of dental development can provide a rough approximation of bone age, but allowance must be made for the wide normal variation in times of dental eruption. Perhaps more helpful is an acquaintance with the *sequence* in which teeth erupt. Both the usual sequence and the dates of dental eruption are outlined in Fig. 4.8.2, but it should be understood that the range of normal eruption times extends several months before and after the median dates shown.

The *tongue* normally occupies all of the space within the lower dental arch, swelling upward gently to partially fill the remaining oral cavity. Under the tongue, folds of oral mucosa meet in the midline to form the *lingual frenulum,* to either side of which lie the *sublingual salivary glands.* The upper and posterior surfaces of the tongue are studded with *taste buds,* and a small pit, the *foramen cecum,* which represents the upper end of the fetal *thyroglossal duct,* lies in the midline posteriorly.

The *palate* forms the elongated dome of the roof of the mouth. A midline *palatal raphe* often marks the line of fusion of the secondary palate, and a small mound, the *incisive papilla,* lies at the spot where the primary palate and the two lateral palatine shelves come together. Seen in cross section, the arch of the palate is rounded and fairly broad from side to side (Fig. 4.8.3A). The soft palate in the posterior third of the oral roof has no underlying bone and dives downward to terminate centrally in the uvula. This structure varies considerably in size and shape in different individuals, from a barely visible midline swelling to a pendulous teardrop-shaped mass hanging down below the posterior curve of the tongue. Laterally, the posterior edge of the soft palate swings downward to meet the pharyngeal wall, forming the *anterior tonsillar pillar.*

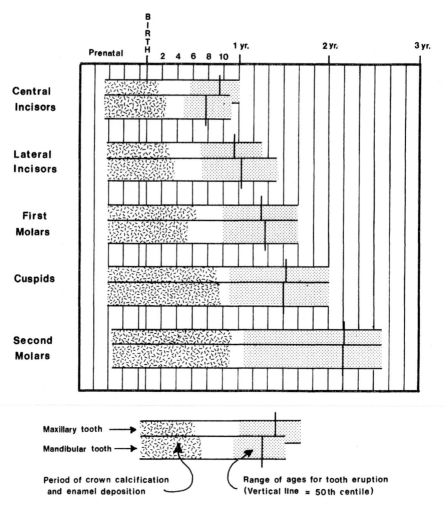

Figure 4.8.2. Development of the primary (deciduous) teeth. The beginning of the stippled area indicates the 10th centile for age of eruption, the vertical line marks the 50th centile, and the end of the bar marks the 90th centile.

4.8.3. Examination Techniques

The lips, gums, and teeth are first inspected for abnormalities. With a tongue depressor or a clean finger, the lips are gently everted and their mucous membranes examined. The patient's mouth is next partly opened, and, using a penlight or otoscope, the buccal mucosa is inspected in the same fashion. Note is also taken of the number, size, and configuration of the teeth. With the patient's mouth fully open, the light is used to help examine the shape of the palate, the size of the tongue, and the inner surfaces of the teeth. If the patient is old enough to do so, he may be asked to "say 'ah'" or to "sing" at this point, which will permit assessment of the movement of the soft palate and the base of

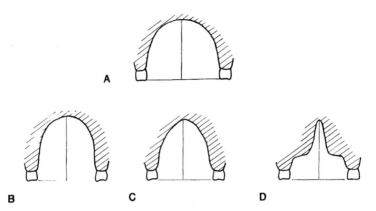

Figure 4.8.3. Diagrams of palatal configuration, coronal sections. (A) Normal palate. (B) Narrow palate of normal height. (C) Gothic palate. (D) Palate narrowed by persistence of secondary palatal ridges.

the tongue. In infants (and rarely in older children), it may be necessary to stimulate a gag reflex to obtain an adequate view of the pharynx. With experience, only a glimpse of the posterior oral structures is enough.

Simply asking an older child to smile allows evaluation of dental alignment and the adequacy of dental coalition.

In newborns and in any other children in whom there may be a question of submucous cleft, palpation of the roof of the mouth should be carried out. The examiner's fifth finger is introduced, palm up, into the mouth, and the length and integrity of the hard palate is determined. Palpation of the alveolar margins in newborns may also be helpful if there is a suggestion of the presence of *natal teeth*.

4.8.4. Minor Variants

4.8.4.1. Spectrum Variants

As mentioned above, there is considerable variability in the time of appearance for both primary and secondary teeth, and **early** or **late dental eruption** may be a familial trait. When teeth are present at birth, they are usually incompletely developed mandibular incisors. Often these natal teeth will be shed, and the remaining primary and secondary dentition will appear at the usual time in childhood.

Minor variations in the size and shape of the teeth are quite common and are usually of no clinical significance. Occasionally, separate inheritance of relatively large teeth along with a relatively small mandible and maxilla may give rise to **dental crowding** and **malalignment**. Primary teeth may be forced into abnormal positions and may interfere with the emergence of elements of the secondary dentition. The term used for an unusually wide space between the upper central incisors is **diastema**.

The surface of the tongue sometimes bears patches of irregular size and shape, seemingly denuded of papillae, which contrast with surrounding areas in which the epithelium is hypertrophic. The patterns on such a **geographic tongue** change slowly with time, and the condition may persist for months or years without producing any difficulty for the affected individual. Similarly, a deeply **furrowed tongue** (*scrotal tongue*) produces an unusual appearance but no symptoms and may be familial.

Occasionally, the lingual frenulum may be unusually thick and short, with insertion close to the tip of the tongue. **Short frenulum** or *tongue-tie* may rarely cause aberrant speech patterns but does not seem to interfere with feeding in infancy.

As might be expected, the width of the palate varies with the breadth of the maxilla, and many individuals with narrow faces will have a **narrow palate** as well. In most cases in which a palate has been described as high arched, it is really only narrow from side to side. A truly high palate is quite rare.

4.8.4.2. Minor Malformations

Some types of narrow palate seem to represent not mere variation of normal but true malformations. The most clearly defined of these is the **gothic palate** seen most frequently in Turner syndrome (Fig. 4.8.3C). This is sometimes associated with a prominent **median palatal raphe** that follows the line of fusion of the hard palate.

Palatal pits are sometimes found in the midline, especially at the point of junction of the primary and secondary palates. A doughnut-shaped swelling over the posterior third of the hard palate is a **torus palatinus**, a benign lesion that may be inherited in a multifactorial pattern.

Too few teeth for the patient's age may be due to delayed dental eruption or to **hypodontia**. **Absent** or **hypoplastic lateral maxillary incisors** can be found as an isolated anomaly but often run in families as an autosomal dominant trait. Rarely, **supernumerary palatal (mesiodens) teeth** will erupt from the primary palate, just behind the upper incisors.

There is a wide variety of minor abnormalities in the shape of the teeth themselves. **Channel** or **shovel teeth** are incisors whose lateral edges curve back toward the tongue, giving them a C-shaped cross section (Fig. 4.8.4). **Notched incisors** have a defect in the incisal edge, representing deficient growth of one of the three dental mammilons; total

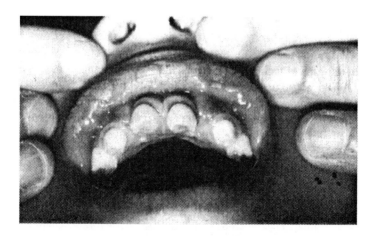

Figure 4.8.4. Channel teeth.

absence of one of these vertical rays produces an incisor narrower at the incisal edge than at the cervix. The classic description of **Hutchinson's teeth**, seen in congenital syphilis, is that of pegged lateral maxillary incisors and notched central incisors resembling the blade of a screwdriver. **Mulberry molars** are almost spherical, with distortion of the cusps into irregular, rounded protuberances. Fusion between two neighboring tooth buds creates a **bigeminal incisor** (Fig. 4.8.5).

4.8.5. Abnormalities

4.8.5.1. Deformations

During postnatal growth, the structures of the mouth normally are subjected to recurring mechanical stress from chewing and tongue movement, and apparently these forces play a role in the configuration of the jaws and palate. Deformation of the mandible is discussed in section 4.7.5.1. **Persistence of the secondary alveolar ridge** causes a remarkably narrow or grooved palate and is caused by inadequacy of tongue thrusting against the roof of the mouth (Fig. 4.8.3D). This movement seems to be required to mold the contours of the palate and prevent overgrowth of tissue lying on the inner aspect of the upper gum line. Tongue thrusting may be impaired by intrinsic factors, such as a *small tongue* or severe neurologic deficit, or by mechanical factors, such as prolonged endotracheal intubation. In the latter instance, direct pressure from the tube itself may also play a small role in deforming the palate. Even in older children whose palates are normal, cessation of tongue movement may lead to gradual narrowing of the palate through overgrowth of the secondary alveolar ridges. This is demonstrated by the boy shown in Fig. 4.8.6, who was normal until he experienced a prolonged period of severe hypoxia and became permanently comatose.

The position of the teeth also can be changed by mechanical forces acting over fairly long periods. This principle is used to advantage in the usual orthodontic procedures in

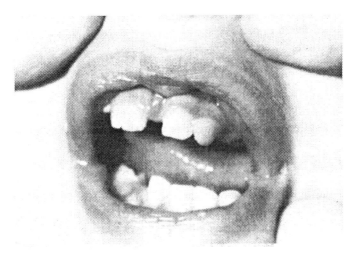

Figure 4.8.5. Bigeminal right central maxillary incisor. Also note wide separation between central incisors (diastema).

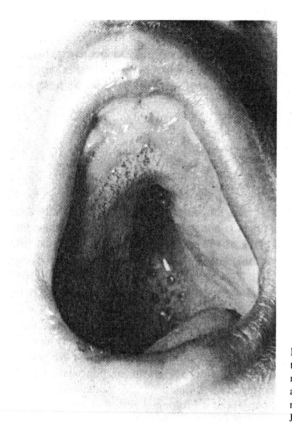

Figure 4.8.6. Palate narrowed by hypertrophy of secondary palatal ridges. Lack of normal tongue thrusting was caused by anoxic brain damage in this previously normal boy. (Photo courtesy of Dr. Kenneth Jones, San Diego, Calif.)

which pressure is applied to the teeth by means of steel braces or other appliances to improve dental spacing or alignment. Unfortunately, **distortion of the dental arch** results just as easily when abnormal mechanical stresses act on the teeth and dental alveoli. For example, the severe anterior open bite shown in Fig. 4.8.7A was caused by pressure from an unusually large tongue, seen in Fig. 4.8.7B.

4.8.5.2. Disruptions

While cysts or other tumors can cause local destruction of tissue, the only major agent of disruption affecting the oral cavity is amniotic bands (see Appendix C).

4.8.5.3. Dysplasias

Lesions of the oral mucous membranes are found in several dysplastic disorders. **Pigmented macules** on the lips and buccal mucosa are clues to the presence of Peutz-Jeghers syndrome; **leukoplakia**, a gray-white plaquelike lesion of the tongue or mucous membranes, may signify dyskeratosis congenita or pachyonychia congenita; and the multiple punctate **telangiectases** of Osler hemorrhagic telangiectasia syndrome may be found on the tongue and mucosa of the lips.

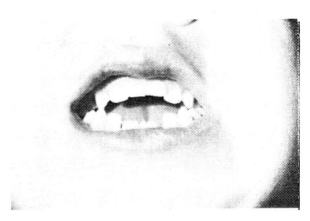

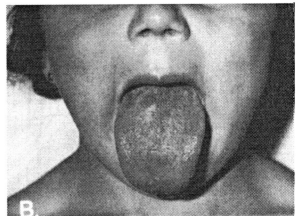

Figure 4.8.7. Deformation of dental arches. (A) Marked anterior open bite in a girl with Beckwith syndrome. (B) Enlarged tongue in the same child, source of the prolonged pressure causing the dental malocclusion.

Intrinsic abnormalities of the teeth may affect only the enamel or the dentin or may involve the structure of the entire tooth. Localized **enamel hypoplasia,** producing grooves, fissures, or pits on the tooth surface, may be caused by nutritional deficiencies such as rickets, excessive dietary fluoride, or some childhood illnesses contracted during the critical period of formation of the permanent dentition. In the many types of **amelogenesis imperfecta,** inadequate calcification results in enamel that is thin, soft, and friable, and the teeth are yellow to brown in color and unusually subject to caries. (Fig. 4.8.8A). A different and somewhat more common disorder is **dentinogenesis imperfecta** or **hereditary opalescent dentin,** in which the teeth have a pearly blue-gray color and wear down very quickly because the normal enamel is inadequately adherent to the underlying dentin (Fig. 4.8.8B).

Oligodontia, with numerous missing, conical, or peg-shaped teeth, is a common feature in several forms of ectodermal dysplasia (Fig. 4.8.8C). The most severe degree of this malformation is **anodontia,** in which there is complete absence of the primary and secondary dentitions.

A **thickened tongue** results from deposition of storage materials in some metabolic diseases, and **gingival hyperplasia** may be produced by some medications, notably

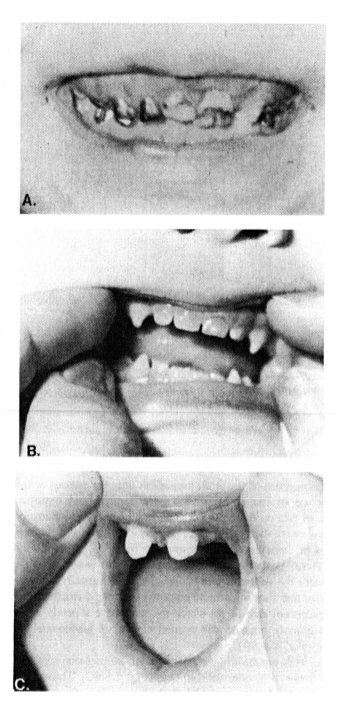

Figure 4.8.8. Dental dysplasias. (A) Fractured, discolored, and absent enamel in amelogenesis imperfecta. (B) Translucent teeth in hereditary opalescent dentin syndrome. (C) Generalized dental hypoplasia in hypohydrotic ectodermal dysplasia syndrome.

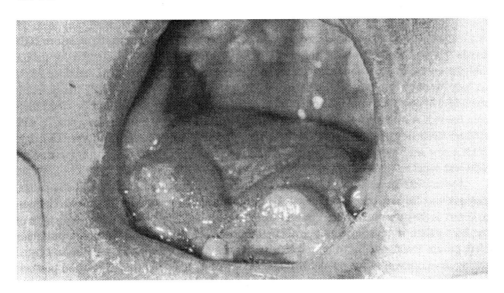

Figure 4.8.9. Lobulated tongue with fibroma of distal tip seen in orofaciodigital syndrome type II.

diphenylhydantoin, taken on a chronic basis. The oral cavity and tongue also may be involved in the localized tissue enlargement caused by lymphangiomas.

4.8.5.4. Malformations

Abnormal overgrowth of the oral mucosa may take the form of **aberrant frenulae** between the gums and the lips. These bands may be quite dense and broad, and the alveolar ridge may be deficient at the site of attachment. More rarely, small **mucosal fibromas** may be found on the surface of the oral or pharygeal mucous membranes.

Microglossia denotes a tongue that is much smaller than normal and may be bound down to the floor of the mouth. This abnormality may be associated with micrognathia or persistence of the secondary alveolar ridges (see Section 4.8.5.1). Conversely, a very large tongue (**macroglossia**), such as is commonly found in the Beckwith-Wiedemann syndrome, can produce breathing difficulties and orthodontic distortion (Fig. 4.8.7B). **Asymmetry of the tongue** may be seen in true hemihypertrophy or, rarely, in hemifacial atrophy. A **lobulated tongue** has a free border that is interrupted by one or more indentations, at the base of which may lie a hamartoma or a fibrous band extending to the floor of the mouth (Fig. 4.8.9). Retention of secretions within the sublingual salivary glands produces a **ranula**, a bluish cystic mass lying under one or both sides of the tongue just lateral to the frenulum.

The most common of the major malformations affecting the oral cavity is cleft palate.* In the most severe cases, often associated with bilateral cleft lip, the mouth

---

*Genetically, there are two classes of palatal clefts: those associated with cleft lip and those occurring in isolation. Although both types show a multifactorial inheritance pattern, they seem to have different mechanisms of pathogenesis and separate risk rates.

communicates with the nasal cavity above through a broad opening, with only vestigial remnants of the palatal shelves laterally. At the other end of the spectrum, a cleft or **bifid uvula** has no clinical significance but indicates that a mild genetic potential for palatal clefting exists, information that may be helpful in genetic counseling. Intermediate forms include **unilateral cleft palate**, in which the palatal shelf on one side of the defect is markedly hypoplastic while the other is virtually normal in size, and *posterior cleft palate* (see below). A midline **palatal fistula** represents a local zone of failed palatal fusion, with normal structures anterior and posterior to the defect. Such openings may vary in length from a few millimeters to one or two centimeters. Figure 4.8.10 illustrates some of the different types of palatal defect.

Incomplete or posterior cleft palate extends from the posterior edge of the palatal mucosa into the hard palate and may take any of three configurations. Mildest and hardest to detect is the **submucous cleft palate** where a palpable defect of the posterior margin of the hard palate is covered with normal oral mucosa. The edges of a **V-shaped posterior cleft palate** usually seem to be under tension, suggesting that inadequate tissue existed during development of the palatal shelves. On the other hand, a broad **U-shaped posterior cleft palate** is a sign of mechanical obstruction of palatal closure. The usual sequence of events causing this kind of defect begins with inadequate growth of the mandible, resulting in a small oropharyngeal cavity. The tongue, rising between the palatal shelves, blocks their upward swing and prevents their approach toward each other in the midline. At birth, the child will be found to have the Pierre Robin sequence, consisting of microg-

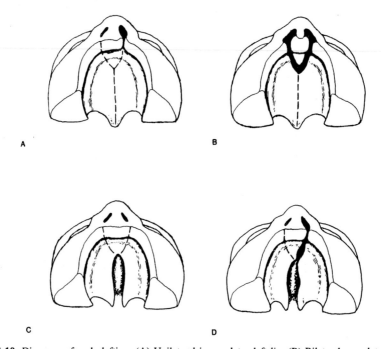

Figure 4.8.10. Diagrams of oral clefting. (A) Unilateral incomplete cleft lip. (B) Bilateral complete cleft lip separating primary from secondary palate. (C) U-shaped cleft palate. (D) Unilateral cleft lip and palate. [After Langman (1969).]

nathia, posterior (U-shaped) cleft palate, and **glossoptosis**. The oral cavity is so small that the tongue falls back into the pharynx, causing partial or complete obstruction.

4.8.6. Summary

Many of the congenital anomalies found in the mouth are both subtle and unfamiliar, and a thorough and deliberate examination of this region will pay disproportionate dividends.

4.9. NECK

The neck serves primarily as a flexible support for the head and as a conduit for all of the vessels, nerves, and other structures passing between the head and the thorax. Aside from these, the most important contents of the neck are the thyroid and parathyroid glands. Embryonic development of this region largely involves a "stretching out" of tissues lying caudal to the primitive pharynx, with most tissue migration occurring along the axis of the body.

4.9.1. Embryology and Development

The neck develops from tissues of the second, third, and fourth branchial arches and the mesenchyme that comes to surround them. In week 4 of gestation, the *pharyngeal pouches* on the inner surface of the oral cavity correspond to the *branchial clefts* on the outer surface; during week 5, the second arch begins to grow caudally, covering and eventually obliterating the branchial clefts externally (Fig. 4.9.1). With continuing growth, components of the second pharyngeal pouches begin to form the palatine tonsils, while third pouch structures migrate downward by week 6 to form one pair of *parathyroid glands* and the *thymus*. The fourth pharyngeal pouches give rise to the second pair of parathyroids at about the same time. The branchial clefts are gradually smoothed over by proliferation of nearby mesoderm, from which are derived the strap muscles of the neck.

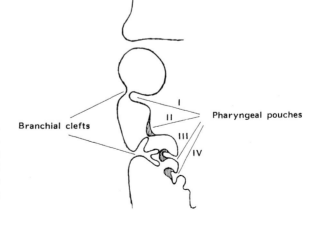

Figure 4.9.1. Coronal section of developing pharynx at 5 weeks of gestation. The shaded regions are the sites of origin of the thymus (third pharyngeal pouch) and the parathyroid glands (third and fourth pouches).

Meanwhile, in the midline, an endodermal thickening develops just behind the earliest rudiments of the tongue at about 3.5 weeks. Growing ventrally, this tissue forms a diverticulum that rapidly plunges downward to take up its final position as the *thyroid gland* on the front of the neck. By the end of week 7, the trailing *thyroglossal duct* is closed, leaving only a dimple at the base of the tongue, the foramen cecum.

4.9.2. Anatomy and Landmarks

The topographical anatomy of the neck is fairly simple: the anterior surface is bounded above by the lower jaw, below by the sternum and clavicles, and laterally by the *sternocleidomastoid muscles* (Fig. 4.9.2). Posteriorly are found the medial borders of the trapezius muscles running parallel from the occiput down to the upper back. The *thyroid* and *hyoid cartilages* are helpful landmarks anteriorly, while the prominent spine of the seventh cervical vertebra defines the base of the neck posteriorly.

4.9.3. Examination Techniques

The neck is first inspected for general configuration, symmetry, and any unusual masses. The relative width and length of the neck are assessed by simple observation. Neck motility can be evaluated by passive rotation and flexion in the infant, while the same motions can be tested in the older child by asking him to touch his chin to his chest and to each shoulder and then to lay each ear on the ipsilateral shoulder.

Next, the neck is palpated, beginning laterally, with special attention to the anterior edges of the sternocleidomastoids and any midline masses, including the thyroid gland.

Auscultation of the neck is rarely necessary but may be helpful in cases of congenital heart disease or suspicion of a cervical arteriovenous malformation.

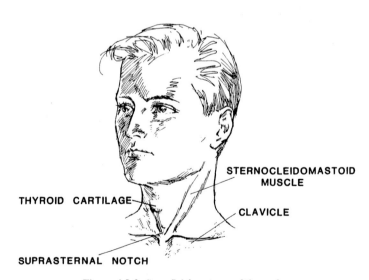

Figure 4.9.2. Superficial anatomy of the neck.

4.9.4. Minor Variants

4.9.4.1. Spectrum Variants

The general dimensions of the neck may vary somewhat in normal individuals, and the appearance of mildly short or long necks may run in families. The "Adam's apple," which becomes more protuberant during puberty, especially in boys, is simply a **prominent thyroid cartilage.**

4.9.4.2. Minor Anomalies

Branchial arch remnants are usually discovered as firm, painless masses lying near the anterior edge of the sternocleidomastoid muscles. These vestiges are made up of branchial cartilage that has failed to undergo normal regression and, when isolated, are of only cosmetic concern. Most commonly unilateral, they may sometimes be associated with a *branchial cleft cyst, sinus,* or *fistula.*

4.9.5. Abnormalities

4.9.5.1. Deformations

At birth, some normal babies have rather **redundant neck skin** posteriorly, probably caused by a prolonged chin-down fetal position. Gradual stretching of the skin results in compensatory overgrowth (see Section 4.15). The same phenomenon may occur over the anterior neck in children with face presentation and then may be associated with *mandibular hypoplasia.*

When an infant's head is held tilted to one side and the chin cannot be turned fully to the same side, torticollis is present. There seem to be a number of causes of this clinical sign: injury and hematoma formation within one sternocleidomastoid muscle has been implicated, as has intrauterine constraint, permitting secondary muscle shortening. As a rule of thumb, if the head is tilted backward as well as to the side, or if there is a palpable mass within the strap muscles, intrinsic injury is most likely. A discrepancy in the size of the ears may be a valuable clue to the presence of prolonged intrauterine constraint as a cause for the unusual head position (see Section 4.3).

Distension of the skin of the neck by underlying edema during intrauterine development causes a type of deformation that persists into adult life even though the edema disappears. This **lateral neck webbing** may be mild, forming small vertical ridges of redundant skin at the sides of the neck; in more severe instances, it may be seen as wide sheets of skin running down from the mastoid area to the tip of the shoulder (Fig. 4.9.3).

4.9.5.2. Disruptions

Rarely the neck may become encircled by amniotic bands or, more frequently, late in gestation, by the umbilical cord. Either of these entrapments may cause breakdown of underlying tissues but, much more important, may impinge on and occlude the large blood vessels of the neck. If severe or prolonged, this compression can result in ischemia, hemorrhage, or thrombosis in the brain, with eventual death of the fetus.

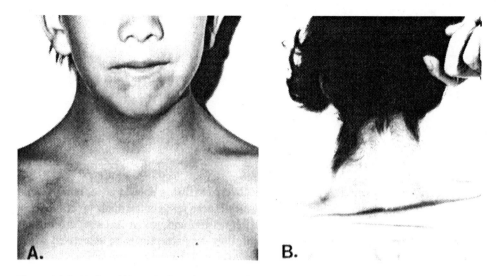

Figure 4.9.3. Neck webbing. (A) Frontal view showing mild webbing. (B) Posterior view of another child demonstrating more severe webbing with downward extension of the nuchal hairline.

4.9.5.3. Dysplasias

Disorders that affect the endocrine glands of the neck are most often dysplastic in nature, such as the **thyroid enlargement** seen in congenital hypothyroidism. **Absence of palpable thyroid** tissue occurs in the athyrotic hypothyroid sequence, which will produce progressive features of cretinism beginning in early infancy. Rarely in such cases, a persisting rest of thyroid tissue in the thyroglossal duct will continue to function and enlarge. This reduces the clinical features of hypothyroidism but produces a midline enlargement of glandular tissue along the course of the tract. Hypoplasia to **aplasia of the thymus** and **parathyroid glands** may be found in the DiGeorge sequence, representing very early failure of tissue differentiation in the third and fourth pharyngeal pouches.

4.9.5.4. Malformations

A **short neck** is usually the result of absence, malformation, or coalescence of one or more cervical vertebrae, often giving the impression that the head is resting directly on the shoulders. Neck mobility usually is limited in all planes of flexion, but rotational movements may be intact (Fig. 4.9.4). *Neck webbing* or *high placement of the scapulas* can produce a similar appearance, but these can be discriminated from a truly short neck by noting the distance between the base of the mandible and the top of the clavicle with the head in a neutral position. Posterior horizontal folds of redundant neck skin sometimes accompany a short neck.

A rare form of neck webbing involves folds of skin extending from the lower margin of the mandible down to the clavicles or sternum. Unlike the lateral neck webbing described above, these **neck pterygia** seem to reflect an underlying abnormality of connective tissue and most often accompany similar webs of skin across large joints in such conditions as multiple pterygium syndrome.

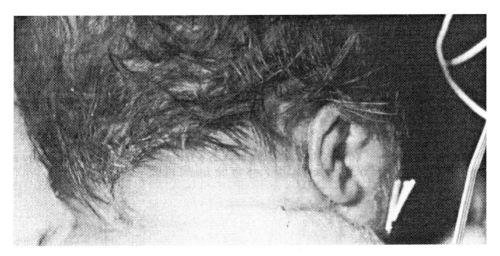

Figure 4.9.4. Upswept posterior hairline. Note shortness of neck.

A number of localized malformations of the neck represent partial persistence of primitive pharyngeal pouch or branchial cleft structures. If a portion of the embryonic cleft becomes pinched off, it may remain as an isolated, fluid-filled branchial cleft cyst. Alternatively, such a remnant may drain into the pharynx or onto the surface of the neck through a branchial cleft sinus. When an open tract extends all the way from the tonsillar fossa to the anterolateral neck, it is called a branchial cleft fistula. Anatomically, the external openings of any of these tracts will lie close to the anterior margin of the sternocleidomastoid muscle (Fig. 4.9.5).

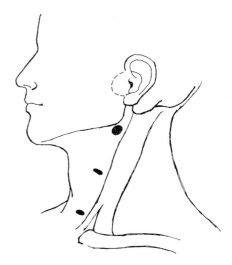

Figure 4.9.5. Diagram showing common locations for branchial cleft cysts and fistulas. The dashed line encloses the zone where preauricular tags are most likely to appear. [After Langman (1969).]

One other embryologic structure, the thyroglossal duct, occasionally fails to undergo complete closure after the descent of the thyroid gland into the lower neck. The resulting **thyroglossal duct cyst** or **sinus** can appear anywhere along a line connecting the sternal notch and the base of the tongue. The midline position of these lesions distinguishes them from branchial cleft abnormalities.

4.9.6. Summary

Anatomically and embryologically, the neck is a fairly simple structure, and only a few characteristic dysmorphic anomalies are to be found there.

4.10. CHEST

The chest "cage" is aptly named, since it acts primarily as an enclosure for the thoracic organs. The ribs, acted on by the intercostal muscles, take part in the movements of breathing but otherwise serve only as static anchor points for muscles of the deep neck and shoulder girdle.

4.10.1. Embryology and Development

During the first month of intrauterine life, the embryo grows rapidly in both the longitudinal and lateral planes. The lateral margins of the embryonic disk grow downward and beneath the central axis, pulling the amniotic membranes with them and incorporating the primitive gut tube (Fig. 4.10.1A). Mesenchymal cells of the *sclerotomes* of each somite migrate medially, above and below the notochord and neural tube, to form the *vertebral bodies* and *arches* as well as ventrally within the thoracic body wall to become the *ribs* (Fig. 4.10.1B). Either from the distal tips of the rib primordia or from an independent focus of mesenchyme arise two parallel *sternal bars* that eventually fuse with each other and the first six or seven pairs of ribs. Later, four *sternal ossification centers* appear in the midline. The *muscles* of the thorax derive from the myotomes that straddle the intervertebral spaces.

The embryology of the nipples and mammary glands is discussed in section 4.15.

4.10.2. Anatomy and Landmarks

For purposes of clinical examination, the chest can be delimited by the clavicles above, the rib margins below, and the posterior axillary lines laterally. (The back is discussed separately in Section 4.14.) The chest is normally broader than it is thick, and the contours of the lower two-thirds of the anterior chest are defined by the rib cage, while the upper third owes its external shape largely to the pectoral muscles of the shoulder girdle. Helpful landmarks include the *sternal notch*, the *xiphoid process*, and the *nipples*, which usually lie between the *midclavicular* and *anterior axillary lines* (Fig. 4.10.2). The *costal angle* is outlined by the rib cartilages as they course laterally below the xiphoid.

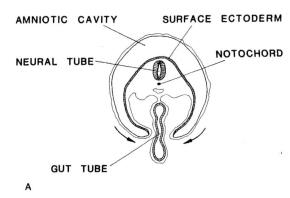

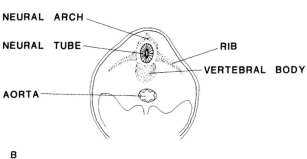

Figure 4.10.1. Embryogenesis of the anterior body wall and vertebrae. (A) Cross section of embryo at 4 weeks of gestation. The lateral body folds are growing ventrally and medially, soon to enclose the gut tube. [After Langman (1969).] (B) By 5 weeks, mesenchymal condensations are forming the primordia of the vertebrae and ribs.

4.10.3. Examination Techniques

Examination of the chest begins with inspection for symmetry, unusual masses, or abnormal configuration. Note should be taken of the general shape of the thorax, the placement of the nipples, and the contour of the ribs and *sternum*. It is important to watch the child breathe for a few moments, looking for symmetry of chest motion and suprasternal or intercostal retractions.

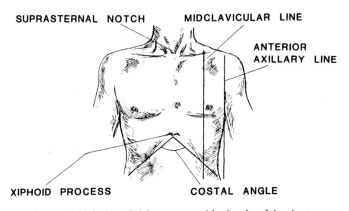

Figure 4.10.2. Superficial anatomy and landmarks of the chest.

Palpation is useful to determine the nature of any unusual masses, to estimate the amount of breast tissue present, and to detect cardiac thrills or heaves. A rough idea of the length of the sternum should be obtained by placing a fingertip in the sternal notch and the thumb of the same hand over the xiphoid process. Estimation of the costal angle may also be accomplished by palpation.

Percussion of the chest may occasionally be helpful in the dysmorphology exam when there is marked asymmetry of rib spacing or respiratory excursion on the two sides. In such cases, it is particularly important to determine which side of the chest has the normal percussion note, since dullness might be heard over a pleural effusion or chylothorax, while a hyperresonant note might indicate pneumothorax or diaphragmatic hernia.

In most pediatric settings, auscultation is the most important mode of examining the thorax and its contents; in dysmorphology, however, this technique is of limited use. While cardiac auscultation remains an extremely important part of any pediatric examination, it is a subject that has been treated in depth by other authors and will not be specifically addressed here.

Only a few measurements of the chest have been standardized; of these, the *internipple distance* and total *chest circumference* are pertinent for the dysmorphology exam. The former is simply the distance between the centers of the nipples, but this measurement should always be supplemented by measurement of the thoracic circumference at the nipple line, since a ratio of the two values is the most practical way to minimize errors caused by variations in chest shape and size.

4.10.4. Minor Variants

4.10.4.1. Spectrum Variants

In some individuals and occasional families, the chest may be flattened from front to back; in extreme cases, the sternum is noticeably depressed below the level of the rib ends. This **pectus excavatum** *(funnel chest)* may be of cosmetic concern but usually produces few functional problems even when quite severe (Fig. 4.10.3A). In contrast, protrusion of the sternum (**pectus carinatum** or *pigeon breast)* increases the depth of the chest from front to back while producing a relative narrowing from side to side (Fig. 4.10.3B). This configuration appears in its most severe form in association with kyphosis of the thoracic spine or other vertebral abnormalities. The term **shield chest** denotes an unusually broad and often short upper thorax, frequently associated with *wide-spaced nipples* (see below) (Fig. 4.10.4).

The costal angle usually reflects the proportions of the height and breadth of the chest; a long, narrow rib cage produces an acute costal angle, and a "barrel chest" is associated with an obtuse one.

The xiphoid process seems to be especially variable in shape and size. In normal individuals it may be bifid, protuberant, unusually long, or so small as to be almost impalpable.

While intrinsic abnormalities of the nipples and *breasts* are discussed elsewhere (see Section 4.15), the placement of the nipples seems largely to reflect the development and conformation of the underlying chest wall. The most commonly seen variant is wide-spaced nipples, in which these structures are displaced laterally to or beyond the anterior

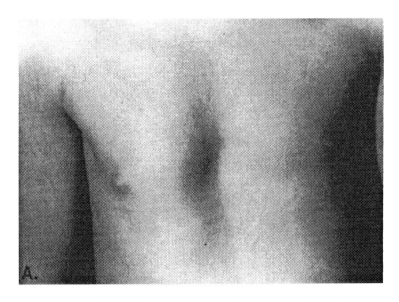

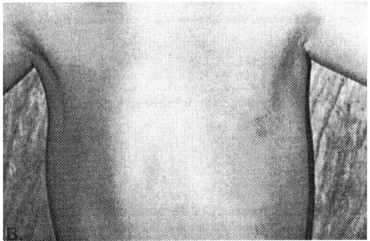

Figure 4.10.3. Sternal anomalies. (A) Pectus excavatum. (B) Pectus carinatum.

axillary lines (Fig. 4.10.4). A deep chest may produce an illusion of lateral placement of the nipples, whereas a broad, flat chest may make them appear to be too close together. In questionable cases, it is best to measure the distance between the nipples and calculate the ratio of this length to the chest circumference, using standard tables for comparison.

4.10.4.2. Minor Anomalies

Occasionally, palpation of the anterolateral chest wall reveals irregularities suggesting **fused** or **bifid ribs.** Radiographs are necessary to confirm such findings and have an

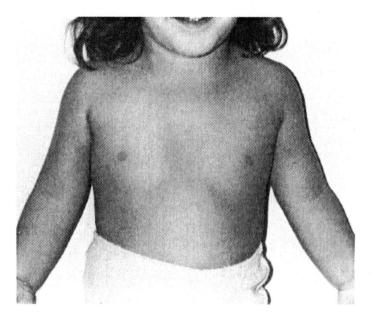

Figure 4.10.4. Broad, shieldlike chest with wide-spaced nipples in Turner syndrome.

additional advantage in providing extra information about possible associated abnormalities of the vertebral bodies.

4.10.5. Abnormalities

4.10.5.1. Deformations

   Scoliosis can produce asymmetry of the thorax that is manifested in the physical exam by intercostal spaces widened on one side and narrowed on the other. The splinting action of the narrowed intercostal spaces may reduce respiratory excursion on that side as well. A moderate degree of pectus excavatum may be produced by sternal retractions in infants with chronic respiratory disease, and this deformity may correct itself only slowly, if at all, once the respiratory problem has disappeared.

   Rarely, the thoracic wall may be deformed by direct pressure during prenatal growth. Uterine fibroids, a twin, or even one of the baby's own limbs may be the deforming object (Fig. 4.10.5).

4.10.5.2. Disruptions

   Disruptive events involving the chest wall are quite rare but, when they do occur, are usually extremely severe both in extent and in injury to underlying body organs and structures (see Section 4.11 for examples).

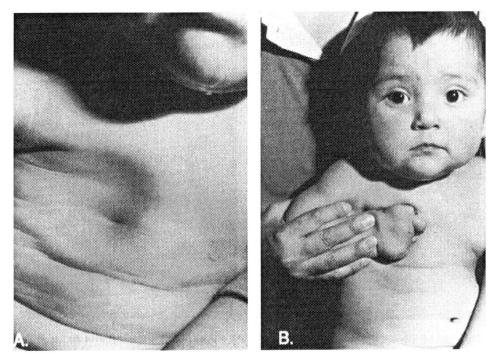

Figure 4.10.5. Chest deformity caused by extrinsic pressure. (A) Localized zone of depression seen during inspiration. On expiration, this region bulges outward slightly. The underlying ribs are extremely thin, irregular, and yielding to palpation. (B) The baby's fist held in the position of comfort, where it had been lodged during the last several weeks of gestation.

4.10.5.3. Dysplasias

The ribs may be involved in a number of bone dysplasias and in the mucopolysaccharidoses, but the changes produced (usually widening and cupping of the distal ends) are not easily detected by physical examination. Indication of splaying or irregularity of the ribs should be confirmed by X-ray examination. Complete **absence of the clavicles** or hypoplasia of their lateral portions as a hallmark of cleidocranial dysostosis.

4.10.5.4. Malformations

Malformations of the bony and muscular elements of the chest wall may be seen in isolation or as parts of various syndromes. The most common of the muscular malformations is **absence of the pectoralis major muscle**. This defect, usually seen in conjunction with distal hypoplasia of the hand in Poland complex, may occasionally involve other muscles of the shoulder girdle. Nipple, areola, and underlying breast tissue may also be absent on the affected side (Fig. 4.10.6A).

Bony abnormalities include **beaded ribs**, in which the costochondral junctions are enlarged and sometimes tender. This sign, once known as the "rachitic rosary" because of

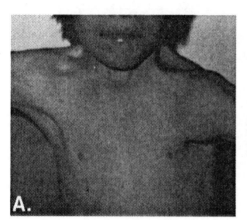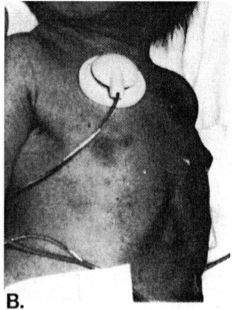

Figure 4.10.6. Chest malformations. (A) Poland anomaly, with aplasia of the sternal head of the left pectoralis major muscle. (B) Short sternum in trisomy 18. Only two sternal ossification centers could be identified on lateral chest X-ray.

its association with severe vitamin D deficiency, is a feature of some chondrodystrophies and hypophosphatasia as well. A noticeably **short sternum** usually implies a failure of development of one or more sternal ossification centers (Fig. 4.10.6B). In early child-hood, these centers can be seen well on a lateral chest X-ray, which is helpful in confirm-ing the clinical impression. The defect in a **cleft sternum** is shaped like a narrow, inverted letter U extending upward from the xiphoid area. Often, the heart can be palpated immedi-ately below the skin covering the cleft. This malformation seems to result from failure of midline fusion of the paired islands of sternal mesenchyme. If the defect is very large, even skin coverage may be incomplete, and mediastinal structures are exposed to the exterior. At birth, the baby presents with **ectopia cordis**, and immediate surgical interven-tion is necessary for survival (Fig. 4.10.7).

4.10.6. Summary

The structures of the bony thorax and its associated musculature are all mesenchymal in origin, and most of the anomalies in this region reflect early interference with migration or differentiation of this embryonic tissue.

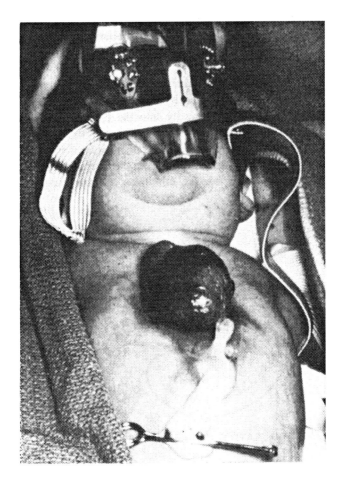

Figure 4.10.7. Ectopia cordis. The entire central chest wall is deficient, and the heart, pericardial sac, and part of one lung lie exposed. (Photo courtesy of Dr. Herb Koffler, Albuquerque, N.M.)

4.11 ABDOMEN

Like the thorax, the abdomen is primarily a container for the viscera. Although the abdominal wall is even simpler in structure than the chest cage, its embryonic history makes it more susceptible to a variety of developmental anomalies.

4.11.1. Embryology and Development

The abdominal wall is formed by first lateral and then ventral migration of mesenchyme from the sclerotomes of the middorsal somites (Fig. 4.10.1). During month 1 of gestation, rapid body growth reduces the relative size of the opening between the primitive gut tube and the yolk sac (the *vitelline duct*). An outpouching of the hindgut, the *allantois,* extends into the connecting stalk that joins the embryo to the developing placenta. Also found there are two veins and two arteries, the *umbilical vessels* (Fig. 4.11.1). All of these structures become enveloped by the amnion as the stalk lengthens to form the *umbilical cord.*

With rapid growth of the liver, primitive kidneys, and midgut during gestational month 2, space within the abdominal cavity is at a premium, and as a result, loops of developing bowel are extruded temporarily into the base of the umbilical cord (Fig. 4.11.1A). During week 10, these intestinal loops once again retreat into the abdomen (Fig. 4.11.1B). By this time, the vitelline duct, allantois, and right umbilical vein have become obliterated. Eventually, mesenchyme from the lateral body walls migrates medially into the zones above and below the umbilicus, forming the muscle layers of the abdominal wall.

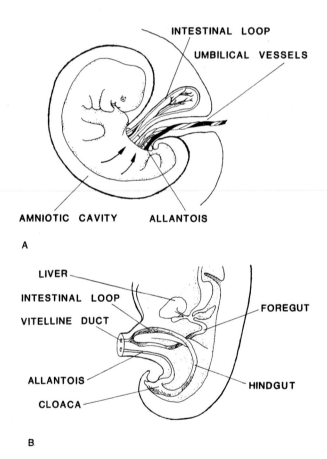

Figure 4.11.1. Embryogenesis of anterior abdominal wall and umbilical cord. (A) Embryo at 5 weeks of gestation, showing ventral migration of lateral body fold mesenchyme above and below the region of the body stalk. [After Langman (1969).] (B) Sagittal section of embryo at 7.5 gestational weeks. The intestinal loop is beginning to retract into the abdomen, and the allantois and vitelline duct are degenerating. (Umbilical vessels omitted for clarity.)

4.11.2. Anatomy and Landmarks

For purposes of the clinical examination, the abdomen can be defined as extending from the lower rib margin to the upper edge of the pelvic bones and laterally around to the paraspinal muscles of the flanks. In infants, the abdomen is large in relation to the rest of the body, as are the *liver* and *kidneys*. At birth, the umbilical cord is normally about 50–60 cm long and 1–1.5 cm in diameter. The umbilical vessels course in an irregular spiral between the placenta and the abdomen, since they are longer than the cord itself (and the vein is longer than the arteries).

The paired *rectus abdominis muscles* normally are separated by only a shallow median groove. The usual position of the *umbilicus* is in the midline about halfway from the *xiphoid notch* to the *pubic symphysis*.

Useful landmarks include the extensions of the midclavicular and anterior axillary lines down from the chest (Fig. 4.10.3), the *costal* (or *rib*) *margins,* the *iliac crests,* and the *anterior superior iliac spines*.

4.11.3. Examination Techniques

The entire abdominal examination is usually performed with the patient supine, but occasionally another position may be found useful for infants and small children.

First, a brief inspection of the abdomen provides information about symmetry, muscle tone, and the presence of major defects of the abdominal wall. Special attention should be paid to the umbilicus, especially in the newborn.

Next, auscultation is used to evaluate the nature and distribution of bowel sounds and to detect any abnormal sounds such as bruits.

In no other part of the examination is palpation more valuable than in evaluating the abdominal contents. Beginning with gentle palpation with the flat of the hand over all four quadrants, the examiner should feel for any defects in the abdominal wall, including an unusually large space between the abdominis rectus muscles. Then move to deeper palpation with the fingertips, beginning in the right upper quadrant, where the liver edge should be sought and the liver evaluated not only for size but for consistency. In infants, special attention should be devoted to trying to feel the kidneys and evaluate their relative size. In younger babies with weak abdominal muscles, the lower pole of the right kidney and the entire left can often be ascertained, but in older children this becomes progressively more difficult. Any unusual masses should be carefully evaluated for size and consistency, and an effort should be made to determine if they are associated with or attached to any other intra-abdominal structures.

When palpating the abdomen of a resistant child, it is often useful to maintain gentle but firm pressure for the space of several respiratory cycles, pushing deeper with each inspiration. In this way, it is often possible to overcome abdominal muscle tension and obtain a better impression of deep-lying structures.

When examining a resistant toddler, a better palpation of the abdomen occasionally can be obtained by having him sit upright in his mother's lap, facing away from you, and reaching around to palpate his abdomen from behind. Here again, gentle persistent pressure with ratchetlike progress made between cries is usually effective.

Abdominal percussion is valuable not only in determining the presence of tympani or fluid levels but also in defining the size of the liver and spleen. Dullness to percussion over the lower ribs provides a rough outline of these organs. The liver size also can be estimated by placing a stethoscope over the right lower ribs and moving it gradually upward while lightly percussing or scratching the skin nearby. The change in sound when the stethoscope bell reaches the level of the lung marks the upper extent of the liver. The distance from this point to the lower hepatic margin is the *liver span*.

If there is a question of enlargement of an abdominal organ, it is helpful to record its approximate measurements. Liver size may be recorded as the distance below the right costal margin where the hepatic edge is palpable, but spurious impressions may be produced in children with extreme respiratory excursions or lung hyperexpansion. It is better to record the measurement of liver span.

4.11.4. Minor Variants

4.11.4.1. Spectrum Variants

The superficial appearance of the abdomen may be modified by the amount of subcutaneous fat present. The term **diastasis recti** refers to a widened space between the rectus abdominis muscles. Varying degrees of separation may be found in normal individuals and in small children may be expressed as a bulge lying between the umbilicus and the xiphoid process which protrudes with crying or straining. Small (3–5 mm in diameter) abdominal wall defects palpable directly beneath the umbilicus, without bulging of the overlying tissues, are fairly common and benign. Small **umbilical hernias** are seen as tense to fluctuant masses covered with intact skin. They range widely in size, and the diameter of the opening in the abdominal wall may be considerably smaller than the size of the hernial sac. At birth, a palpable defect smaller than about 1 cm in diameter may be considered a normal variant and can be expected to close spontaneously by 2 –3 years of age. *Incarcerated umbilical hernias* cannot be reduced into the abdomen and constitute a surgical emergency (see also Section 4.12).

In the newborn, the first few centimeters of the umbilical cord may be covered with skin extending from the abdominal wall. This **skin umbilicus** results in an "outie" in later life. More rarely, the membranes of the cord extend out onto the surrounding skin, resulting in a very flattened, smooth, **membranous umbilicus**.

4.11.4.2. Minor Anomalies

Protrusion of a bulge of peritoneum through a defect in the muscular wall of the abdomen lateral to the midline is a **ventral hernia**. These are usually unilateral and are quite variable in size, and the margins of the defect may be difficult to feel, in contrast with the sharp-edged ring of connective tissue found in umbilical hernias.

The presence of a **single umbilical artery** is noted in about 1% of all newborn babies but in a much higher proportion of children with congenital abnormalities, especially congenital heart disease and renal anomalies. It is not, however, pathognomonic of any of these conditions.

Unusual **umbilical position** is a rare clue to abnormal early development. A caudally placed umbilicus (Fig. 4.11.2) suggests inadequate migration of mesenchymal tissue into

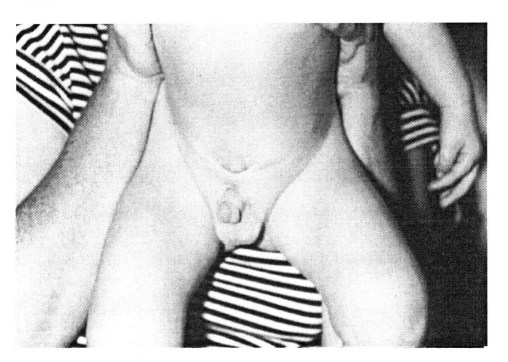

Figure 4.11.2. Extreme downward displacement of umbilicus.

the zone between the body stalk and the cloacal membrane in the first 2 months of life. This minor anomaly probably has the same pathogenesis as does *exstrophy of the bladder* (Section 4.12) but a milder degree of expression.

4.11.5. Abnormalities

4.11.5.1. Deformations

Without bone or cartilage, the abdominal wall and the intra-abdominal organs do not demonstrate deformational abnormalities. *Umbilical cord length,* however, is strongly influenced by the amount of tension produced in the cord by fetal movement. Thus, a **long umbilical cord** (over 90 cm) usually has been stretched by the movements of an extremely active fetus. The combination of an unusually long cord and vigorous intrauterine movement can result in fetal entanglement or the creation of a **true knot** in the cord. Conversely, extreme intrauterine immobility from any cause can result in a **short umbilical cord** with a total length as small as 20 cm, carrying the danger of early placental separation or even avulsion of the cord at the time of delivery.

4.11.5.2. Disruptions

Extreme distension of the abdomen during prenatal time, from whatever cause, can destroy all of the muscles of the abdominal wall. The **absence of abdominal mus-**

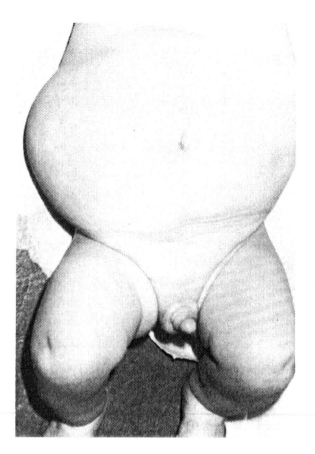

Figure 4.11.3. Lax, thinned abdominal wall with redundant skin in uretheral obstruction sequence. Also note skin dimples on lateral knees caused by intrauterine compression.

culature or *prune belly sequence* (Fig. 4.11.3) is most frequently the result of obstruction of the distal urethra, which causes immense distension of the bladder and subsequent ablation of the abdominal muscles. Other causes include intra-abdominal tumors, severe prenatal ascites, and cystic hygromas of the mesentery. The common clinical findings are a flaccid, thin abdominal wall, through which the outlines of loops of bowel and their peristaltic movements can be seen easily. The abdomen has a doughy consistency on palpation, and the abdominal viscera can be felt with unusual ease. Older patients will be unable to sit up or support themselves in a sitting position.

4.11.5.3. Dysplasias

The signs of dysplastic disorders to be found during the abdominal examination are changes in the size and consistency of the liver and spleen. In most of the storage diseases, **hepatosplenomegaly** is an early and consistent feature and may progress to massive proportions with time. The enlargement of the liver may cause its lower edge to "dive" deeply into the abdomen, making difficult an accurate estimate of its size. A huge liver may distend the abdomen, occupying all but the left lower quadrant. A **shrunken liver**, quite firm in consistency, may be found in the late stages of some metabolic disorders such as Wilson disease.

4.11.5.4. Malformations

Malformation of the anterior abdominal wall produces three major types of peri-umbilical herniation, clinically similar in appearance, that have different embryologic origins and significance.

An **omphalocele** is caused by failure of complete return of the intestines from the *connecting stalk* to the abdominal cavity during week 10 of gestation. For this reason, *intestinal malrotation* is a very frequent associated finding. The umbilical vessels run down one side of the hernial sac, which consists only of a fragile layer of amnion, often ruptured before or at the time of birth (Fig. 4.11.4A). The sac may contain a single loop of bowel or the liver and most of the intestines, in which case it can be differentiated from *abdominal eventration* only by the relative size of the body wall defect.

Hernia into the umbilical cord results from a defect in the abdominal wall permitting extrusion of abdominal contents into the base of the cord. In this case, the intestinal loops have retracted normally during embryogenesis only to reemerge through the defect during fetal life. Thus, the hernial sac is made up of both peritoneum and the amniotic sheath of the umbilical cord, making surgical repair somewhat easier. This condition is caused by inadequate ventral migration of body wall mesenchyme, and if the defect is quite large, eventration of the abdominal viscera takes place, with the intestines and liver lying free in the amniotic cavity.

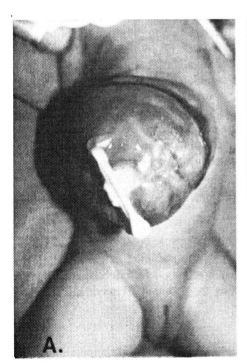 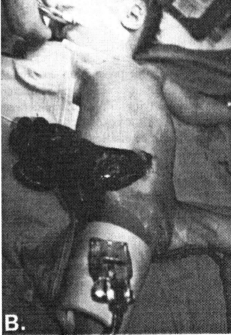

Figure 4.11.4. Major defects of the abdominal wall. (A) Massive omphalocele. Note umbilical cord emerging from apex of omphalocele sac. (B) Gastroschisis. Note absence of covering membrane and position of defect lateral to umbilicus. (Photos courtesy of Dr. Patrick Jewell, Albuquerque, N.M.)

The third type of herniation, **gastroschisis**, also involves extrusion of abdominal contents through an anterior defect, but in this case the opening is paramedian rather than lying in the position of the umbilical stump, the umbilical cord lies to one side of the defect, and there is no covering membrane (Fig. 4.11.4B). The cause of gastroschisis might be a unilateral deficit of mesenchymal migration in early embryogenesis.

Weakness or deficiency of connective tissues in the lower abdominal wall may lead to **inguinal hernias**. In the *indirect* type, failure of complete closure of the internal inguinal ring and *processus vaginalis* after testicular descent allows protrusion of a peritoneal sac, sometimes containing loops of bowel, down along the spermatic cord. This creates a fluctuant swelling in one side of the scrotum or, rarely, in the labium majus in females. A *direct* hernia in the inguinal region resembles other anterior herniations in that weakness of the connective tissue of the abdominal wall permits peritoneum to bulge out to one side of the rectus abdominus muscle close to its insertion on the pubic bone. In either type of hernia, incarceration or volvulus of the contained bowel may occur, necessitating immediate surgical intervention.

Palpation of a liver edge that seems to run horizontally across the entire abdomen or that is larger on the left side than the right may signify **situs inversus.** In the *totalis* form, the heart will lie on the right side of the chest as well; in the *abdominus* version, only those organs lying below the diaphragm are found in a mirror-image relationship. *Polysplenia* or *asplenia* may be found with either type.

A remnant of the vitelline duct may persist as **Meckel's diverticulum**, outpouching from the middle portion of the ileum. Rarely, such a diverticulum extends as a patent tract connecting the bowel and the umbilical stump, and small amounts of fecal material may find their way to the surface, producing an immediate clue to the existence of this anomaly.

In a similar way, persistence of a remnant of the allantois as a **patent urachus** may result in a tract leading from the bladder to the umbilicus, where the presence of urinary drainage signals the presence of this anomaly. A **urachal cyst** may be left behind as a fluid-filled remnant of the primitive allantois. It will sometimes be palpable as a firm, spherical mass lying in the midline between the umbilicus and the symphysis pubis. A **urachal fistula** is a blind tract that opens at the umbilicus and is quite susceptible to infection. It can be discriminated from a patent urachus by administering an oral dose of methylene blue, which is promptly excreted in the urine and will stain the umbilical drainage if the urachus is patent.

4.11.6. Summary

Most of the dysmorphologic abnormalities of the abdomen fall into one of two classes: early embryonic malformations primarily involving defective body wall closure, and later disruptive or dysplastic events affecting the abdominal viscera and umbilical cord.

4.12. GENITALIA

The developmental complexity of the genitourinary system is second only to that of the face and brain, and therefore the variety of congenital anomalies affecting this region is equally broad. Some few abnormalities of the external genitalia have significance in relation to occult malformations of the urinary tract, but the majority represent localized aberrations of development, and their causes range across the entire gamut of pathogenetic mechanisms discussed in Chapter 1. For these reasons, this section begins with an especially thorough review of embryology as an aid to understanding the individual anomalies of this region.

4.12.1. Embryology and Development

The development of the external genitalia begins by about week 4 of gestation, when the primordial germ cells are just beginning to migrate from the yolk sac to the dorsal wall of the abdominal cavity. Externally, a midline *genital tubercle* and symmetric lateral *urogenital folds* appear surrounding the *cloacal membrane* at the lowest point of the ventral abdominal wall (Fig. 4.12.1A). Internally, the *urorectal septum* is growing downward, dividing the cloaca into an anterior *urogenital sinus* and, posteriorly, the rectum (Fig. 4.12.1B).

When the urorectal septum reaches the cloacal membrane during embryonic week 6, the two structures fuse, forming the *perineum* and dividing the cloacal membrane into an anterior *urogenital membrane* and the smaller posterior *anal membrane,* both of which soon rupture (Fig. 4.12.1C). Lateral *labioscrotal swellings* become evident at this point and gradually enlarge during the next 2–3 weeks, as does the *phallus,* formed from the genital tubercle and the distal portions of the urogenital folds.

Until week 9, there is no real distinction between the appearance of the genitalia in the two sexes, but at this point the influence of the distant *gonads* begins to be felt. In the strictest sense, the "normal" pathway of genital development in the human produces a female phenotype. The presence of a Y chromosome in male embryos, however, allows the early production of androgens in the *testis,* which diverts genital development onto the sidetrack leading to a male phenotype.

In the female developmental pathway, phallic growth slows after week 9 to keep pace with the gradual enlargement of the urogenital folds as they form the *labia minora.* The labioscrotal folds grow somewhat more rapidly, eventually to fuse both anteriorly and posteriorly, forming the *labia majora.* The *vaginal vestibule* arises from the outermost portion of the urogenital sinus; further within, paired outgrowths from the dorsal wall fuse to form a solid *vaginal plate,* which grows upward to make contact with the tip of the descending Müllerian ducts, which will form the uterus and cervix. Later, the central cells of this endodermal cylinder will break down to form the vaginal lumen, temporarily separated from the cavity of the urogenital sinus by the membranous *hymen.* Growth of the solid vaginal plate ventrally and caudally helps to narrow the lower segment of the urogenital sinus into the tubular *urethra,* which opens to the surface just caudal to the phallus, now called the *clitoris,* at the upper junction of the labia minora (Fig. 4.12.2A).

Embryos possessing a Y chromosome undergo somewhat more rapid and extensive development of the external genitalia. By week 10, fusion of the urogenital folds has begun, closing over the *urethral groove* on the inferior surface of the phallus. At the same time, the labioscrotal folds are enlarging and fusing posteriorly to form the early *scrotum.* The phallus continues to grow rapidly, and by the end of month 3, the urogenital folds have completely enclosed the urethral groove to form the *penile urethra.* Extension of the urethra through the *glans penis* takes place by way of a groove that forms in a plate of

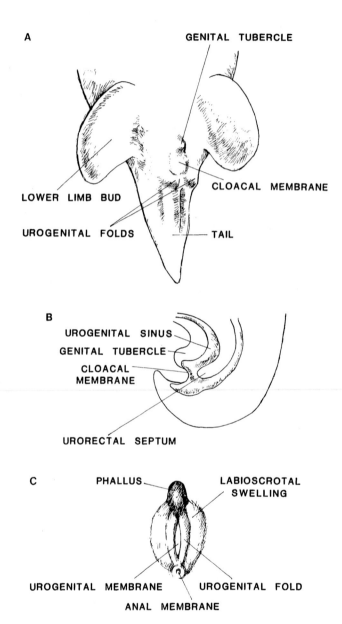

Figure 4.12.1. Embryogenesis of external genitalia and hindgut. (A) Ventral view of posterior embryo at 4.5 gestational weeks, showing earliest genital primordia. [After Jirasek (1983).] (B) Sagittal section of posterior embryo at 6 weeks of gestation, showing impending septation of the cloaca by the urorectal septum. (C) External genitalia at the "indifferent" stage, gestational week 7. [After Moore (1982).]

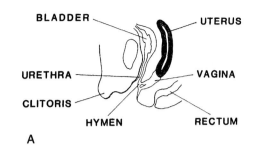

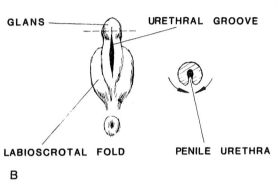

Figure 4.12.2. Early sexual dimorphism of the genitalia. (A) Sagittal section of female embryo at 11 weeks of gestation. [After Langman (1969).] (B) Male external genitalia at about gestational week 9. The urogenital groove is beginning to close, and the labioscrotal folds will soon meet and fuse below the phallus.

epithelial cells extending vertically from the lower surface (Fig. 4.12.2B) and whose edges eventually fuse in a fashion similar to the urogenital folds.

The final event in the prenatal development of the male genitalia is the completion of the descent of the testes from their position high on the dorsal wall of the pelvic cavity to their eventual location within the scrotum. This process seems to be facilitated by androgenic hormones, but the exact mechanism for testicular descent remains in question. By the end of month 3, differential growth of the body has brought the testis close to the inner end of the inguinal canal. There it remains until the end of month 7, when, over the course of just a few days, it traverses the length of the canal to the external ring, carrying with it a pouch of peritoneum, the *processus vaginalis*. By month 8, the testis has reached the scrotum, and the processus vaginalis has become obliterated, leaving a fluid-containing space, the *tunica vaginalis,* alongside the testis.

4.12.2. Anatomy and Landmarks

In the male, the base of the *penis* rests just below the lower edge of the *pubic symphysis;* in infants or obese children, it may be partially buried in a *suprapubic fat pad.* The penis itself consists of the *shaft* and the *glans,* which in uncircumcised boys is covered by the *foreskin (prepuce).* At the tip of the glans, the *urethral meatus* opens as a small vertical slit. A *median raphe* runs down the underside of the penile shaft, merging with the *scrotal raphe* which demarcates the two sides of the scrotum (Fig. 4.12.3A). Within the scrotum are found the *testes* and *spermatic ducts.* The testes are normally somewhat uneven in degree of descent, with one (more commonly the right) lying a little

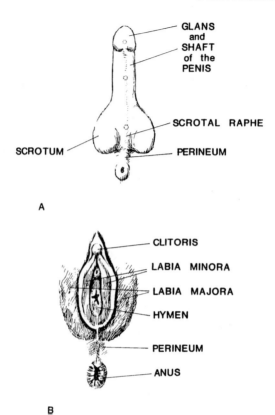

Figure 4.12.3. Anatomy of the external genitalia. (A) Male genitalia showing midline raphe. Dashed circles indicate typical sites of hypospadias on the glans, penile shaft, and base of the penis. (B) Female genitalia.

lower in the scrotal sac. Testicular size remains relatively stable during early childhood but increases rapidly at the onset of puberty, reaching adult size by 14–17 years.

The female external genitalia are marked by the skin-covered labia majora surrounding the labia minora, which are surfaced with mucous membrane. At the upper junction of the labia minora lies the clitoris, hooded by a membranous fold and protecting the urethral meatus at its base (Fig. 4.12.3B). Just within the labia minora lies the *vaginal introitus*, where remnants of the hymeneal membrane may be seen in infants and prepubertal girls. Beyond the hymeneal ring lies the vault of the *vagina*, with the uterine *cervix* projecting into its most proximal portion.

4.12.3. Examination Techniques

Inspection serves to detect the great majority of congenital abnormalities of the female external genitalia. Only rarely will internal palpation or inspection of the vagina be required during the dysmorphology evaluation, and such examinations should be reserved for those instances in which a strong suspicion of internal anomalies exists. The usual examination involves only the spreading of the labia majora to permit visualization of the labia minora and clitoris. The urethral meatus usually is not well seen in female children.

Examination of the male genitalia involves inspection of the penis and scrotum, with special attention to the site of the urethral meatus. The testes should be palpated within the scrotum, and their size and consistency should be estimated. If a testis is undescended, an attempt should be made to detect it in the inguinal canal. A forefinger is pressed flat against the skin just above the lateral pubic bone, and two fingers of the other hand are used to stroke gently from this point downward along the course of the canal. Often the testis can be felt as a rounded, mobile mass that can be coaxed temporarily to a position below the *external inguinal ring.*

When the testes or penis seem unusually small or large, measurements may be helpful. Testicular size can be estimated by measuring the length and width of the testis as it is held steady by gently pinching beneath it until the overlying scrotal skin is taut. A somewhat better estimate of testicular volume can be obtained by comparison with the set of graded ovoid shapes of an *orchidometer.* Penile length is measured along the upper surface of the shaft to the tip of the glans, with the measuring tape or ruler pressed firmly into the soft tissues over the symphysis pubis and the penile shaft gently stretched. In obese boys it is important to measure carefully, since an apparently small penis may simply be partly engulfed by a large suprapubic fat pad.

In examining *ambiguous genitalia,* it is important to note the size and texture of the phallus, the location of the urethral meatus, and the presence or absence of a vaginal introitus. The labia majora should be palpated for masses that might represent a testis or ovotestis. If a vaginal opening exists, a skilled examiner can sometimes ascertain by palpation whether uterine structures are also present, but this determination is more frequently made with radiographs or other special studies.

4.12.4. Minor Variants

4.12.4.1. Spectrum Variants

Female. The labia majora, the clitoris, and especially the labia minora may vary considerably in size among individuals. At birth, the labia minora may be temporarily engorged and edematous from maternal hormonal influences during late pregnancy.

In prepubertal girls, **hymeneal remnants** usually are an incidental finding in the physical examination. Free tags or strands of hymeneal tissue may protrude between the labia minora and are especially prominent in the newborn. Less frequently, bands or a lacelike multiperforate sheet of membrane extends across the vaginal introitus (see also Section 4.12.5.4).

Male. As is true of most other anatomic structures, the size of the various elements of the male external genitalia vary independently and over a rather wide range. **Macro-** and **microorchidism** are best defined by comparisons of measurements from the patient with published standards of normal; sizes falling more than two standard deviations from the mean often have pathological significance. The same considerations apply to penile size. An unusually **large phallus** for age usually indicates abnormal androgenic stimulation of testicular or adrenal origin, while true **micropenis** may represent either deficient hormonal stimulation during growth or a failure of early morphogenesis (see Section 4.12.5.4).

4.12.4.2. Minor Anomalies

Female. Small zones showing **adhesions between the labia minora** are sometimes seen in female infants and often can be separated by gentle traction with the fingers. Their cause is obscure.

Male. At birth, as many as 15–20% of infant males have some degree of **hydrocele**, caused by the accumulation of fluid in the tunica vaginalis around the testis. Even when the volume of fluid is enough to distend the scrotum severely, causing apparent discomfort to the baby, complete spontaneous resolution over a few weeks to months is to be expected. Another cause of a fluctuant intrascrotal mass is **hydrocele of the cord**, which occurs when the proximal and distal closures of the processus vaginalis take place but a cystic dilatation of the intervening duct remains. Both types of hydrocele must be discriminated from *inguinal* and *scrotal hernias.*

Mild **hypospadias** is relatively common in surveys of newborn boys and usually involves only a small displacement of the urethral meatus onto the ventral surface of the glans. More severe forms no longer fall under the heading of minor abnormalities, since surgical correction is usually necessary, and the risk for associated abnormalities becomes much higher (see Section 4.12.5.4).

Since testicular descent occurs late in gestation, it is no surprise that babies of the youngest gestational ages have the highest rates of *undescended testis* or **cryptorchidism**. Even at term, however, about 3% of male infants have an incompletely descended testis on one side (on the right nearly twice as often as on the left). More than half of these cryptorchid testes descend into the scrotum during the first month of life, and 99% will be normally situated by the end of the first year.

Prolonged cryptorchidism is neither normal nor a minor anomaly because of high frequency of two associated complications. First, retention of a testis within the abdomen beyond late childhood greatly increases the risk of testicular malignancy. Second, failure of the testis to descend leaves the empty inguinal canal as a ready passageway for an *indirect hernia* during any episode of increased intra-abdominal pressure.

4.12.5. Abnormalities

4.12.5.1. Deformations

The soft tissues making up the external genitalia can be distorted transiently by direct pressure from tumors, cysts, and other masses, but there are no characteristic types of congenital deformation of these structures.

Sexual abuse in childhood can produce a pattern of deformational and disruptional abnormalities that is becoming recognized as a help in diagnosis. These changes include increased diameter of one or more body orifices (vagina, anus, and even urethra) with patulous sphincters and, often, scars of soft tissue stretching or tearing. These findings occasionally have been mistaken for anomalies of morphogenesis, but their differentiation from birth defects is important because of the great differences in approach to these two sets of problems.

4.12.5.2. Disruptions

Although there are no characteristic developmental disruption abnormalities affecting the external genitalia, they may be affected by amniotic band disruptions that involve the lower abdominal wall or pelvic structures.

4.12.5.3. Dysplasias

The size of the male genitalia is governed by hormonal influences, which may be upset in some dysplastic disorders and disease states. **Testicular hypoplasia** and associated functional *hypogonadism* is seen in some dysmorphic syndromes. The testes are usually smaller than normal for age and soft in consistency. **Macroorchidism** after puberty is a feature of the fragile X syndrome.

True *micropenis* is usually caused by inadequate androgenic stimulation or end-organ unresponsiveness during late fetal life but is also found in boys with a number of chromosomal and other dysmorphic disorders without known endocrine abnormalities. Otherwise normal in structure, the penis is small in diameter and length, the latter measurement falling below the 2nd percentile for age (Fig. 4.12.4A). Some instances of **ambiguous genitalia** also fall in this category. Such changes may be caused by partial masculinization, as in girls with adrenogenital syndrome, and in boys with one variant of the feminizing testis syndrome, or with prenatal exposure to certain estrogenic compounds.

4.12.5.4. Malformations

The complex embryogenesis of the genital system and the external genitalia sets the stage for a bewildering array of structural anomalies, most of which are quite rare. This is fortunate, because some external genital anomalies can be associated with life-threatening malformations of the urinary tract, and most will require extensive surgical repair. A majority of these severe abnormalities have their origins earlier than week 12 of gestation, before sexual dimorphism becomes apparent to gross examination. For this reason, it is possible to discuss the physical diagnosis of these abnormalities in a generic sense, applicable to both sexes. Later, the anomalies specific to each sex will be addressed.

Failure of formation of the genital tubercle leads to **absence of the phallus.** In females, absence of the clitoris may not be diagnosed during childhood unless urinary complications associated with an aberrant course of the urethra lead to specific investigations. In males, absence of the penis is immediately apparent at birth, although the scrotum is usually present and the testicles are descended. Frequently, the bladder drains through a fistula into the rectum or onto the perineum (Fig. 4.12.4B).

The term *ambiguous genitalia* encompasses a rather wide range of abnormalities having their origin before week 12 of gestation. Usually, there is some degree of retention of the undifferentiated genital state present in the 8- to 9-week embryo (Fig. 4.12.1C), and the same phenotype can be seen in children of either genetic sex. The phallus commonly shows hypospadias with chordee formation and appears large in proportion to the persisting labioscrotal folds, which may or may not contain gonads (testis, ovotestis, or rarely a well-defined ovary). If a vaginal orifice is present, it is often small, and the vaginal vault

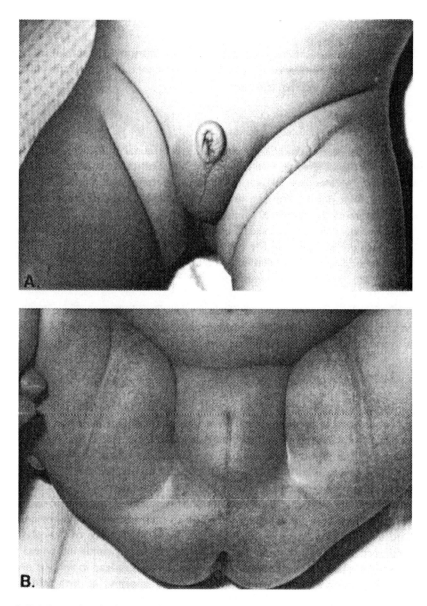

Figure 4.12.4. Incomplete development of the phallus. (A) Micropenis, with the hypoplastic penile shaft partly buried in the pubic fat pad. (B) Penile agenesis. The urethra opens at the top of the scrotal raphe. Note hypoplastic, unrugated scrotum. (Photo courtesy of Dr. Herb Koffler, Albuquerque, N.M.)

may be shallow or atretic. Variations toward the "male" end of the spectrum tend toward a picture of hypospadias with a bifid scrotum (Fig. 4.12.5A), while a more feminized pattern includes a vaginal introitus and labia minora that extend to the base of the phallus (Fig. 4.12.5B).

   Asymmetry of the genitalia results from unequal early development of the paired

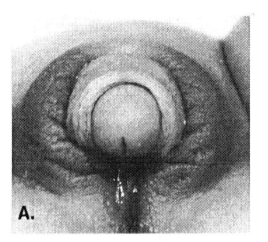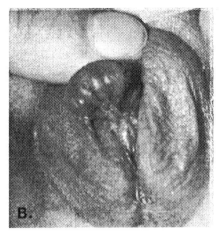

Figure 4.12.5. Ambiguous genitalia.

structures lying to either side of the genital membrane and may be manifested as hypoplasia or aplasia of one labium majus or one side of the scrotum. The most marked and remarkable form of asymmetry is **true hermaphroditism,** in which both the internal and external genitalia are divided at the midline, with one side of the body having a male configuration and the other that of a female. This extraordinarily rare abnormality is probably best explained by sex chromosome mosaicism involving one vertical half of the body.

Duplication of external genital structures, while extremely rare, has been reported as part of an apparent sagittal mirror-image doubling of the posterior axis of the embryo. Partial or complete duplication of the vagina, labia, penis, or scrotum may be seen, accompanied by a variety of internal rearrangements of genital organs and bladder outlet(s).

In **epispadias,** the external urethral orifice is found on the upper surface of the phallus. As in hypospadias, the opening can be located anywhere along the dorsum, from the glans to the base. This rare anomaly is sometimes seen as an isolated defect in either sex but more frequently appears in conjunction with **exstrophy of the bladder.**

Exstrophy of the bladder really represents a failure of complete closure of the caudal portion of the abdominal wall, probably brought about by incomplete migration of mesenchyme into that area during weeks 4 and 5 of gestation. This leaves the unsupported surface ectoderm in direct contact with the entodermal lining of the urogenital sinus. This fragile double membrane soon ruptures, and the urogenital sinus is laid open to the amniotic cavity. At birth, the posterior bladder wall is seen as a reddened, granulomatous mass lying just above the pubic symphysis (Fig. 4.12.6). The ureteral orifices can often be discerned laterally, exuding urine onto the surface of the thickened and hypertrophic bladder mucosa. Bladder exstrophy is almost invariably associated with epispadias, and the pubic bones are widely separated.

It is thought that the etiology for **exstrophy of the cloaca** is similar to that for exstrophy of the bladder but that the deficiency of mesenchymal migration is more severe and that rupture of the anterior body wall occurs earlier, before partitioning of the cloaca.

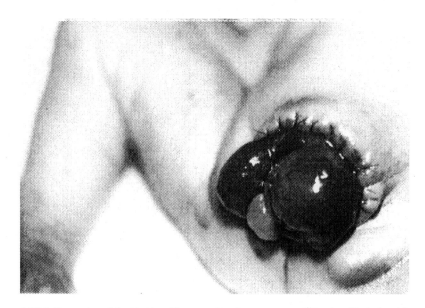

Figure 4.12.6. Exstrophy of the bladder. (Postoperative photo courtesy of Dr. Ann Kosloske, Albuquerque, N.M.)

Thus, the bladder is present only as lateral remnants, which along with the interior of the rectum are exposed on the surface of the lower abdomen. In addition, the abdominal viscera, including the liver, may herniate through the infra-abdominal defect. Once again, there is a wide gap between the pubic bones.

Male-Limited Genital Defects. Mild degrees of hypospadias (those with the meatus on the ventral surface of the glans) are quite common and of minimal significance (see Section 4.12.4.2 and Fig. 4.12.3A). However, **severe hypospadias with chordee** has more important implications, both for urological repair and for association with other malformations. The pathogenesis of hypospadias is essentially similar for all degrees of severity: a failure of complete fusion of the margins of the urogenital folds to form the penile urethra. In one form, the defect is localized to a small segment, with normal urethra both proximally and distally, creating a **double meatus.** More commonly, the urethra lies wide open down to the level of the displaced orifice. The penile shaft is shortened and the ventral portion of the foreskin is missing. *Chordee* refers to the ventral curvature of the penile shaft caused by associated partial agenesis of the corpus spongiosum.

A **bifid scrotum** indicates failure of the testosterone-induced fusion of the two labioscrotal folds at about 10–11 weeks of gestation. Genitalia in which the urethral meatus opens between the halves of a bifid scrotum (**scrotal hypospadias**) constitutes one form of ambiguous genitalia, especially worrisome if the testes cannot be palpated. In **perineal hypospadias,** the meatus opens near the anal orifice, and the appearance of the genitalia is pseudovaginal. Both of these forms of hypospadias have a strong association with structural abnormalities of the urinary tract, which should receive prompt evaluation.

In the earliest stages of development of the external genitalia, the genital tubercle may be displaced backward from its usual site at the cranial junction of the urogenital

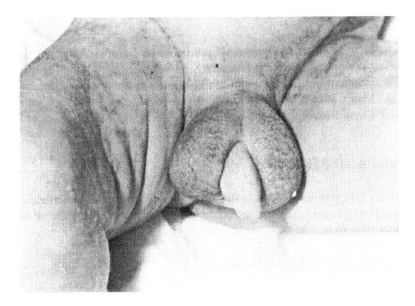

Figure 4.12.7. Shawl scrotum.

folds. A **shawl scrotum** is the mildest sign of this developmental anomaly; a continuation of the skin of the scrotum arches over the base of the penis (Fig. 4.12.7). If the embryo-logic displacement is more severe, the penis may give the appearance of emerging from the center of the scrotum or being embedded in it. The most extreme and least common example of this same process is **transposition of the penis and scrotum,** in which the penis comes to rest between the scrotum and the anus.

Female-Limited Genital Defects. A totally **imperforate hymen** is not a minor abnor-mality because it may occlude the vaginal opening completely, obstructing the outward flow of normal vaginal secretions. In such instances, the hymeneal membrane can be seen bulging out into the vaginal vestibule, often under considerable tension (**hydrocolpos**). After puberty, the obstruction of menstrual flow on the same basis is called **hydro-metrocolpos,** and the retained menstrual fluid has a distinct blue color behind the intact hymen.

Total **absence of the vagina** invariably has been associated with extreme hypoplasia or absence of the structures derived from the Müllerian system and often bilateral agenesis of the kidneys. A **shallow vagina** may indicate partial failure of Müllerian development, with preservation of the lower two-thirds of the vagina, derived from the urogenital sinus.

Hypospadias in females simply implies an opening of the urethra posterior to its usual site, sometimes in the anterior vaginal wall. The condition is very rare and probably represents incomplete septation of the urogenital sinus. Meatal stenosis and recurrent urinary tract infections frequently complicate this anomaly.

Duplicated or **septate vagina** represents incomplete fusion of the Müllerian ducts and is always accompanied by partial or complete duplication of the uterus as well. The exact embryogenesis of this anomaly is obscure.

4.12.6. Summary

Developmental defects of the external genitalia may occur at almost any time during the embryonic period and may be produced by failures of cell proliferation, tissue migration or differentiation, programmed cell death, end-organ unresponsiveness, or hormone imbalances. Many of the resulting abnormalities constitute genuine dysmorphologic emergencies when discovered in the newborn.

4.13. ANUS AND PERINEUM

The anus and perineum share in the developmental processes described in Section 4.12 for the external genitalia. The important anomalies in this region are all variants on the theme of imperforate anus.

4.13.1. Embryology and Development

By the end of week 6 of gestation, the *urorectal septum* has divided the cloacal membrane transversely into two unequal portions: the urogenital membrane ventrally and the anal membrane dorsally (Fig. 4.12.1B). During the following week, two lateral mounds of tissue, the *anal hillocks,* coalesce to form a ring around the anal membrane, which thus becomes located at the bottom of the *anal pit* (*proctodeum*). At about the end of week 7, this membrane ruptures, forming the *anal canal,* which permits open communication between the lumen of the hindgut and the amniotic cavity surrounding the embryo. The distal one-third of the anal canal develops from the anal pit and is lined with stratified squamous epithelium, while the proximal two-thirds has a lining of columnar epithelium derived from mesenchyme within the anal hillock.

The *perineum* (*perineal body*) represents the site of fusion of the urorectal septum with the cloacal membrane.

4.13.2. Anatomy and Landmarks

The puckered margin of the anal orifice, lying at the base of the *gluteal crease,* may be more or less darkly pigmented in the newborn. The perineum extends to the anterior edge of the anus to the base of the scrotum in boys and from the posterior junction of the labia majora in girls. The length of the perineum ranges from approximately 1 cm in neonates to 5 cm or more in adults (Fig. 4.12.3).

4.13.3. Examination Techniques

The perineum and anus are first inspected directly, with attention to the location and size of both structures. In males, especially in the newborn period, it is often necessary to lift the scrotum to see the perineum adequately. If the anus seems small, displaced, or actually imperforate, it is helpful to determine the position of the anal sphincter by lightly stroking the skin in the area with a sharp object such as a pin or broken tongue depressor. When the sphincter is stimulated in this way, it will contract, and the movement this imparts to the overlying skin gives a good indication of the position and potential function of the sphincter itself. Rarely is digital examination of the anal canal and rectum necessary as part of the dysmorphology evaluation, but it can provide valuable information about anal sphincter tone and the presence of masses in the lower abdomen. A well-lubricated glove or finger cot and use of the smallest available finger is mandatory for rectal examination in children.

4.13.4. Minor Variants

4.13.4.1. Spectrum Variants

There is some normal variability of anal placement in the anterior–posterior plane, but this falls between rather narrow limits. The relative length of the perineal body provides the best measure of anal placement (see above).

4.13.4.2. Minor Anomalies

Anal tags are small (1–4 mm) outgrowths of mucosa arising from the anal margin. They are relatively common and have no pathological significance. **Rectal polyps,** on the other hand, may signify the presence of a genetic disease such as Peutz-Jeghers syndrome. Such polyps are usually pedunculated, several millimeters to 1 cm in diameter, and deep red in color. They may rarely extend out of the anal orifice from a base on the mucosa of the lower rectum. **Hemorrhoids** are quite uncommon in children but, just as in adults, may indicate impedance of blood flow in the inferior vena cava or compression of pelvic veins.

A mild degree of **anal stenosis** is relatively common in newborn babies but seems to resolve spontaneously within the first three to six months of life. Rarely, persisting problems with ribbonlike stools will necessitate artificial dilatation or surgery to relieve the stenosis. Embryologically, this probably represents hypoplasia or incomplete rupture of the anal membrane at the end of week 7.

4.13.5. Abnormalities

4.13.5.1. Deformations

Although a **patulous anal sphincter** may denote an abnormality of innervation to the perineum, it can also be produced by repeated sexual abuse (see Section 4.12.5.1.).

4.13.5.2. Disruptions

There are no characteristic disruptive abnormalities of the perineum and anus except, perhaps, for the mucosal tearing and scarring associated with sexual abuse.

4.13.5.3. Dysplasias

Few examples of tissue dysplasia are seen in this region. The anal mucosa may rarely bear the characteristic lesions of multiple mucosal neuroma syndrome, which easily can be mistaken for small polyps or hemorrhoids, and the angiokeratomas of Fabry disease may appear first over the perineum.

4.13.5.4. Malformations

As can be appreciated from the discussion of embryology outlined above, the major malformations of this portion of the body are related to abnormalities of septation of the cloaca and formation of the anal canal. An **ectopic anus** occurs when there is an abnormality of fusion between the urorectal septum and the cloacal membrane during week 6 of gestation. If there is inadequate development of the urorectal septum, if its junction with the cloacal membrane is too far anterior, or if tissue proliferation is inadequate in the developing perineal body, the anus is displaced forward and may open anywhere along the perineum (Fig. 4.13.1.). The anal opening is generally much smaller than normal. Usually, the anal sphincter has been "left behind" and can be detected by an anal wink at the normal site. In all such cases, fecal incontinence is present. In the most severe form of this malformation, **persistent cloaca,** developmental arrest at about 5–6 weeks totally prevents the descent of the urorectal septum, and hence the hindgut and the vagina open into the same common cavity.

Anal ectopia may also be seen in the form of *posterior* displacement of the anus, producing an abnormally long perineum, but this is much rarer than the anomalies outlined above (Fig. 4.13.2).

True **imperforate anus** appears in two forms: the rare **membranous atresia** probably results from failure of perforation of the anal membrane at the end of gestational week 7; much more common is **anorectal atresia,** in which the rectum ends blindly some distance above the perineum. In the latter type, a fistula usually joins the rectal cul-de-sac with the vagina or the urethra. On the surface, a remnant of the anal canal may be seen in the form of a shallow dimple; once again, the anal sphincter is usually intact and in its normal location. A third abnormality, **rectal agenesis,** features a very high blind-ending

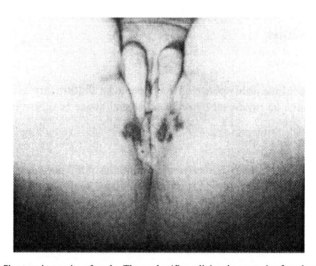

Figure 4.13.1. Short perineum in a female. The anal orifice adjoins the posterior fourchette of the vagina.

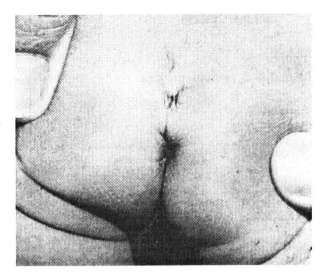

Figure 4.13.2. Posteriorly displaced anus, lying just below the coccyx.

rectum, with a well-formed but blind anal canal below. Embryologically, this defect is caused not by abnormal cloacal septation but by true intestinal atresia, similar to that found elsewhere along the length of the intestinal tract and possibly of vascular origin.

4.13.6. Summary

Abnormalities of anal placement may signify the presence of rectovaginal fistulas, and the possibility of imperforate anus justifies the examination of this area in every newborn baby.

4.14. BACK

Examination of the back is frequently neglected or performed in a cursory fashion, but several important dysmorphologic features occur in this region. Those of most significance involve the spine and can be readily detected clinically. Since many of these abnormalities arise before week 5 of gestation, the back should be examined with special care in children with evidence of other anomalies occurring very early in embryogenesis.

4.14.1. Embryology and Development

The development of the back as an anatomical region begins with the closure of the *neural tube,* which is completed midway through week 4 of gestation (Fig. 4.14.1B). Within the next few days, mesoderm from the adjacent sclerotomes migrates from each side over the dorsum of the neural tube, surrounding the remnants of neural crest tissue, as well as ventrally, where it engulfs the notochord (Fig. 4.14.1C). Condensation of the ventral mass of sclerotome cells around the notochord forms the *vertebral body,* while

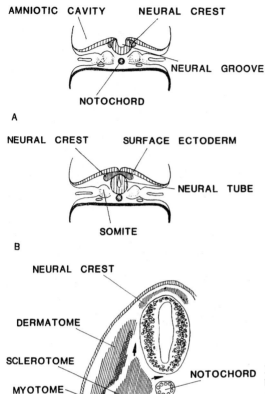

Figure 4.14.1. Embryogenesis of the posterior body wall and neural tube. (A) Cross section of embryonic plate at 2 weeks of gestation. (B) Cross section of 2.5 week embryo, showing closure of neural tube. (C) Cross section of embryo at 4 weeks. Mesenchyme from the sclerotome is beginning to extend around the neural tube and notochord (cf. Fig. 4.10.1B).

those lying dorsally make up the *neural arch* of each vertebra (Fig. 4.10.1B). Meanwhile, a third branch of mesenchymal migration takes place in a ventrolateral direction as the costal processes. In the lumbar zone, these remain rudimentary, but in the thorax they elongate rapidly, forming the ribs.

The *muscles* of the back are derived from the myotomes, distinct concentrations of mesenchymal cells within each somite of the embryo. Migrating with the ribs, one group of cells makes up the segmented intercostal muscles, while others travel dorsally and cross somitic divisions to become the paraspinal and posterior muscles of the shoulder girdle. The *scapula* arises at the base of the developing upper limb bud by week 6 of gestation, while the *pelvic girdle* begins to appear slightly later.

4.14.2. Anatomy and Landmarks

Extending from the tops of the shoulders to the gluteal folds, the back is not really the featureless plane that it seems at first glance (Fig. 4.14.2A). In the midline, just below the

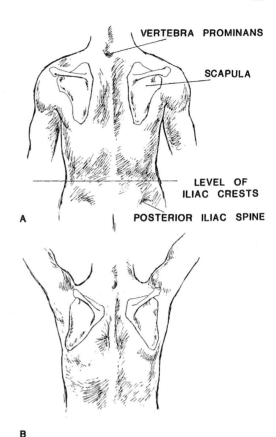

VERTEBRA PROMINANS

SCAPULA

LEVEL OF
ILIAC CRESTS

A

POSTERIOR ILIAC SPINE

B

Figure 4.14.2. Superficial anatomy and landmarks of the back, showing normal rotation of
scapulae upon elevation of arms.

skin, are found the *spinous processes* of the neural arches, the most prominent of which is
that of the seventh cervical vertebra (*vertebra prominans*). The spine is flanked by a thick
column of *paravertebral muscles* on either side. Further laterally in the thoracic region,
the lower edges of the scapulas reach down to about the level of the seventh rib, moving
upward and laterally to about the fifth rib when the arms are raised (Fig. 4.14.2B).

A horizontal line drawn across the upper margins of the *iliac crests* will fall between
the spinous processes of the third and fourth lumbar vertebrae, which is the level of the
body of the fourth lumbar vertebra. The *sacrum* and *coccyx,* covered only by skin and
subcutaneous tissue, provide useful landmarks in the lower back, as do the *posterior iliac
spines,* over which the skin is usually dimpled.

Viewed from the side, the spine is not perfectly straight but shows a series of gentle
curves (Fig. 4.14.3A). Beginning at the base of the skull, the cervical vertebrae show a
mild *lordosis* or concavity, followed by the shallow convexity of the thoracic spine. The
lumbar region is again lordotic. Finally, the sacrum conforms to the slight forward tilt of
the pelvis, whereas the coccyx is quite variable, its tip projecting posteriorly in some
individuals and curling anteriorly in others. These normal spinal curvatures in the sagittal
plane may be indistinct in infants, but their absence in older children often has diagnostic
significance (Fig. 4.14.3B).

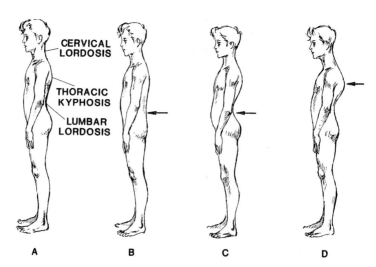

Figure 4.14.3. Lateral views of a standing subject showing spinal curves. (A) Normal spine. (B) Loss of normal lumbar lordosis. (C) Accentuated lumbar lordosis. (D) Thoracic kyphosis.

4.14.3. Examination Techniques

The back is first inspected for general configuration and symmetry. Infants and toddlers can be examined in the mother's arms; older children may be asked to stand on the floor, facing away from the examiner. Any unusual mass over the spine should be noted, and special attention should be paid to depressions, pits, or tufts of hair occurring in the midline, especially over the sacrum. Changes in texture or pigmentation of the skin may also be appreciated best during the examination of the back because of the large area being observed.

While viewing a standing child from behind, look for any lateral curvature of the spine (scoliosis). Such a curve in the lumbar region might be produced by leg length discrepancy, so a finger should be placed on the iliac crest on each side to determine whether the pelvis is level. Younger children may stand in unusual attitudes, and it helps if they clasp their hands together in front and raise them to shoulder level. Sometimes it is necessary to make several observations at different times during the examination before one can be sure whether scoliosis is present. Inspection from the side can reveal an unusual concavity (lordosis) or convexity (*kyphosis*) of the spine (Fig. 4.14.3C and D) If an abnormal curvature is found, its location and approximate severity should be recorded; in the case of scoliosis, an indication is made as to which side of the body the convexity of the curve is directed. Next, the child is asked to bend forward completely at the waist, and a "skyline view" is obtained along the axis of the spine. If fixed thoracic scoliosis is present, its rotary component will usually produce a "rib hump" in this position* (Fig. 4.14.4).

---

*A useful instrument called the Scoliometer has been developed to provide a clinical measure of the severity of rotoscoliosis, based on the principle of the bubble level.

Inspection of the back is followed by palpation of the spinous processes and the sacrum in search of detectable defects of the axial skeleton. An attempt should be made to see the bottom of any dimples over the sacrum or coccyx. It may be necessary to separate the buttocks with the fingers to determine the presence of lesions over the distal coccyx.

4.14.4. Minor Variants

4.14.4.1. Spectrum Variants

Overall trunk length in proportion to height may vary considerably from individual to individual and family to family, producing "short-waisted" and "long-waisted" phenotypes.

During the first year or two after learning to walk, many children will have a noticeable **lumbar lordosis** and a protuberant abdomen. This "toddler's swayback" seems to be caused by relative weakness of the abdominal muscles leading to a forward tilt of the pelvis. The condition improves rapidly with age and needs no special treatment.

A **bifid spinous process** is sometimes found on palpation over the thoracic spine. This represents a mild degree of incomplete fusion of the paired lateral portions of the neural arch and is of no consequence (but see *spina bifida* below).

4.14.4.2. Minor Anomalies

Blind **sacral dimples** are quite common, usually appearing in the midline but occasionally found a bit to one side and, more rarely, at multiple sites. These should not be confused with the shallow skin depressions found over the posterior superior iliac spine. Sacral dimples are benign but must be discriminated from minor degrees of *spinal dysraphism* (see below).

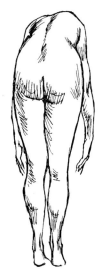

Figure 4.14.4. Posterior view of patient with thoracic scoliosis, showing rib hump on the right.

Some minor anomalies of skin pigmentation or hair distribution may be seen overlying the spine (see Section 4.15).

4.14.5. Abnormalities

4.14.5.1. Deformations

Rarely, children subjected to severe intrauterine constraint are found to have variable degrees of *scoliosis* at birth. Despite the expected tendency for such deformations to correct themselves after removal of the aberrant mechanical force, some children experience persisting scoliosis and may require bracing or surgical treatment. In such cases, there are invariably other deformations involving joints or other structures, yielding the clinical picture of *arthrogryposis multiplex congenita.* Because this is a heterogeneous diagnostic category, however, a number of other etiologic possibilities must be considered before attributing such abnormalities to simple intrauterine constraint (see Chapter 5).

4.14.5.2. Disruptions

There are no major disruptions that characteristically involve structures of the back.

4.14.5.3. Dysplasias

Several metabolic storage diseases produce changes in the shape of the vertebral bodies. While these anomalies can best be defined by X-rays of the spine, some will cause distinctive clinical abnormalities evident on physical examination. The most common abnormality, *wedging of the vertebrae,* reduces the height of the anterior portion of the vertebral bodies, causing a thoracic or thoracolumbar **gibbus,** a localized dorsal protrusion indicating a fixed forward flexion of the spine. A more extensive thoracic kyphosis is seen in older adults with osteoporosis. Some of the genetic osteodystrophies also produce kyphosis but more often cause flattening of the entire vertebral body (*platyspondyly*), which leads to a clinical appearance of a **short trunk.** Some degree of associated scoliosis may be found with either type of spine abnormality.

The normal lumbar lordosis may be accentuated to a pathological degree in some types of bone dysplasia. There is a deep concavity of the lumbar spine with an excessive forward tilt of the pelvis so that the sacrum lies almost in the horizontal plane when the patient is standing (Fig. 4.14.3C). This abnormal positioning puts unusual stress on the hip joints and the ligamentous support of the lumbar vertebrae, and eventual development of arthritis of the hips and, more rarely, spondylolisthesis of the lumbar vertebral bodies can be anticipated.

Unusual protrusion of the medial border of the scapulas may be seen in certain types of muscular dystrophy. Such **winged scapulas** are also a feature of cleidocranial dysplasia caused by absence of the lateral clavicles, allowing the scapulas to swing unusually far upward and forward (Fig. 4.14.5).

Hyperadrenocorticism (Cushing disease) is often marked by a **hypertrophied dorsal fat pad** lying high on the back between the scapulas. This easily can be distinguished from kyphosis by palpation.

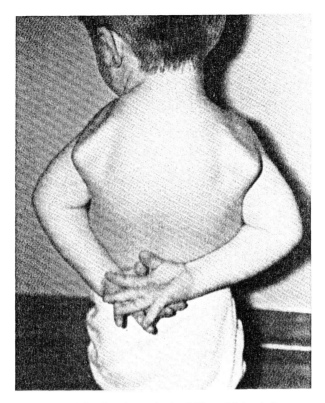

Figure 4.14.5. Winged scapulas in cleidocranial dysplasia.

4.14.5.4. Malformations

Scoliosis is the commonest type of spinal malalignment, involving lateral curvature of the spine into a C- or S-shaped configuration when viewed from behind. Its usual cause is asymmetric strength and tone of muscles acting on the spinal column. This muscular imbalance, in turn, often results from neurologic deficit produced by trauma, infection, or hypoxic damage to the brain or spinal cord. A rarer cause for such distortion of the spine is intrinsic bony abnormality of the vertebral bodies, such as *hemivertebrae.*

In *simple scoliosis,* the shoulder and the hip on one side are demonstrably closer to each other than are those on the other side, and the plane of the shoulders is tilted upward on the convex side of the curve (Fig. 4.14.6A). More complex distortion may arise when compensatory curves of the spine develop over time. For example, a lumbar scoliosis, convex to the left, may eventually result in a compensating thoracic scoliosis, convex to the right, as the child unconsciously attempts to bring his eyes and shoulders to a horizontal plane (Fig. 4.14.6B).

Most scoliosis is accompanied by a twisting of the spine around its own axis, so that the ribs on the convex side of the curve protrude backward while those on the concave

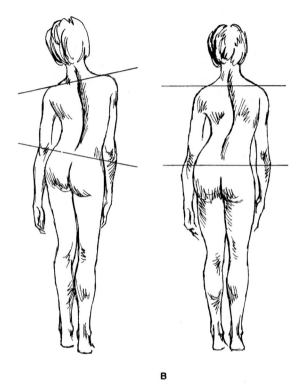

A   B

Figure 4.14.6. Scoliosis. (A) C-shaped thoracic scoliosis, showing convergence of planes of shoulders and hips on concave side of curve. (B) S-shaped curve; thoracic scoliosis convex to the right, compensatory lumbar curve convex to the left. The shoulder and hip planes are parallel.

portion of the curve are directed more anteriorly than usual. This **rib hump** can be detected by sighting along the spine as outlined in Section 4.14.3.

Abnormalities of the scapula may affect its position or size as well as its configuration. In the Sprengel sequence, a unilateral or bilateral **high scapula** also may be smaller than normal and relatively immobile. This anomaly, associated with abnormal segmentation of the cervical vertebrae, forms part of the Klippel-Feil sequence. Unusually **small scapulas,** having normal mobility and position, are features of a few chondrodystrophies and chromosomal disorders.

In contrast to a blind *pilonidal dimple,* a **pilonidal sinus** may connect with the underlying distal end of the spinal canal. This condition should be suspected when the bottom of a midline pit over the sacrum cannot be seen, if there is any fluid emerging from the depths of such a pit, or when the pit contains dark hairs (even one). An overlying hemangioma or pigmented nevus is also a danger signal. Besides the obvious implications for ascending infection presented by communication between the spinal canal and the exterior, such a lesion may signify the presence of a **tethered cord.** In this anomaly, the caudal part of the spinal cord is bound by a stout connective tissue band to the interior of the bony canal. With growth, the spinal canal normally grows more rapidly than the spinal cord, resulting in a recession of the cauda equina upward with age in relation to the vertebral bodies. With a tethered cord, the neural tissue is firmly attached at its caudal end, and growth of the spine puts gradually increasing traction on the cord, which may gradually pull the lower end of the brainstem down into the foramen magnum, like a cork into a bottle. This is the **Arnold-Chiari** malformation, which may be productive of severe neurologic impairment.

The presence of a palpable mass over the spine at any level is a cause for concern. A soft, poorly defined midline mass that is fairly firm and seems to move with the skin may be a **lipoma** (see Section 4.15). Although such tumors are benign, they may signify an underlying *spina bifida* (see below) and may even extend into the spinal canal. Further evaluation, including X-ray studies and surgical exploration, may be needed. A firm or fluctuant mass that lies just lateral to the midline over the sacral area is likely to represent a **sacrococcygeal teratoma.** These primitive tumors, which may reach immense size (Fig. 4.14.7A), are made up of contributions from all three germ layers of the embryo and may contain identifiable muscle, bone, hair, and teeth in a chaotic mix. Some of these embryonal tumors will extend into the abdomen or pelvis in a "dumbbell" shape, and all require urgent surgical attention. Their malignant potential is rather small, but their size and continuing growth can disrupt adjacent structures and can interfere with bowel and bladder function by mass effect.

The most common cause for *midline* masses over the spine in newborn infants is some type of **spinal dysraphism.** The neural tube fails to close completely over a variable portion of its length, resulting in a spectrum of abnormality of the spinal cord and its surrounding structures. The mildest form of dysraphism, **spina bifida occulta,** usually has no clinical manifestations whatever but occasionally may be marked by an irregularity of the spinous processes or an overlying lipoma, hemangioma, or patch of dark hair. This failure of complete closure of the bony neural arches does not involve the spinal cord itself and is usually discovered incidentally in X-rays of the spine.

A **meningocele** occurs when the membranes surrounding the spinal cord bulge outward through a dorsal defect in the bony spinal canal (Fig. 4.14.8A). The resulting mass may be tense or fluctuant and is covered by intact skin. Meningoceles occur most frequently over the lower lumbar and sacral spine and usually create no neurologic problems.

The more severe **myelomeningocele** also is seen most commonly in the lumbar region but may affect the neural tube at almost any level. Again, the posterior elements covering the spinal canal fail to form, but in this type of defect the cystic mass that bulges out posteriorly contains neural tissue, and the surface of the meninges is exposed to the exterior, with no skin covering (Fig. 4.14.7B and 4.14.8B). Small defects spanning one or two vertebral bodies in the lower lumbar zone may contain only a few components of the cauda equina, while larger lesions, lying higher on the spine, may incorporate a large segment of the spinal cord itself. The meningeal sac often ruptures before birth or during delivery, exposing the neural tissues to direct injury and the risk of infection. Even if the sac remains unruptured or is closed promptly by the best available surgical procedures, loss of neurologic function distal to the lesion is the rule. Absence of control of the urinary and anal sphincters, bladder paralysis, and variable degrees of sensory and motor deficit to the lower limbs may be found. Furthermore, secondary *hydrocephalus* frequently

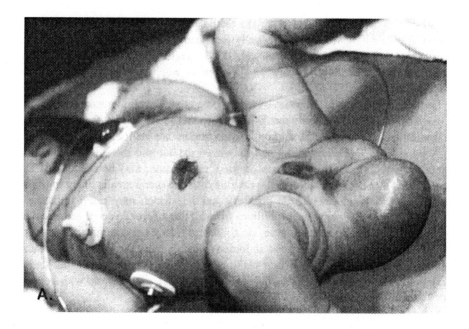

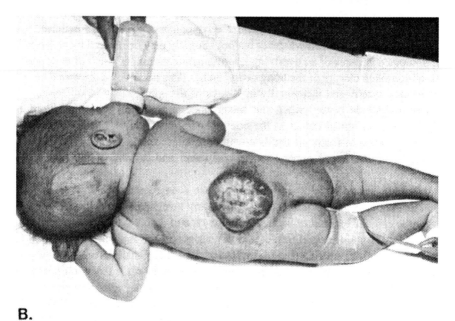

B.

Figure 4.14.7. Major anomalies of the lower back. (A) Sacrococcygeal teratoma. (Photo courtesy of Dr. Ann Kosloske, Albuquerque, N.M.) (B) Large lumbar myelomeningocele. Note hydrocephalus with subcutaneous shunt tubing, bladder catheter.

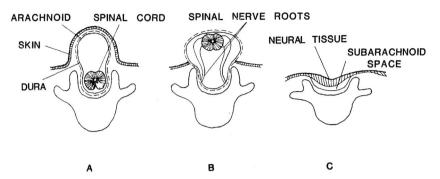

Figure 4.14.8. Types of incomplete neural tube closure. (A) Myelocele with defects of neural arch and dura, but intact skin and spinal cord. (B) Myelomeningocele with intact meningeal sac containing neural elements. (C) Rachischisis with a completely open neural tube, no overlying perineural membranes or skin. [Modified after Moore (1988).]

develops, either as a result of interference with the flow of cerebrospinal fluid by the Arnold-Chiari malformation or from other causes not well understood.

The most severe degree of dysraphism is **spinal rachischisis,** in which there was complete absence of fusion of the embryonic neural tube spanning several vertebral segments, with subsequent failure of development of any of the overlying structures, including meninges, the bony neural arches, and skin (Fig. 4.14.8C). The poorly organized neural structures are widely open to the exterior, with no covering membranes. Rachischisis involves the thoracic region more commonly than the other types, is frequently associated with *anencephaly* and *iniencephaly,* and is incompatible with extra-uterine survival.

4.14.6. Summary

Most of the dysmorphologic anomalies of the back arise either from malformation or malalignment of the vertebral bodies, which frequently has a syndromic basis, or from failure of complete closure of the neural tube, usually an isolated malformation.

4.15. SKIN

The skin is not only the largest but also the most easily examined organ of the body, and it may be for this reason that such a large number of cutaneous abnormalities has been described. Though it is simple in structure, literally dozens of primary developmental anomalies of the integument are known, and it is secondarily involved in some aberrations of underlying tissue as well. Many skin anomalies are localized, benign, or inconsequential, but others may provide valuable clues to the identity of dysmorphic syndromes.

4.15.1. Embryology and Development

Only the most superficial layer of the skin, the *epidermis,* is derived from the surface ectoderm of the embryo. A small number of ectodermal cells lying close to the neural tube proliferate rapidly, and their offspring migrate laterally, forming circumferential bands of epidermal cells, until they meet at the anterior midline. Each band represents a clone derived from one ectodermal precursor cell, and their course bears no constant relationship to the somitic divisions of the body wall. The underlying *dermis* is made up of connective tissue originating from mesoderm. Initially, the cells of the epidermis form a single layer of simple squamous epithelium, keeping pace with the growth of deeper tissues (Fig. 4.15.1A). As these superficial cells keratinize, they are shed from the surface of the embryo and replaced by cells from the *basal layer,* where cell division is quite rapid. By 10 weeks of gestation, this layer has become several cells thick; with further growth, its lower margin becomes corrugated into *epidermal ridges,* which extend down into the developing dermis. At about the same time, *melanoblasts* of neural crest origin are making their way into the dermis (Fig. 4.15.1B), coming to rest at the dermal–epidermal junction by about week 12.

Between gestational weeks 16 and 18, hair follicles have begun to invaginate into the dermis (see Section 4.16), and the epidermal ridges have become prominent enough to become visible on the surface of the skin as *dermal ridges* over the palms and fingertips as well as the plantar aspects of the feet and toes. The overall pattern of these dermal ridges is dictated by the contours of the soft tissues clothing these areas. The formation and significance of these patterns are discussed in Appendix B.

Skin development continues throughout intrauterine life. By the time of birth, all of the components of adult skin are present (Fig. 4.15.1C). The melanoblasts have matured

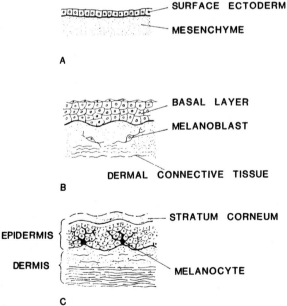

Figure 4.15.1. Embryogenesis of the skin. (A) Single-cell layer of surface ectoderm at 4 weeks of gestation. (B) Skin development at gestational week 11. Melanoblasts from the neural crest are migrating through the dermis. (C) Mature skin. [After Moore (1982).]

into *melanocytes,* which in dark-skinned individuals will already be filled with granules of melanin pigment. Actual incorporation of melanin into epidermal cells does not occur until after birth, however. Retention of large sheets of pigment-filled melanocytes deep in the dermis produces the gray-blue color of *Mongolian spots* (see Section 4.15.4.2). Desquamated epidermal cells, shed fetal hair, sebum, and amniotic cells make up the *vernix caseosa,* the white, soapy coating that covers the baby's skin at birth.

The *sebaceous glands* begin as lateral diverticula from the sheaths of the hair follicles. Growing into the connective tissue of the dermis, each gland develops into a raspberry-shaped cluster of alveoli (Fig. 4.16.1C), discharging an oily secretion (*sebum*) into the follicle. The only hairless areas in which sebaceous glands are found are the glans penis and the labia minora. *Sweat glands* originate as solid cylinders of surface epithelium growing down into the dermis. With further elongation, the free end begins to form a coil, while cell death at the core of the cylinder creates a lumen, and secretory cells differentiate at the periphery. Sweat glands tend to develop in relation to epidermal ridges, especially on the palms and soles. *Mammary glands,* which are highly modified sweat glands, first can be detected at about 6 weeks of development as solid bulbs of epithelium growing down into the dermis. Earlier, at about week 4, a *mammary ridge* (*milk line*) extends from the axilla to the inguinal region bilaterally (Fig. 4.15.2A), but by the time of the first epithelial budding, only a small segment of skin with potential to form mammary glands remains in the pectoral area on each side. At this site, the downgrowth and branching of the mammary primordium is accompanied by canalization of the epithelial buds to form the lactiferous ducts (Fig. 4.15.2B). Fat and connective tissue from the surrounding mesenchyme add bulk to the developing breast. Late in gestation, the *nipple* and a circular zone of skin around it, the *areola,* are elevated slightly above the level of the skin by mesenchymal proliferation. The mammary gland remains quiescent, with only the major ducts in place, until puberty, when in females a second stage of rapid growth occurs. Marked proliferation of secondary and tertiary ducts takes place, along with deposition of fat and connective tissue, under the influence of ovarian hormones.

Skin pigmentation is under multifactorial genetic control and therefore varies over a wide range, even in members of the same racial group. Pigmentation is a function of the incorporation of melanin within cells of the epidermis, and two forms of this pigment are

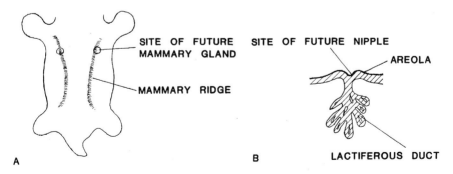

Figure 4.15.2. Embryogenesis of the mammary glands. (A) Diagram of ventral surface of embryo at 4 weeks of gestation, showing mammary ridges. (B) Early stage of mammary development, showing proliferation of lactiferous ducts. [After Moore (1982).]

produced. The eumelanins are the dark brown substances responsible for pale tan to almost black skin color. A second group of yellow-red pigment called pheomelanins are produced in smaller amounts but may be the primary pigmentary component in individuals with pale skin and blonde or red hair. It is the ratio between these two types of pigment and the total number of melanin granules per unit area that provides the many gradations of normal skin color. *Tanning* stimulates melanocytes to produce more melanin but also to distribute it more widely through elaboration of more numerous cellular processes extending between the skin cells at the dermal–epidermal junction. Tanning can occur from sun exposure or chronic mild trauma in any skin with functioning melanocytes capable of producing normal melanin pigment.

After the embryonic period, *skin growth* seems to be mostly passive, with only a mild intrinsic tendency to reach a certain expanse. When underlying tissues grow slowly, cutaneous growth keeps pace, but if the size of a structure increases rapidly, the expansile forces stimulate rapid proliferation of overlying skin cells. Only in instances of explosive increase in tissue size, as with some tumors, will the skin's growth potential be exceeded, causing excessive stretching and thinning of the integument.

4.15.2. Anatomy and Landmarks

The *texture* of the skin is normally smooth, soft, and resilient. With a magnifying lens, a fine pattern of linear depressions can be seen, dividing the surface of the skin into tiny polygonal islands. Cutaneous pigmentation varies gradually from area to area, with no sharp demarcations in color. The *thickness* of the skin is influenced by subcutaneous connective tissue and fat and varies in different areas of the body, being thinnest over the dorsum of the hands and feet, the shins, and the nasal bridge and thickest on the back. The skin is freely movable over underlying tissues, but in some areas, such as the fingertips, this *mobility* is limited to a few millimeters in any direction. The inherent *elasticity* of the skin enables it to fit over irregular surfaces, smoothly covering the contours of underlying structures, and also to stretch with muscle expansion and contraction and joint movements. This property is derived from abundant elastic fibers in the dermis. A second set of dermal connective tissue fibers is interwoven like a wickerwork basket, providing most of the structural *strength* of the skin.

There are few clinical landmarks detectable in normal skin beyond those provided by underlying structures. The only ones helpful from the dysmorphologic point of view are the *creases* that occur around the joints, especially where the skin is thin or tightly bound down as over the interdigital joints and the palms (see Section 4.20). These creases are the result of mechanical stresses produced by repeated joint movement. The circumferential creases seen in chubby babies or in the limbs of individuals with some kinds of chondrodysplasia are produced by skin growth that exceeds the growth rate of the underlying limb, in the first case because of the rapid deposition of subcutaneous fat, in the second because of inadequate linear growth of the underlying bones.

The *dermatoglyphic ridges* of the palms and soles are unchanging relics of the soft tissue configurations of these regions that existed during late embryonic time. The patterns that they form sometimes have diagnostic value (see Appendix B).

In some pathological states, otherwise invisible landmarks may prove helpful in diagnosis. The *anterior midline* of the trunk seems to provide a boundary to some types of ichthyosis and other vascular and pigmentary changes. The surface outline of embryonic *dermatomes* defines the distribution of lesions associated with spinal nerve roots. A third type of patterning of skin abnormalities is produced by *Blaschko's lines,* which demarcate certain nevi and dermatoses. These lines represent the course of early migration of primordial skin cells progressing from the dorsal to the ventral midline. When made visible by the presence of a pathological process such as incontinentia pigmenti, these bands of epidermal cells can be seen to have very irregular margins, with a roughly V-shaped configuration over the back, a wavy or S-shaped distribution on the anterior trunk, and a longitudinal orientation over the limbs (Fig. 4.15.3).

The distribution of the *skin appendages* may provide helpful diagnostic clues. Hair patterning, the most valuable of these features, is discussed in Section 4.16. Sweat glands are normally found everywhere on the surface of the body except the glabrous skin of the mucocutaneous junctions of the lips and genitalia. The spacing of sweat pores, however, varies considerably from one area to another. On the palms and soles, the sweat pores surmount the dermal ridges, where they are spaced about 1 mm apart, but they are much more widely spaced in the skin of the back. Sebaceous glands are found in all hair-bearing zones of the skin and are most active in producing sebum where the hair is the most abundant, especially on the scalp.

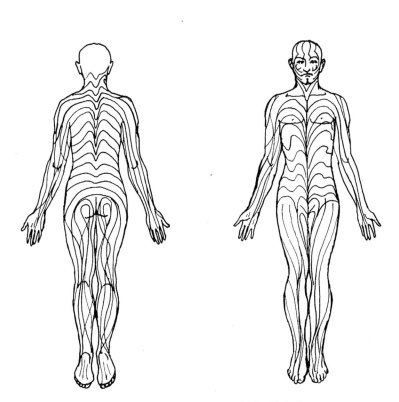

Figure 4.15.3. Stylized depiction of Blaschko's lines.

4.15.3. Examination Techniques

Since the skin is so superficial and essentially two dimensional, it is the one organ of the body that can easily be examined in its entirety. For adequate inspection of the skin, the patient must be disrobed, but usually this can be done in stages as the general examination progresses. If a generalized skin abnormality is suspected or detected, however, it is most advantageous to have the patient disrobe completely or nearly so in order that the distribution and continuity of skin changes can be documented. Inspection of the skin provides an impression of the general degree of pigmentation, the presence of discrete nevi or other skin lesions, and an estimation of the adequacy of subcutaneous tissues. In addition, any unusual creases or wrinkling of the skin can be detected, and more severe degrees of skin laxity can be seen.

Palpation of the skin provides information about the texture, moisture, and temperature of the skin. Skin mobility may be assessed by pressing a fingertip firmly on the skin surface and moving it in a circular fashion. The size of the circle that can be traced in this way gives a rough indication of how tightly the skin is bound to underlying tissues. Elasticity can be judged by gently pinching up the skin, pulling it away from subjacent tissues. If hyperelasticity is suspected, this maneuver should be carried out in a place where skin is normally not very distensible, such as over the forehead. The thickness and consistency of subcutaneous tissues can also be determined by palpation. Rarely, firm stroking of the skin will cause almost immediate development of small blisters in the traumatized area (the *Koebner phenomenon*) or even localized separation and tearing of the epidermis (the *Nikolsky sign*). Both of these abnormalities are indicative of severe skin disease.

Special examination techniques to assist in detecting hypopigmented zones and determining sweat gland distribution and function are described in Appendix A. Methods for recording and analyzing dermatoglyphic patterns are outlined in Appendix B.

4.15.4. Normal Variants

4.15.4.1. *Spectrum Variants*

General *skin pigmentation* is under the control of a number of genes of small effect, and, of course, varies widely among racial groups. Even in individuals within the same family, however, considerable variation in skin color is possible. The skin of newborn infants usually is lighter in color than would be expected for their genetic background, but it gradually darkens during the first year of life with the establishment of normal melanocyte function. Therefore, judgments concerning eventual skin color probably should be postponed until the child has reached the toddler stage.

A moderate amount of *skin drying* and superficial desquamation of the skin is present in many people during the winter months, involving primarily the lateral aspects of the arms and legs and areas under constrictive clothing.

Breast size in adolescent and adult women also is subject to considerable variation, although genetic factors play a major role. Unusually small or overly large breasts at puberty may be the source of considerable concern but in most cases will be found to fall within the broad limits of the normal range. Similarly, mild to moderate degrees of breast asymmetry in women is not abnormal, nor is mild hyperplasia of breast tissue beneath the areola in pubescent boys.

4.15.4.2. Minor Anomalies

A wide variety of **nevi** can be found in normal individuals and, when isolated, usually have no diagnostic significance. A few, however, may have malignant potential (see Section 4.15.5.4). The benign nevi can be conveniently divided into pigmented, hamartomatous, and vascular types.

Benign Pigmented Nevi. The common pigmented nevi all have in common a localized abnormality in either distribution or function of melanocytes. The so-called *Mongolian spot* is a transient minor anomaly frequently found in infants of darkly pigmented racial groups. The dull blue-gray patches are usually found over the sacrum and lower back but rarely extend as far as the shoulders and neck. Usually a few centimeters across, they occasionally cover most of the skin of the back and even can be found on the proximal limbs. These spots have no dysmorphologic significance but sometimes are mistaken for bruises, raising a suspicion of child abuse.

Cafe-au-lait spots range in size from a few millimeters to several centimeters in diameter and have a color only slightly darker than that of the surrounding skin. The most common type has edges that are fairly regular and quite clearly demarcated ("coast of California") (Fig. 4.15.4A). About 5% of white individuals have one such spot, but the figure for blacks approaches 15%; in that population, about 2% have three or more. The presence of more than five cafe-au-lait spots greater than 1 cm in diameter should be

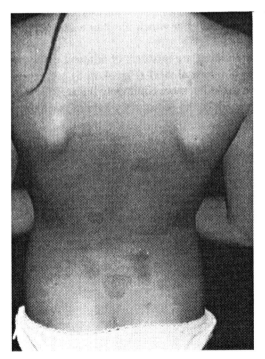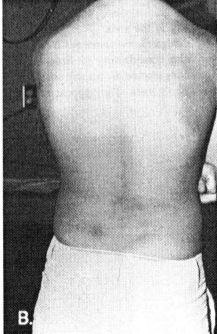

Figure 4.15.4. Cafe-au-lait spots. (A) Discrete, smooth-edged coast-of-California spots in neurofibromatosis. (B) Diffuse, poorly demarcated lesion with irregular coast-of-Maine borders over right scapula and lower back in Albright polyostotic osteodystrophy.

considered to indicate a diagnosis of neurofibromatosis until proved otherwise. A second type of cafe-au-lait spot has a much more irregular border ("coast of Maine") and is usually larger and solitary (Fig. 4.15.4B). Such lesions are often seen in children with Albright polyostotic dysplasia and tend to be found more frequently over regions whose bones show fibrous dysplasia.

Freckles are smaller, slightly more darkly pigmented spots of varying sizes up to 2 cm in diameter. They may be found in clusters or distributed over a wide area, usually in sun-exposed zones. Freckles normally do not occur in the axillae, and their presence there is another strong indication of neurofibromatosis. **Lentigines** are quite similar but smaller and darker. They are present at birth or soon after and do not fade in winter.

Junctional nevi are the common macular pigmented spots that become more numerous with age. They are caused by excessive numbers of melanocytes (nevocytes) at the dermal–epidermal junction. Somewhat larger and darker than freckles, they also occur in sun-exposed areas but in a solitary fashion. In some instances, proliferation of nevocytes down into the dermis occurs, giving rise to a raised, more or less darkly pigmented papular or verrucous lesion. These **intradermal nevi** often form the base for several dark hairs and seldom grow larger than 1 cm in diameter. They are rare on the palms, soles, and genitalia, where they must be differentiated from true melanomas. A **compound nevus** is a combination of the preceding two forms. **Halo nevus** is the term given to a darkly pigmented junctional or intradermal nevus that is surrounded by a pale zone of depigmented skin. This halo reflects the body's immune response to the nevocytic cells, which is affecting melanocytes in the surrounding normal skin for a short distance as well. Quite often the pigmented zone of a halo nevus will show mild inflammatory changes and undergo gradual disappearance over several months, after which the skin will repigment normally in the area.

Benign Hamartomatous Nevi. These skin lesions are mixtures of different cell types and vary considerably in size and location. **Epidermal nevi** (Fig. 4.15.5) are raised, verrucous lesions of variable size, sometimes round but more commonly linear, following Blaschko's lines. They appear at birth or in infancy and are slightly hyperpigmented or

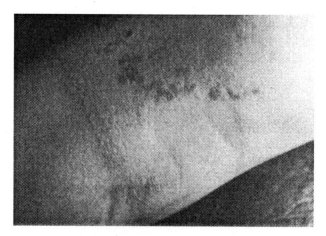

Figure 4.15.5. Linear epidermal nevus.

yellowish in light-skinned individuals, while appearing dark brown to black in more pigmented children. The appearance of linear epidermal nevi on the face (*coup de sabre*) has a more ominous significance, often being associated with seizures and mental deficit. **Angiofibromas** are small (1–2 mm), smooth-surfaced lesions ranging in color from bright red to deep purple. Occurring more frequently with age, they are insignificant if their numbers are few, but if numerous, especially around the genitalia and perineum, they may indicate the presence of disorders such as Fabry syndrome or fucosidosis (Fig. 4.15.6).

Vascular Nevi. The most common minor anomalies in this category are the flat **salmon patches** (*nevus flammeus*) that affect almost half of newborn babies. These zones of dilated superficial capillaries are usually found in the skin over the nape of the neck (*stork bite*), the midforehead, glabella, philtrum (*angel's kiss*), or eyelids. Multiple sites are often affected. These diffusely outlined patches range in color from salmon pink to deep red and are more evident when the baby cries. They gradually fade and disappear over the first few years of life, although those on the nape tend to persist.

Another macular hemangioma is the **port wine stain** (Fig. 4.15.7A), which represents a regional dilatation and engorgement of mature capillaries. Usually affecting the skin of the face and neck, these lesions are sharp bordered and range in color from pale purple to deep burgundy. Although they may be of considerable cosmetic importance, these nevi do not necessarily indicate underlying abnormalities unless they extend into the area of distribution of the ophthalmic branch of the trigeminal nerve that serves the facial skin over the upper eyelid and brow. In this zone, a port wine stain may signal the presence of the intracranial vascular anomalies of Sturge-Weber syndrome (Fig. 4.15.7B).

Flat, bright red lesions from the size of a pinpoint to a pinhead are called **telangiectases** and are formed by local dilatation of arterioles in the skin. Progression may occur to a "spiderlike" form in which several small vessels seem to emerge from a central point. A few isolated telangiectases are not unusual, but when present in large numbers on the skin of the face and upper trunk, as well as in the bulbar conjunctiva, they are usually signs of one of several genetic disorders.

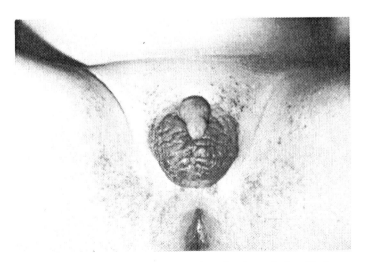

Figure 4.15.6. Angiokeratomas over groin and perineum in fucosidosis.

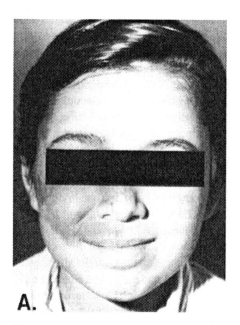
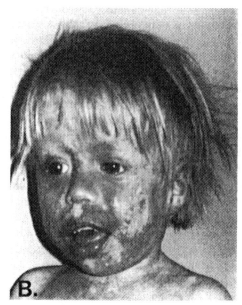

Figure 4.15.7. Vascular nevi: port wine angiomas. (A) Facial port wine stain that does not extend into the area of distribution of the ophthalmic segment of the fifth cranial nerve. (B) Extensive port wine stain involving most of the face in Sturge-Weber syndrome.

Vascular abnormalities causing *raised nevi* include **capillary hemangiomas** (*strawberry marks*), which appear at birth as pale or slightly reddened zones of skin a few millimeters to several centimeters across. During infancy, rapid growth occurs, and the lesions become elevated above the surrounding skin with a spongy consistency and attain a bright red to purple color that blanches with gentle pressure (Fig. 4.15.8A). This

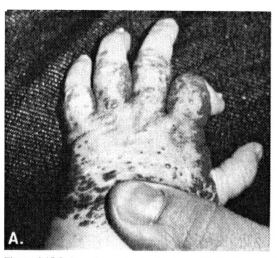
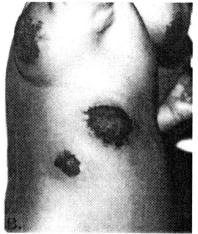

Figure 4.15.8. Vascular nevi: raised lesions. (A) Capillary angioma over dorsum of hand, undergoing spontaneous regression. (B) Large cavernous angiomas over trunk and scapula. Note lesion on chin.

vascular tumor is apparently caused by a local persistence of angioblastic cells that give rise to a plexus of thin-walled capillaries with poor venous drainage. Their natural history is usually one of continued rapid enlargement during the first few months of life, followed by gradual spontaneous regression over the next several years. Rarely, such hemangiomas may expand sufficiently to interfere with function or may evidence bleeding or superficial infection. In such instances, treatment with steroids, sclerosing agents, or surgery may be necessary. More usually, these lesions can be allowed to follow their normal regressive course. Apparently based on the same localized failure of normal angiogenesis, deep **cavernous hemangiomas** (Fig. 4.15.8B) grow slowly after birth, have a blue color because of their site below the dermis, and feel like a bag of worms. Blood flow through these tumors is very slow, and therefore they do not compress easily or blanch with pressure. Sometimes such angiomas are associated with overgrowth of subjacent tissues, including bone.

Other Minor Anomalies. **Supernumerary nipples** are found rather frequently at birth, especially in members of darkly pigmented racial groups. They may be found anywhere along the milk line but most often appear below the usual site of breast placement as an oval pigmented spot, less than half the size of the normal nipple (Fig. 4.15.9). Occasionally these rudimentary structures are symmetrically paired or multiple, but they are more often solitary. Supernumerary nipples can be distinguished from other pigmented skin spots by their location, by their slightly elevated and rugated surface, and by the frequent presence of a short horizontal fold of skin transecting their center.

Normal skin dimples can be found over the acromion process, the lateral elbows, and the sacrum, where the skin is relatively tightly bound to underlying bony prominences. In the sacral area, such dimples may be crease shaped or multiple and should be distinguished from a pilonidal sinus (see Section 4.14.5.4).

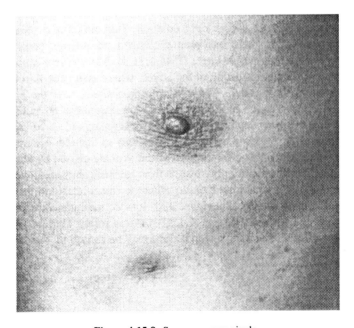

Figure 4.15.9. Supernumerary nipple.

4.15.5. Abnormalities

4.15.5.1. Deformations

Because of its inherent elasticity and growth potential, the skin is quite easily deformed, especially by stretching caused by unusual enlargement of underlying structures. Once localized skin growth has taken place, however, it does not easily reconstitute itself if the distending forces are removed. A small amount of *redundant neck skin* may be seen in normal children, but when there is enough to cause visible folds or webs on the lateral neck, prenatal edema in the region is almost certain to be the cause. Extensive redundancy of the neck skin is seen in a number of dysmorphic conditions, including Turner and Noonan syndromes (Fig. 4.9.3). A more extreme example of this phenomenon is seen in the **redundant abdominal skin** caused by massive abdominal distension in the urethral obstruction sequence (Fig. 4.11.3).

Like the normal creasing of skin that takes place over the joints, **aberrant skin creases** can be formed if joints move in an unusual plane, as in congenital hip dislocation or clinodactyly. Atypical crease patterns of the palms and fingers are discussed in Section 4.20.

Hyperplasia of the horny layer of the epidermis in response to repeated mild trauma results in typical **callus formation.** Instead of being shed gradually, the cornified epithelial cells are formed more rapidly and adhere to the basal layer in a thick, firm plaque, providing protection to the dermis below. The skin of the palms and soles is particularly subject to callus formation, but such thickening can occur anywhere on the body if prolonged trauma takes place.

4.15.5.2. Disruptions

Severe or prolonged pressure on the skin may cause loss of subcutaneous tissue or even breakdown of the dermis, with ulcer formation. Skin dimpling is seen frequently in a relatively mild form when there has been prolonged intrauterine pressure upon bony prominences such as the elbows or knees (Fig. 4.11.3). More severe examples are found in cases of extreme prenatal distortion of the bones, where **aberrant skin dimples** appear over abnormal bony prominences. The most common site is over the apex of a severe curvature of the tibia in cases of fibular hypoplasia, but other areas can be similarly affected. Broader, shallower depressions are found over sites of loss of subcutaneous fat, such as those caused by repeated subdermal injections in diabetic patients.

The most severe examples of disruption of the skin are caused by amniotic bands. It is still unclear whether this abnormality results from intrinsic abnormality of the skin itself or whether aberrant bands of amniotic tissue adhere to intact fetal skin; in either case, the result is circumferential constriction rings, with loss of subcutaneous tissue sometimes extending down to the periosteum (Fig. 4.15.10). More rarely, aberrant superficial clefting of the face or extensive cicatrical skin lesions may be caused by this same mechanism (see Appendix C).

4.15.5.3. Dysplasias

By definition, skin dysplasias are generalized abnormalities that affect virtually the entire integument of the body. For convenience, they will be separated into (1) those

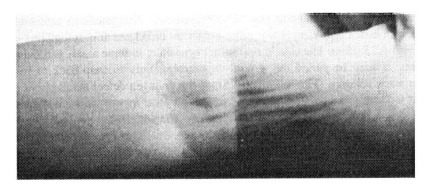

Figure 4.15.10. Circumferential constriction ring above the elbow, caused by an amniotic band.

disorders causing primary structural changes in the dermis and epidermis and (2) the pigmentary abnormalities of melanocyte distribution and function.

Generalized Structural Abnormalities. Absence or diminution in number of the elastic fibers of the dermis results in **cutis laxa.** The strength of the skin is unaltered, but without its normal elasticity, it sags in response to gravity, producing an abnormally wrinkled appearance, and sometimes hangs in folds over joints (Fig. 4.15.11). The sagging is especially noticeable in the face, where it resembles premature aging, since it mimics the changes seen with normal loss of elasticity with advancing years (Fig. 4.21.1C). In other disorders, primarily those of the Ehlers-Danlos group, **skin fragility** and **hyperelasticity** cause problems. Histologically, the elastic fibers are intact, but the supporting collagen tissue is defective, leaving the skin unusually thin and fragile. The

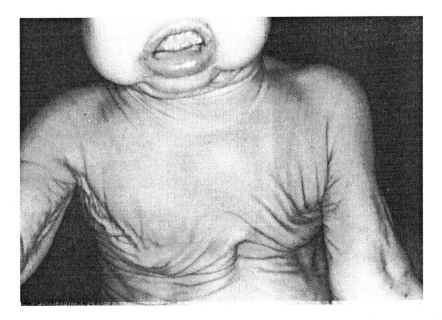

Figure 4.15.11. Extreme skin redundancy in cutis laxa syndrome (also see Fig. 4.21.1C). (Photo courtesy of Dr. M. Tottori, Honolulu, Hawaii.)

loss of connective tissue support may result in extensive ecchymosis or actual tearing of the skin with minor injury, and the resulting scars are broad and thin, resembling cigarette paper (Fig. 4.15.12A). The skin is also quite distensible; in some areas, particularly over the joints, it may be pulled out several centimeters, only to snap back to its normal position when released (Fig. 4.15.12B). Since the collagen defect involves not only the skin but tendons and ligaments as well, remarkable *joint hypermobility* is often present. Several generations ago, individuals with these characteristics were exhibited as the "India rubber men" in circuses and carnivals.

Thickened skin is found in several metabolic disorders, including the oligosaccharidoses and mucolipidoses. The accumulation of metabolic byproducts within cells results in a skin texture that is firmer than normal, and the increase in thickness causes coarsening of the facial features and contributes to limitations of joint movement.

Thinning of the dermal layer yields diffusely **thin skin** that appears translucent and somewhat waxy, with easily visible subcutaneous veins (Fig. 4.2.3B). The normal contours of the skin are strongly influenced by underlying adipose tissue. Disorders in which there is widespread diminution or absence of subcutaneous fat (**lipoatrophy**) are notable for an emaciated appearance in which the outlines of the muscles are clearly visible, especially over the face.

A number of different abnormalities of the stratum corneum are included under the general heading of **ichthyosis.** These conditions all involve faulty keratinization, and the name is derived from the small plates of thickened epidermis seen in many forms, yielding a pattern similar to the scales of a fish. **Ichthyosis vulgaris,** the mildest (and most common) type, most frequently involves the back and the extensor surfaces of the limbs. **Ichthyosis congenita** produces large sheets rather than small scales of adherent epidermis. In the newborn period, this disorder often is manifested by a "collodion membrane"

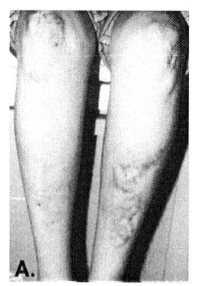 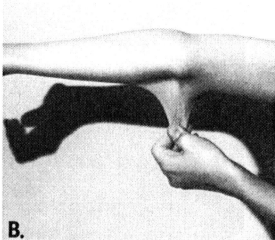

Figure 4.15.12. Skin changes in Ehlers-Danlos syndrome(s). (A) Thin, hypoplastic (cigarette paper) scars over the shins. (B) Extreme skin distensibility over the elbow.

covering the skin of the entire body as if coated with a layer of dried varnish (Fig. 4.15.13A). The most severe form of congenital ichthyosis goes by the name of **harlequin fetus.** Invariably fatal, this disorder produces a tight, constricting integument with a leatherlike consistency. The body is so tightly encased that the joints become fixed in position, and the lips and conjunctiva protrude (Fig. 4.15.13B). Late fetal growth usually results in deep cracking and fissuring of the unyielding skin.

Several types of **epidermolysis bullosum** have been described, all of which have a histological basis quite different from that of the ichthyoses: inadequate bonding between the epidermal and dermal layers. The epidermis separates easily from the stratum lucidum or the basal membrane, and the intervening space fills with fluid, producing large bullae. Blebs may form with gentle rubbing of the skin (the Koebner phenomenon). When the blisters break, the denuded areas resemble second-degree burns. In the more severe forms of this disease, scarring occurs, sometimes to the extent that the fingers and toes are bound together with loss of the distal digits to form a mittenlike mass (Fig. 4.15.14).

Other Dysplasias. **Premature thelarche** is, in the strictest sense, a functional rather than a structural anomaly in that normal breast tissue is reacting to abnormally early hormonal stimulation. This produces enlargement and pigmentation of the nipples and proliferation of glandular tissue within the breast. The resulting breast enlargement may be symmetric or asymmetric and may be accompanied by lactation and a growth spurt. Endocrinologic consultation should be sought, since even if this condition is part of a syndromic disorder, it often can be treated, alleviating concern on the part of the child and her family and avoiding complications that might otherwise ensue.

Congenital **absence of the sweat glands** is found primarily among the large group of disorders classified as ectodermal dysplasias. Sweat glands may be missing everywhere

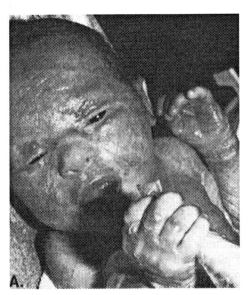 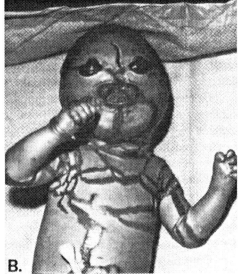

Figure 4.15.13. Congenital ichthyosis. (A) Lamellar ichthyosis (collodion baby). (B) Harlequin fetus. The indistensible skin has been ruptured by continued fetal growth. Note joint constrictions and mucosal eversion of the mouth and conjunctivae. (Photo courtesy of Dr. Nelson Ordway, Phoenix, Ariz.)

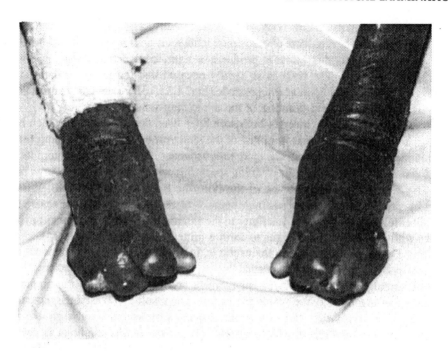

Figure 4.15.14. Scarring of hands and fingers in epidermolysis bullosum. (Photo courtesy of Dr. Walter Burgdorf, Albuquerque, N.M.)

on the skin or may be deficient only in certain regions. Individuals with generalized absence of sweating will experience recurrent fevers in response to high environmental temperatures. Several of the conditions in this category are X linked, and Lyonization in carrier females often produces a mosaic pattern of distribution of sweat pores that may be detected by special testing (see Appendix A).

Generalized Pigmentary Abnormalities. The **hypopigmentation** of classical oculo-cutaneous albinism (Fig. 4.15.15) is caused by inability of the melanocytes to elaborate melanin pigment. The skin is pale, dry, and highly susceptible to sunburn. Lightly pigmented freckles are frequently found in affected individuals from darker racial groups. A number of variant forms of albinism have been discovered, with defects in different parts of the metabolic pathway leading to melanin; in some of these, partial pigmentation gradually takes place during childhood. A milder degree of pigmentary dilution occurs in some other metabolic disorders, including phenylketonuria. The skin and hair color in these patients is lighter than would be expected for their family and racial backgrounds but not to the extent seen in the different forms of true albinism.

Generalized **hyperpigmentation,** a feature of a few rare conditions such as *Fanconi syndrome,* may have a slightly gray or green tint. The skin color in acute jaundice is yellow to orange, whereas chronic (especially obstructive) jaundice produces a greenish or bronze hue.

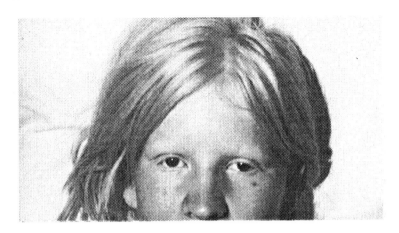

Figure 4.15.15. Oculocutaneous albinism. The skin and hair are pale, and the irises are hypopigmented. Horizontal nystagmus was present.

4.15.5.4. Malformations

In this section, localized developmental anomalies are discussed, again divided into subcategories addressing structural and pigmentary abnormalities and concluding with disorders of the cutaneous glands.

Localized Structural Abnormalities. Full-thickness **absence of skin** is most commonly seen as a single small defect of the scalp, 1–2 cm across, located close to the normal site of the parietal hair whorl (*aplasia cutis congenita verticis*) (Fig. 4.15.16). The lesions have a well-defined edge and resemble a fresh cigarette burn. Such defects occasionally may be multiple or involve a larger portion of the scalp. Their etiology is unknown, and they heal with scarring, leaving a zone of permanent alopecia. Extremely large areas of skin aplasia may be found on the scalp in conjunction with amniotic bands. Aplasia of skin in other parts of the body is quite rare, affecting the trunk or limbs, often in a symmetric fashion. Its cause is presently unknown, although some cases have been associated with prenatal infections with the chickenpox virus (Fig. 4.15.17). Small zones of thinning or **absence of the dermis,** with intact epidermis, occur in focal dermal hypoplasia (Goltz syndrome). Subcutaneous fat herniates up through the dermal defects, appearing on the surface as yellow-tan excrescences beneath a thin membrane of epidermis (Fig. 4.15.18).

Skin tumors of various types are features of several dysmorphic syndromes. Best known are the lesions of neurofibromatosis. **Neurofibromas** may occur before birth but usually are recognized during and after puberty. Having the color of the overlying skin, neurofibromas range in size from 3–4 m to several centimeters in diameter and in shape from soft subcutaneous nodules to pedunculated masses (Fig. 4.15.19A). Often one can push the tumor down through a skin defect immediately below it (the "buttonhole" effect). Larger, **plexiform neurofibromas** may undergo rapid growth and be covered with dark, thickened, and sometimes hairy skin (Fig. 4.15.19B). The misnamed "adenoma sebaceum" of tuberous sclerosis is actually an angiofibroma arising in hypertrophied hair

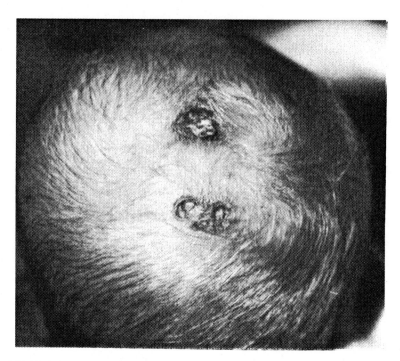

Figure 4.15.16. Aplasia cutis verticis. Posterior view of scalp, showing multiple zones of full-thickness skin aplasia lying close to the midline.

follicles. These fibromas characteristically appear first in the nasolabial folds of the face as small pink papules that gradually increase in number and size, spreading into the "butterfly area" over the nose and medial cheeks (Fig. 4.15.20). **Lipomas** are benign, usually solitary overgrowths of fat cells. They are soft, freely movable, and symmetrically rounded, measuring from 1 to several centimeters in diameter. The overlying skin is normal in color and texture, lacking the central duct opening seen in sebaceous cysts, with which these tumors are sometimes confused. A single lipoma is of no clinical consequence unless it is located in the midline over the sacrum or low lumbar spine, when it might indicate spina bifida occultum. One final skin tumor of diagnostic significance is the **xanthoma.** These lesions derive their yellow color from the lipid-laden cells which they contain and are characteristically found on the palms, soles, upper eyelids, and extensor surfaces of joints (Fig. 4.15.21). Cosmetically unattractive, xanthomas are harmless in themselves, but they may signify the presence of potentially lethal hyperlipidemia.

Several types of *nevi* have been described as features of dysmorphologic syndromes. *Epidermal nevi* are described in Section 4.15.4.2. The **nevus sebaceus of Jadassohn** is a hamartomatous lesion with mixed tissue components that most commonly appears on the scalp or face. These nevi are seen at birth as flat or slightly raised yellow-brown patches with a greasy or waxy, hairless surface (Fig. 4.15.22). They may enlarge rapidly during

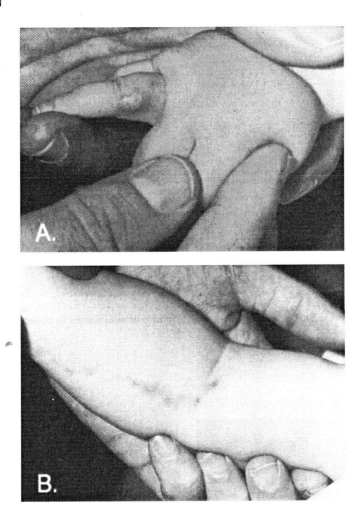

Figure 4.15.17. Skin disruption from intrauterine varicella virus infection. (A) Scarred, thickened lesion on fourth finger. (B) Similar deep scarring in a linear distribution over the forearm.

puberty and have a high potential for malignant change. **Giant hairy nevi** may be pale at birth, with fine vellus hairs, but increasing pigmentation takes place during the first year of life, often with the growth of dark, coarse hair. The hyperpigmented zones may be extremely large, covering the lower trunk ("bathing suit nevus") with numerous satellite lesions (Fig. 4.15.23). The tan to brown skin is roughened and thick, and it frequently includes darker brown to black patches. The presence of one or more of these giant nevi entails a high risk of malignancy (4–10%) and is the most common precursor of *melanoma* in childhood. Similar in appearance but with quite different significance, the so-called **faun-tail nevus** is an elongated patch of dark skin bearing abundant long, dark hair, located in the midline over the lumbar spine or sacrum (Fig. 4.15.24). It is a rare but helpful indicator of a tethered spinal cord.

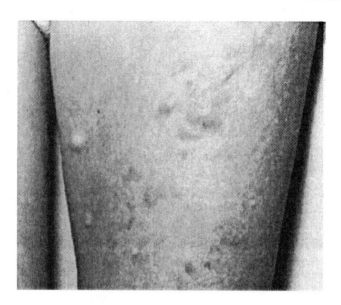

Figure 4.15.18. Focal dermal hypoplasia with herniation of subcutaneous fat in Goltz syndrome.

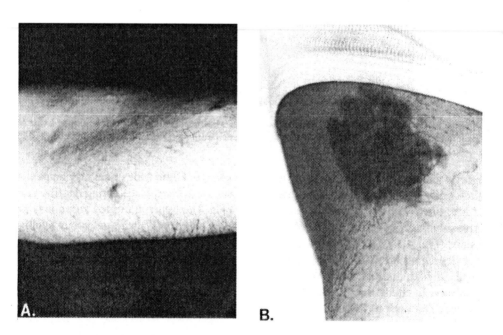

Figure 4.15.19. Skin lesions of neurofibromatosis. (A) Scattered sessile neurofibromas. (B) Plexiform neurofibroma. The thickened, hyperpigmented skin bears numerous dark hairs.

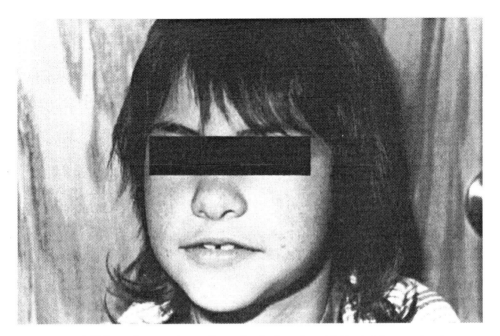

Figure 4.15.20. "Adenoma sebaceum" over the cheeks and nasal bridge in tuberous sclerosis.

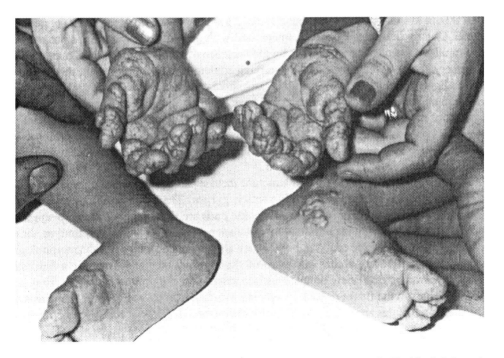

Figure 4.15.21. Severe palmar and plantar xanthomas in familial hypercholesterolemia. The blood cholesterol level in this child was 1200 mg/dl. (Photo courtesy of Dr. Alberto Hayek, La Jolla, Calif.)

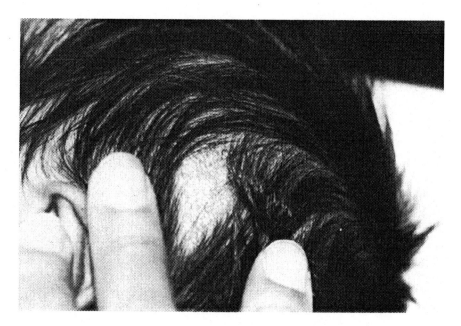

Figure 4.15.22. Nevus sebaceus of Jadassohn on the scalp. The lesion has a greasy, "orange peel" appearance.

About 1% of newborns are found to have a small **nevocellular nevus** or **congenital mole.** Usually less than 1 cm in diameter and with a sharp border, these lesions can be distinguished from cafe-au-lait spots by the presence of speckles of darker pigment at the periphery and an accentuation of the overlying epidermal ridges. At present, the potential for malignant change in these smaller congenital nevi remains controversial. In older children and adolescents, **dysplastic nevi** have ominous implications for eventual development of melanomas. Dysplastic nevi have four helpful diagnostic features: asymmetry, irregular borders, variegated color, and a diameter greater than 0.6 cm. The presence of even one such lesion in an individual with a family history of malignant melanoma calls for immediate dermatologic consultation.

Other regional changes in skin structure include the thickened, indurated, and convoluted scalp skin referred to as **cutis verticis gyrata.** The entire scalp or only a small patch may be involved (Fig. 4.15.25). **Knuckle pads** are firm, hypopigmented plaques of thickened skin overlying the proximal interphalangeal joints. As an isolated finding, these pads are of only cosmetic concern, but they are also associated with a few dysmorphologic syndromes. **Shagreen patches** are zones of slightly thickened and firm skin a few centimeters across, with a finely dimpled surface resembling the peel of an orange. They are usually found on the flanks or back in patients with tuberous sclerosis. **Hyperkeratosis of the palms and soles** appears as thick, horny yellow-brown plates of calluslike skin, which may be deeply furrowed and fissured (Fig. 4.15.26).

Localized Pigmentary Abnormalities. **Hypopigmented macules** may be found on the skin of the trunk in children with tuberous sclerosis. These dull white areas may be linear or oval, measuring 1 cm or more across the short axis, and tend to be sharply

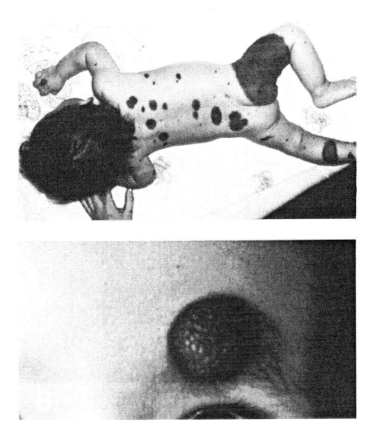

Figure 4.15.23. Multiple giant pigmented nevi. (A) Variable distribution of large nevi with various degrees of pigmentation. Note thickening of skin within lesion on right thigh. (B) Closeup view of giant nevus on eyebrow. Note rugated surface and coarse dark hair emerging from the nevus.

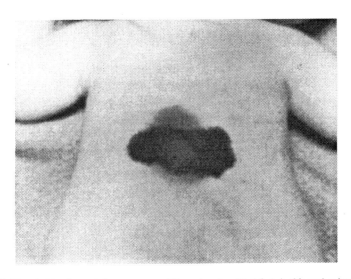

Figure 4.15.24. Flat, darkly pigmented nevus over midthoracic spine. Dark hair in this region is poorly visible.

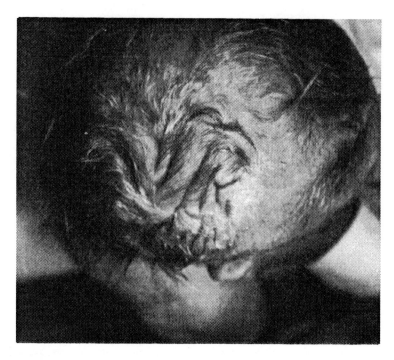

Figure 4.15.25. Cutis verticis gyrata. Large, parallel folds of scalp skin can be seen over the posterior parietal zone.

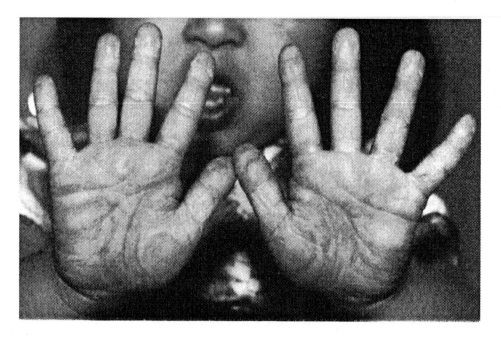

Figure 4.15.26. Hyperkeratosis palmaris. The volar skin is thickened and yellow-tan in color.

pointed at one end and rounded at the other (**ash-leaf spots**) (Fig. 4.15.27). They are most easily seen under ultraviolet light in a darkened room (see Appendix A). **Piebaldness** refers to zones of hypopigmented skin present at birth, which remain constant in shape and relative size. Often associated with a *white forelock,* piebaldness is an occasional feature of the Waardenburg syndrome. **Vitiligo** is a condition in which marked hypopigmentation of the skin gradually develops in a patchy but roughly symmetric distribution over the body (Fig. 4.15.28). The whitened zones may continue to enlarge over a period of several years. In a rare disorder called hypomelanosis of Ito, there is found an irregular distribution of **swirled hypopigmentation** that forms streaks and whorls on the skin. These bizarre patterns look like a photographic negative of the hyperpigmented streaks seen in incontinentia pigmenti, and the two conditions may be difficult to distinguish at first glance (see below).

Regional hyperpigmentation of skin takes several forms. **Multiple lentigines** are usually present at birth but may become more numerous and darker with increasing age and are concentrated on the neck and upper chest (Fig. 4.15.29A). Very similar small, dark brown to **black macules** are distributed around the mouth, on the fingers and toes, and especially on the lips and buccal mucosa in Peutz-Jeghers syndrome (Fig. 4.15.29B). The pattern of **swirled hyperpigmentation** of the skin seen in incontinentia pigmenti has been compared to the appearance of a marble cake. The pigmented zones have very irregular margins and follow the path of Blaschko's lines (Fig. 4.15.30). The pigmentation in **acanthosis nigricans** begins as a light brown to dirty gray discoloration over the axillae, groin, or neck and slowly progresses to a dark brown or almost black area whose edges fade gradually into the surrounding skin (Fig. 4.15.31A).

Poikiloderma is a most unusual pattern of pigmentation in that zones of both hyperpigmented and hypopigmented skin are intermingled with skin of normal color. The

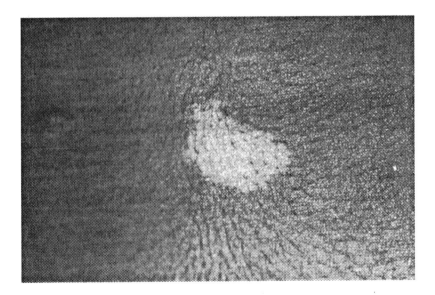

Figure 4.15.27. Hypopigmented ash-leaf spot in tuberous sclerosis.

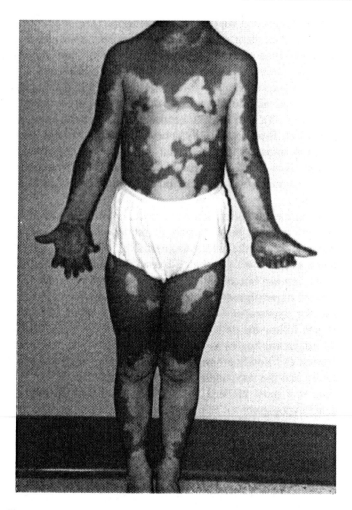

Figure 4.15.28. Vitiligo. Note symmetric distribution of hypopigmented zones.

mottled pattern of light and dark patches, which range from a few millimeters to 1 or 2 cm in diameter, resembles a mosaic floor (Fig. 4.15.31B). On close inspection, the skin appears thin and atrophic. In some poikilodermatous disorders, warty hyperkeratoses may be present over the joints of the hands, knees, and elbows.

Abnormalities of Cutaneous Glands. The breasts in both sexes may be anomalous in structure, size, placement, and number. Supernumerary nipples are relatively common (see Section 4.15.4.2), but the presence of potentially functional **supernumerary breasts** is much more rare. Like extra nipples, these structures appear along the embryonic milk line, unilaterally or bilaterally, usually just below the normal site of breast placement (Fig. 4.15.32A). The nipple and areola are quite well developed, distinguishing this anomaly from simple supernumerary nipples even during early childhood. Pubertal enlargement of the aberrant mammary tissue takes place, and lactation may occur after pregnancy. Aside

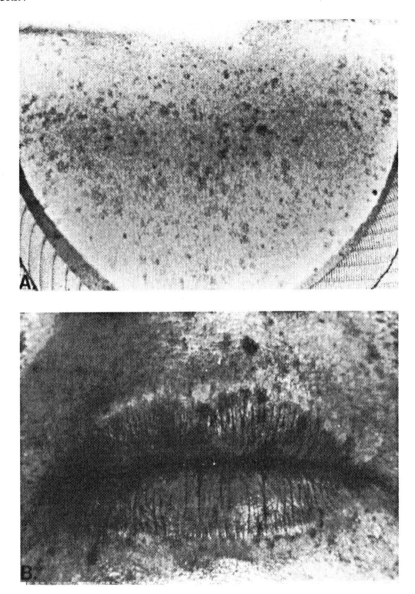

Figure 4.15.29. Punctate hyperpigmentation. (A) Multiple lentigines on the neck in LEOPARD syndrome. (B) Perioral pigment in Peutz-Jeghers syndrome.

from their cosmetic significance, these anomalous rests of mammary tissue are potential sites for the later development of breast cancer. Wide-spaced nipples (see Section 4.10.4) only rarely occur in children with a normal chest configuration. **Hypoplastic nipples** are usually poorly pigmented, with a narrow or absent areolar zone and little palpable breast tissue. Both sides are equally affected, and they may be somewhat wide spaced as well. **Absence of the nipple** (*athelia*) is quite rare but may be seen unilaterally in children with

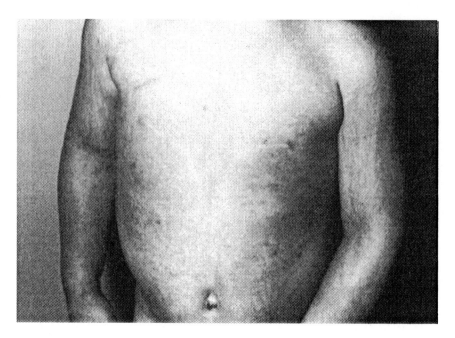

Figure 4.15.30. Linear hyperpigmentation following the distribution of Blaschko's lines in incontinentia pigmenti syndrome.

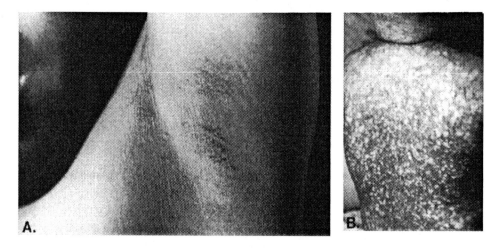

Figure 4.15.31. Other pigmentary abnormalities of skin. (A) Acanthosis nigricans. Hyperpigmented and slightly hyperkeratotic zones are most commonly found in the axillae. (B) Poikiloderma. Macular hypo- and hyperpigmented zones are intermixed with normally pigmented skin in a mosaic pattern.

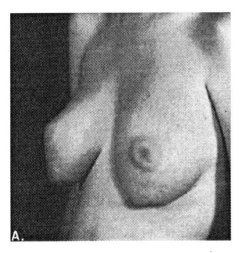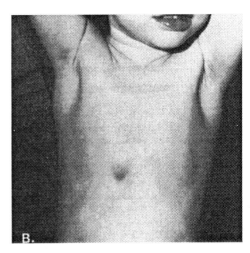

Figure 4.15.32. Anomalies of breast development. (A) Polymastia. Supernumerary nipples and underlying breast tissue lying beneath the curve of the normal breast are visible bilaterally. (Photo courtesy of Dr. M. Schidlower, El Paso, Tex.) (B) Amastia. No visible or palpable nipple or areola is present. (The dark area over the sternum is a bruise.)

the Poland sequence or bilaterally in certain forms of ectodermal dysplasia. Even rarer is complete **absence of the breast** (*amastia*), in which there is no sign whatever of nipple, areola, or deep mammary tissue (Fig. 4.15.32B).

4.15.6. Summary

The skin is basically simple in embryogenesis and structure but is subject to an astonishing array of intrinsic abnormalities, many of which have implications for syndrome diagnosis.

4.16. HAIR

Hair follicles are distributed over the entire surface of the skin except the palms, soles, and zones surrounding the knees, elbows, and digital joints. Variations in the caliber, pigmentation, and patterning of body hair may be influenced by intrinsic factors acting on the hair follicles as well as by aberrant development of the skin and underlying structures.

4.16.1. Embryology and Development

Hair development begins by about week 14 of gestation, when localized thickenings of the lowermost layer of the epidermis bud downward into the dermis (Fig. 4.16.1A). The advancing end of this cell mass soon achieves a teardrop shape to become the *hair bulb*, invaginating at the tip to accommodate mesoderm which forms the *hair papilla*,

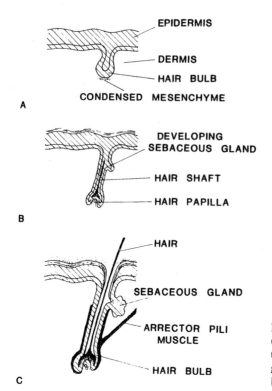

Figure 4.16.1. Embryogenesis of hair follicles. (A) Early hair bulb formation at 14 weeks of gestation. (B) First appearance of hair shaft at about gestational week 16. (C) Mature hair follicle. [After Moore (1982).]

containing a small nutrient blood vessel. The cells in the core of the developing hair cylinder become spindle shaped and keratinize to form the *hair shaft,* while surrounding epithelial cells take on a cuboidal configuration as the *hair sheath* lining the follicle (Fig. 4.16.1B). The cells of germinal matrix in the hair bulb proliferate rapidly, incorporating melanin granules from resident melanocytes, and the growing hair is eventually forced upward through the epidermis. Each hair follicle is normally provided with two additional structures: a sebaceous gland (see Section 4.15) and an arrector pili muscle, which originates at the lower end of the dermal sheath of the hair root and inserts nearby in the papillary layer of the dermis. (It is contraction of these muscles which causes the hair to "stand on end" and produces "goose pimples") (Fig. 4.16.1C).

The hair primordia begin their downgrowth in a direction perpendicular to the surface of the skin, but the skin itself is growing rapidly and is subjected to lateral stresses imposed by growth of underlying tissues. For this reason, the inclination of hair follicles from the vertical reflects the growth patterns of subcutaneous structures during approximately weeks 15–19 of gestation.

From gestational week 20 until birth, the body is covered with fine *lanugo* hair, which is gradually replaced during the first months of postnatal life with coarser, more darkly pigmented *vellus* hair. Within any one body area, these hairs normally reach a predetermined length during the *anagen* or growth phase of their life cycle, which lasts for about 3 years. Thereafter, the follicle becomes quiescent for about 3 months in the resting or *telogen* phase. The hair bulb gradually atrophies, and growth of a new hair then begins in the remaining epithelial cells atop the hair papilla, eventually forcing the old hair shaft up and out of the papilla to be shed.

When examined under the microscope, mature hair can be seen to consist of a central unpigmented core covered by overlapping scales containing melanin (Fig. 4.16.2). The caliber is normally uniform for the entire length of a single hair but varies considerably in different areas of the body.

4.16.2. Anatomy and Landmarks

For clinical purposes, the most important anatomical feature of hair is its *distribution* over the skin. Hair growth is most luxurious where hair follicles are most closely spaced: on the scalp (which bears about 100,000 hairs), the brows, the beard area in males, and the pubic and axillary regions. In sparsely haired areas, the follicles may be 1 cm apart. Except for the brows and lashes, hair growth is suppressed in a wide circular zone around the eyes and in a smaller region around the ears. Scalp hair ends abruptly at the margins of these zones but has a less distinct border over the posterior and lateral neck.

During the early fetal period when downgrowth of scalp hair buds is taking place, the calvarium has not yet developed, and the growing brain itself stretches the overlying skin. As outlined above, this influences the direction of the slant taken by the hair follicles as they penetrate into the dermis. The result is the formation of a *hair whorl,* situated over the part of the brain growing most rapidly from about 16–19 weeks of gestation. The normal position of the scalp hair whorl is slightly lateral to the midline, in the posterior parietal zone. A similar whorl sometimes may be found over the midline of the back.

Unless altered by cosmetics, the *color* of the scalp hair, brows, and lashes is normally uniform. Axillary and pubic hair is usually more darkly pigmented, while the fine vellus hairs over the rest of the body are paler.

The position of the *eyebrows* seems to be influenced by the development of the brow ridges. Medially, the brows lie over the anterior surface of the bony orbit, rising slightly above the orbital margin as they course laterally. The hair follicles of each eyebrow are oriented so that their bases are directed toward a point just medial to the inner canthus of the eye on the same side (Fig. 4.16.3A).

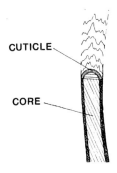

CUTICLE

CORE

Figure 4.16.2. Section of hair shaft.

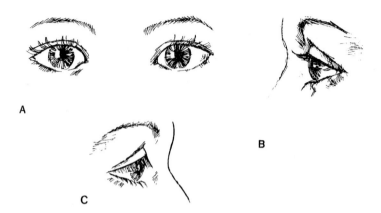

Figure 4.16.3. Periocular hair patterning. (A) Normal brow configuration. (B) Lateral view showing normal upward curve of eyelashes on upper lid. (C) Straight lashes.

The *eyelashes* emerge from the edges of the lids in a gentle outward curve so that when the eye is closed, the upper and lower lashes meet but do not cross or interweave (Fig. 4.16.3B). The eyelashes are normally longest and densest in children between the ages of 6 months and 5 years.

Pubic and *axillary hair* begins to develop at the start of puberty and becomes quite coarse, curly, and darkly pigmented. At maturity, the normal distribution of pubic hair in the male (male *escutcheon*) has a diamond-shaped pattern, extending upward onto the lower abdomen, while the female escutcheon attains an inverted delta configuration.

4.16.3. Examination Techniques

Evaluation of hair distribution is carried out as part of the examination of the skin. Important features include the configuration of the scalp hairline, the presence of pubic and axillary hair, and any unusual patches of hair elsewhere on the body. At the same time, any local variations of hair color are noted. Next, the scalp is inspected to determine the general density of the hair, the position of the hair whorl(s), and any areas of hair loss.

The hair should be rubbed between the fingers to determine its *texture*. If the hair is unusually *fragile*, this maneuver (or simply rubbing the fingers rapidly over the scalp) often will produce fractures of individual hair shafts. In such instances, the hair is often sparse and of uneven length, and an irregular pattern of tiny dots may be found on the scalp, representing the ends of emerging hairs broken off flush with the skin.

In a number of genetic disorders, structural abnormalities of the hair shaft are evident upon examination with low-power microscopy. Special techniques for gathering and examining the hair are described in Appendix A.

4.16.4. Minor Variants

4.16.4.1. Spectrum Variants

Normal hair color varies within wide limits, ranging from almost blue-black to pale yellow-white. As in the skin, the pigmentation of the hair is under multifactorial genetic control and therefore may show considerable variation even within the same family. As a rule, hair color is lighter in the first decade than in young adult life. After about the mid-30s, some hair follicles begin to lose the ability to produce melanin pigment, producing gray or white hairs. The number of such unpigmented hairs gradually increases with age, producing *canities* (the normal graying of the scalp and beard hair).

Several other properties of hair also vary over a continuous spectrum and contribute to detectable differences in appearance. The *density* of hair on the scalp is a function of the spacing of the hair follicles, and exceptionally thick or sparse hair may run in families. Another variable clinical characteristic, hair texture, depends largely on the average caliber of the hair shafts. Hair of smaller diameter is fine and limp and tends to "fly away" after combing, whereas larger-caliber hair is coarse and wiry. A third familial attribute is the relative degree of hair *curliness*. In at least some instances, this characteristic seems to be related to the cross-sectional configuration of the hair; cylindrical hair shafts are quite straight, whereas those with an elliptical or flattened section show a greater tendency to curl. A final biological characteristic of hair is its *potential length,* which is determined by the duration of the anagen phase of the growth cycle. In some individuals, follicles continue to extrude a single hair for a prolonged period, perhaps as much as 6 or 7 years, before entering the telogen phase. Since hair grows at a relatively uniform rate during the anagen phase (approximately 10 mm per month), this may result in scalp hair as long as a meter or more. Each of these four characteristics is independently inherited in a multifactorial fashion, and together with hair pigmentation, they form innumerable combinations that produce the wide normal variability of hair appearance seen in humans.

4.16.4.2. Minor Anomalies

A **low anterior hairline** is especially notable at the sides of the forehead, where the hair-bearing portion of the scalp hair extends unusually far downward, approaching the lateral eyebrows (Fig. 4.16.4). A **widow's peak** is a midline prolongation of scalp hair downward onto the forehead. It is frequently seen in normal individuals with a moderate degree of hypertelorism because the circular zones of hair suppression around the eyes do not overlap completely (Fig. 4.16.5). **Male-pattern baldness** is a very common progressive change of scalp hair distribution in which hair follicles gradually disappear, beginning on both sides of the anterior hairline. The median frontal zone is initially spared, but thinning of the hair over the vertex slowly spreads in all directions until only a fringe of hair remains posteriorly and over the ears. Males with a genetic predilection for this condition may experience hair loss as early as late adolescence. Also relatively common is an **upswept posterior hairline** (Fig. 4.9.4). This may be indicative of some prenatal swelling of the tissues at the back of the neck, changing the angle of hair follicle downgrowth in the region. The presence of a **supernumerary scalp hair whorl** probably indicates a subtle alteration of brain growth during early fetal life (see Section 4.16.1). The usual site for an accessory whorl is just across the midline from the normal one, but it may appear anteriorly as a *cowlick* (Fig. 4.16.6A). Rarely, three or four such whorls may be found over various parts of the scalp (Fig. 4.16.6B). A combination of fine hair texture and unusually perpendicular penetration of the hair follicles into the scalp produces **electric hair** in infants and toddlers (Fig. 4.16.7). More common in boys, this minor anomaly in some instances has been correlated with later learning difficulties.

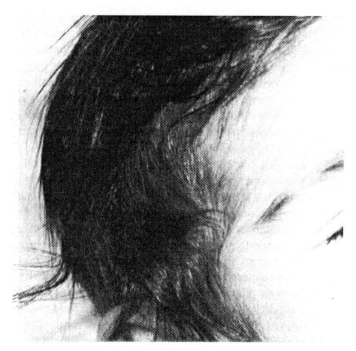

Figure 4.16.4. Low anterior hairline. Note especially the widened "sideburn," so that the lateral hairline approaches the outer end of the eyebrow.

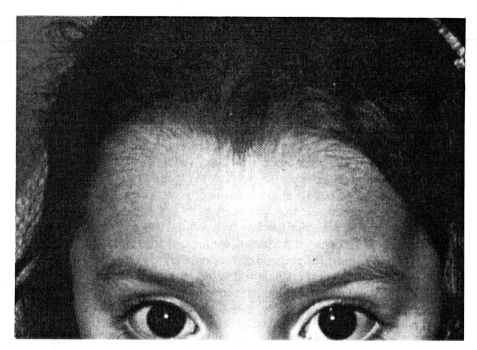

Figure 4.16.5. Widow's peak. A triangular zone of scalp hair extends downward onto the middle of the forehead.

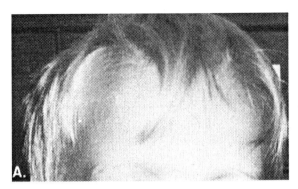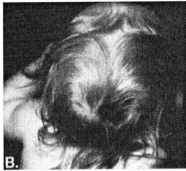

Figure 4.16.6. Scalp hair whorl patterns. (A) Accessory frontal hair whorls causing unusual sweep of anterior hairline. (B) Four symmetric hair whorls (two frontal and two occipital) producing confluent scalp hair patterns.

The skin between the eyebrows usually bears only fine vellus hairs. When the brows encroach on this area, producing the appearance of a single band of hair above the eyes, **synophrys** is present (Fig. 4.16.8A). Somewhat similar in appearance is **medial flare of the eyebrow,** in which the central third of the eyebrow is unusually wide from top to bottom, with the hair follicles radiating from a central point (Fig. 4.16.8B). In older adults, there is normally some gradual hair loss or **thinning of the lateral eyebrows.** In younger individuals, this may be a sign of hypothyroidism.

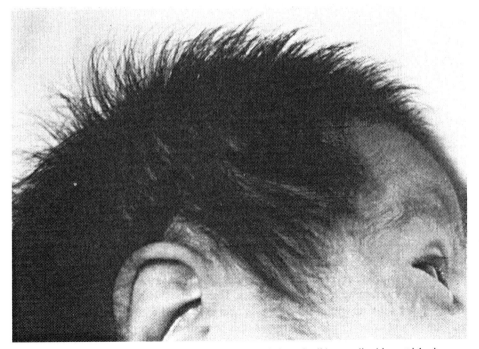

Figure 4.16.7. Electric hair in a child with microcephaly and mild generalized hypertrichosis.

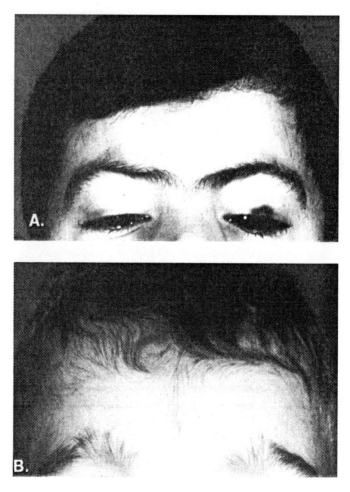

Figure 4.16.8. Unusual eyebrow configuration. (A) Mild synophrys in Cornelia de Lange syndrome (also see Fig. 4.4.9). Note too the irregularly spaced and tangled eyelashes. (B) Widened medial brows. The usual pattern of hair direction is lost, and individual eyebrow hairs are unusually long. Note also the midline frontal hair whorl and low anterior hairline.

Local areas of unusual hair growth may be seen in some normal individuals, often as a familial feature. Dark, curly hair in a zone surrounding the ear and extending into the sideburn area has been called **whisker hair** because of its resemblance to the normal texture of the full male beard. Seen almost exclusively in young men, it may be completely lost in later years, creating a wide hairless region around the ear. It seems to be associated with severe male-pattern baldness. **Hairy ears,** with growth of long dark hair over the upper helix or within the pinna, is also associated with baldness; because it has been seen almost invariably in adult males, this anomaly was long thought to be caused by a Y-linked gene (Fig. 4.16.9). In a very rare condition, **hairy elbows,** unusual growth of long curly hair is noted in early childhood over the extensor surface of the lower arms and

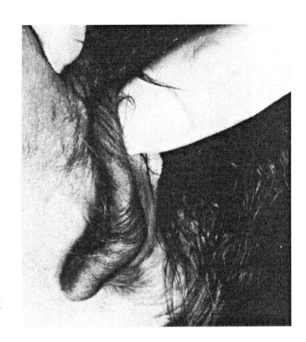

Figure 4.16.9. Hairy ears. Long, coarse, dark hair emerges from the lateral and posterior surfaces of the pinna.

upper forearms. There are no associated abnormalities, and the hypertrichosis gradually resolves over several years. A prominent **dorsal hair whorl,** usually located in the center of the back, may sometimes be seen in children or adults with mild generalized hypertrichosis.

4.16.5. Abnormalities

4.16.5.1. Deformations

No deformational abnormalities of the hair itself seem to exist except, perhaps, for the temporary effects of cosmetic treatments.

4.16.5.2. Disruptions

Hair is usually permanently absent from areas of disrupted skin in conditions such as aplasia cutis congenita or in the severe scalp lesions caused by amniotic bands. After birth, normal hair can be fractured and lost through *chronic trauma,* which most commonly is caused when a baby spends a great deal of time with the head resting in one position on the bed. This **frictional alopecia** usually occurs over the occipital region, is poorly circumscribed, and resolves completely once the infant becomes able to change position at will (Fig. 4.16.10). Other sources of trauma, such as compulsive head rubbing in mentally deficient patients, may produce similar zones of hair loss. In **trichotillomania,** a habit of pulling or twisting the hair results in irregular patches of the scalp where the hair is sparse and broken off at different lengths, but complete alopecia is not seen. Mental deficiency or psychiatric disturbances may be present.

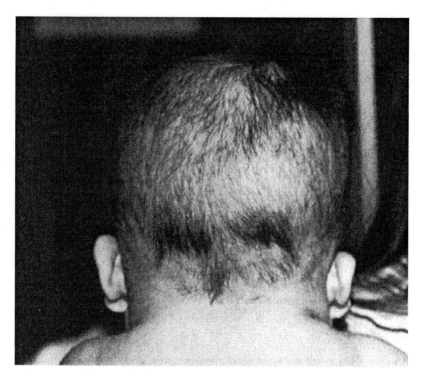

Figure 4.16.10. Frictional alopecia over the right occiput.

4.16.5.3. Dysplasias

The hair shares with the skin an involvement in several forms of ectodermal dysplasia. This usually produces some degree of **generalized alopecia,** in which hair is sparse over the scalp, brows, and lashes, virtually absent on the trunk and limbs, and variably developed in the axillary and pubic regions (Fig. 4.16.11A). This pattern may also be seen as a rare isolated genetic trait. Less severe hypotrichosis, primarily involving the scalp, simply produces the appearance of **sparse hair** in some other dysmorphic disorders, such as cartilage-hair hypoplasia and trichorhinophalangeal syndrome (Fig. 4.16.11B).

Hypopigmentation of hair over the entire body is part of oculocutaneous albinism syndrome and may be seen in other conditions in which pigmentary dilution is a feature (Fig. 4.15.15). **Premature canities** refers to early graying of the scalp hair. Gradual loss of pigment may begin to occur before adolescence, with the hair becoming completely white by the mid-20s. This condition is most often found in families in an autosomal dominant distribution but also is a part of many dysmorphic diseases, including Seckel syndrome, cri-du-chat syndrome, and the mucopolysaccharidoses.

Endocrine and metabolic disorders are at the root of most forms of **generalized hypertrichosis,*** in which hair growth is abnormally luxurious all over the body. Some

---

Hypertrichosis refers to overgrowth of hair in any area of the body, while the term *hirsutism* should be reserved for abnormal hair growth in regions under the control of androgenic hormones, such as the face, anterior chest, shoulders, and lower abdomen.

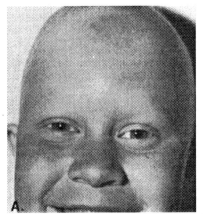 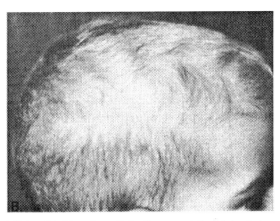

Figure 4.16.11. Widespread hypoplasia of hair follicles. (A) Alopecia totalis in Clouston ectodermal dysplasia. Note absence of brows and lashes. (B) Sparse, fine scalp hair in trichoosseous dysplasia.

types are familial and relatively mild in severity, but one variety results in profuse growth even in normally "forbidden" areas, such as around the eyes and over the nose. Hypertrichosis is seen as a feature of a number of dysmorphic syndromes (Figs. 4.16.4 and 4.16.8B) and also occurs as the result of administration of certain drugs (e.g., diphenylhydantoin, cyclosporin, and minoxidil). Interestingly, generalized increase in body hair also occurs in children with some types of statural growth deficiency as well as in severely brain injured, comatose, or chronically ill patients. In such cases, the growth of profuse body hair, in particular extremely long eyelashes, may occur over a period of several weeks (Fig. 4.16.12). The cause for this phenomenon remains unknown.

4.16.5.4. Malformations

Localized abnormalities of hair generally have only cosmetic significance for the patient but may have great diagnostic value. For example, the presence of an **elongated sideburn** of scalp hair projecting down and forward onto the cheek strongly suggests the diagnosis of Treacher Collins syndrome. A **low posterior hairline** is often a sign of prenatal edema over the back of the neck. The skin in this region is stretched by the underlying distension during the period of hair follicle development. When the edema subsides, the redundant skin may persist as folds or webbing of the neck, while the hair that has been carried along with the distended skin remains behind, reaching farther down the posterior neck than normal (Fig. 4.16.13A). Often, the lower margin of the nuchal hair shows a pronounced M-shaped outline (Fig. 4.16.13B). A patch of dark **hair over the lower midline spine,** even in the absence of an underlying vascular or pigmented lesion, may indicate a tethered spinal cord.

The term **alopecia areata** refers to localized absence of hair from any cause. The most common type can occur suddenly at any age and produces one or more sharply defined round or oval patches of complete hair loss with smooth borders and normal underlying skin (Fig. 4.16.14). On the scalp, these lesions may slowly recover or may enlarge and coalesce until the scalp hair is completely lost (*alopecia totalis*). Some cases

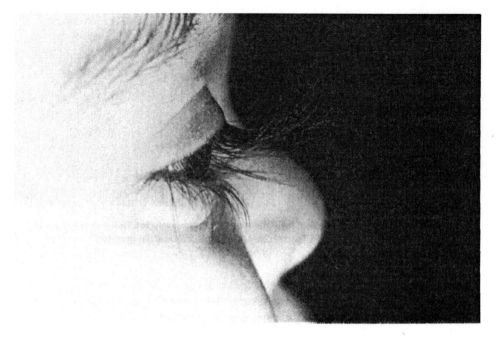

Figure 4.16.12. Luxurious lashes in a 14-month-old boy.

are familial, whereas others may be associated with various endocrine disorders, vitiligo, and a number of rare dysmorphic conditions. Local hair loss also occurs over pigmented, vascular, and hamartomatous nevi.

Patches of decreased hair pigmentation or **poliosis** are most often seen close to the anterior hairline, either centrally or just to one side of the midline. The classic *white*

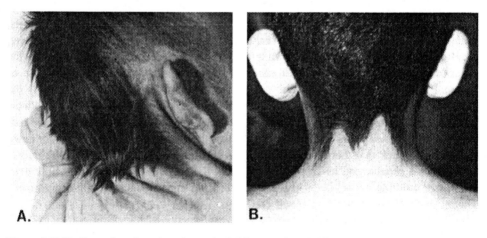

Figure 4.16.13. Unusual configuration of posterior hairline. (A) Low hairline in Turner syndrome, with skin bearing "scalp" hair extending down to the upper back. Note persisting redundancy of neck skin. (B) M-shaped nuchal hairline in a boy with Noonan syndrome. Minimal neck webbing is present. Note protruding ears. (Also see Fig. 4.9.3.)

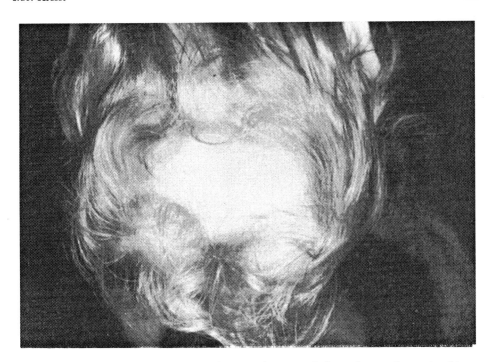

Figure 4.16.14. Localized alopecia. The hairless area is composed of smooth, normal-appearing skin.

forelock of Waardenburg syndrome is one example of this phenomenon, but it may also be seen with other forms of partial albinism (piebaldness) and in normal individuals, following an autosomal dominant inheritance pattern (Fig. 4.16.15).

The configuration of the eyelashes may provide helpful diagnostic clues. **Straight lashes** emerge from the the lid margin at a steep angle and extend straight downward rather than exhibiting the usual gentle upward curve (Fig. 4.16.3C). Such lashes are often seen in children with severe neuromuscular disease or ptosis and may be caused by lack of normal muscle tone in the levator palpebri superioris muscle. Abnormally curly or **tangled lashes** may also be especially long and are found primarily in disorders with generalized hypertrichosis (Fig. 4.16.16). Another rare abnormality of the eyelashes is **distichiasis,** in which an extra row of accessory cilia arises behind the normal staggered double row of lashes at the lid margin. This gives the eyelashes an unusually luxurious appearance.

Excessively **curly hair,** particularly when it is not a familial trait, may serve as a clue to dysmorphologic diagnoses. It is associated with several congenital disorders that also involve the teeth and other ectodermal structures.

Hair fragility is manifested by hair that seems short, fine, and sparse. The hair shafts may be broken off at the skin surface or fractured at irregular lengths, and the hair may have a "woolly" or "kinky" appearance. Various abnormalities of hair shaft development such as *trichorrexis nodosa, monilethrix,* and *pili torti* produce excessive fragility and can be diagnosed by microscopic examination (see Appendix A).

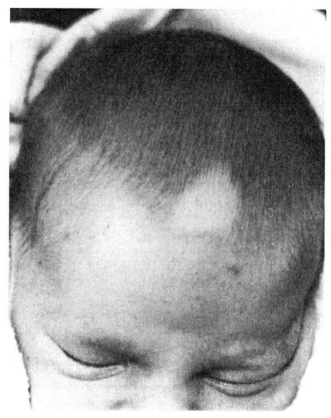

Figure 4.16.15. White forelock. Both skin and hair are hypopigmented in the frontal midline.

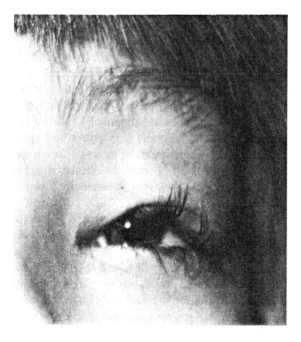

Figure 4.16.16. Tangled, irregularly spaced eyelashes. Note also the redundancy of the upper lid without true epicanthic fold.

4.16.6. Summary

It is usually the distribution rather than the composition of hair that yields the most helpful diagnostic clues, but many dysplastic disorders affect hair makeup in diagnostically distinctive ways.

4.17. NAILS

The nails, like the hair, are skin appendages of ectodermal origin, and their abnormalities often reflect generalized dysplasias of this tissue layer. The more severe nail anomalies may cause great cosmetic concern for the patient but have virtually no functional significance.

4.17.1. Embryology and Development

By gestational week 10, the fingers are separated and well proportioned, and epidermal thickenings can be seen over the dorsal surface of the fingertips. These become better defined by slight elevations of the skin (*nail folds*) bordering the lateral and proximal margins of the developing *nail bed* (Fig. 4.17.1A). Beneath the proximal nail fold, epidermal cells differentiate into the *nail matrix,* which begins to produce a three-layered sheet of compacted and keratinized epithelial cells, the *nail plate* (Fig. 4.17.1B). For the next several weeks, the nail plate is gradually extruded out over the nail bed, to reach the tip of the finger by about 32–33 gestational weeks. Toenail development proceeds in a similar fashion but lags behind that of the fingernails by some 3–4 weeks.

Although the nails are in many ways homologous to hair, they do not undergo a cyclic growth pattern but increase in length at a slow but relatively steady pace throughout life. The average linear growth rate for fingernails is about 1–2 mm per week but normally varies with the seasons, the sex of the subject, or even the time of day. Chronic diseases and nutritional deficiency tend to slow the growth rate, whereas unusually rapid longitudinal nail growth is a feature of several dermatologic conditions.

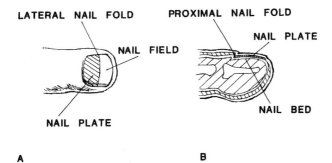

Figure 4.17.1. Development and landmarks of the nails. (A) Dorsal view, showing nail plate growing distally over nail field. (B) Longitudinal section of fingertip, showing relationship of nail to distal phalanx. [After Moore (1982).]

4.17.2. Anatomy and Landmarks

The *shape* of the fingernails as viewed from above ranges from an irregular oval outline to that of a squat rectangle; toenails (except for that of the first toe) are shorter and broader in relation to their length. The shape of a nail and its overall dimensions provide a rough approximation of the size and configuration of the underlying distal phalanx. The pale *lunula* at the proximal end of the nail bed may be partially or completely obscured by *cuticle*, more so in each successive finger progressing from the radial to the ulnar side of the hand (Fig. 4.17.2A). The pink color of the nail bed, seen through the translucent nail plate, is produced by numerous capillary loops. Where the distal edge of the nail rises free from the nail bed, there is an abrupt change in color from pink to white. To either side, the edges of the nail dive beneath the lateral nail folds.

Viewed from the end of the fingertip, children's fingernails form a smooth, low arch, whereas those of adults are often flattened (Fig. 4.17.2D). The edge of the nail appears to be a thin, single layer, and the width of the nail occupies about two-thirds of the width of the dorsum of the finger.

A side view of the finger shows that the nail has a gentle convex curve; from the distal margin, it slopes gently upward, then downward to its junction with the posterior nail fold. This creates a shallow *nail angle* with the skin of the dorsum of the phalanx (Fig. 4.17.3A).

4.17.3. Examination Techniques

Any clinically important abnormalities of nail color, size, shape, or thickness can be detected by simple inspection. In examining the hands, the fingernails are inspected both from the dorsal surface and end-on.

Palpation of the region between the distal interphalangeal joint and the proximal nail fold often reveals a "spongy" consistency when there is significant *nail clubbing*.

4.17.4. Minor Variants

4.17.4.1. Spectrum Variants

Like the texture of the hair (and possibly related to it), the thickness and *strength* of the nails show variability from person to person. The nails are more subject to cracking

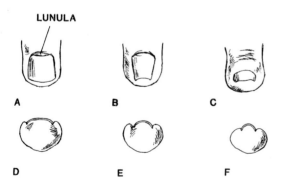

LUNULA

A   B   C

D   E   F

Figure 4.17.2. Normal and abnormal nail configurations. (A) Dorsal view of normal nail. (B) Tapering nail. (C) Short, hypoplastic nail. (D) End-on view of normal fingertip, showing usual low arch contour of nail. (E) Narrow nail. (F) Extremely narrow, hyperconvex nail.

NAIL ANGLE

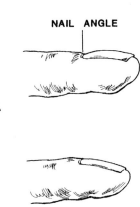

A

Figure 4.17.3. Lateral view of fingertip to show nail conformation. (A) Normal nail and nail angle. (B) Loss of nail angle seen in early clubbing of the fingertips.

B

and splitting during the dry winter months, but individuals with thin nail plates experience fragility of the fingernails year round. As mentioned above, the *growth rate* of the nails can be influenced by a number of factors and is normally slower in the feet than the hands. In infancy, the toenails may be quite small, often with an upturned distal edge.

4.17.4.2. Minor Anomalies

Several distinct alterations in nail configuration may be seen in normal individuals, and some are familial. The most common is the **koilonychia** ("spoon nails") seen in many infants. The nail plate is thin, its center is depressed below the level of the periphery, and the free margin of the nail is turned upward. When isolated, this anomaly normally resolves spontaneously during early childhood. Similar findings in later life may be produced by a number of disease states, the best known of which is *hypochromic anemia*. **Transversely grooved nails** reflect a transient slowing or cessation of nail plate production in the nail matrix, frequently caused by a febrile illness. A shallow depression runs partway or completely across the nail, often with a low ridge at its proximal border (Fig. 4.17.4A). The position of the groove moves distally with nail growth, leaving behind a normal nail. **Longitudinally grooved nails** are also fairly frequent, often occurring as a result of trauma to the nail matrix (Fig. 4.17.4B). **Hippocratic nails** (*onychauxis*) are very broad, covering almost the entire dorsum of the fingertip, and have a doubly convex configuration with loss of the proximal nail angle (Figs. 4.17.3B and 4.17.8C). These changes are benign and frequently familial but strongly resemble the clubbing of the nails seen in severe cardiac or pulmonary disease. The two conditions easily can be differentiated by the presence of cyanosis of the nail beds and a spongy consistency of the proximal nail matrix in true clubbing. One other variant of nail formation is seen in **potter's thumb** (*murderer's thumb, racquet nail*). The distal phalanx and nail are shortened and disproportionately wide, with diminished transverse curvature (Fig. 4.20.8C). Predominantly affecting the first digits, this condition may be asymmetric and can also involve the toes. The trait often occurs in families in an autosomal dominant distribution. A similar nail configuration is seen in Rubinstein-Taybi syndrome, but there it is associated with radial or tibial deviation of the affected digits.

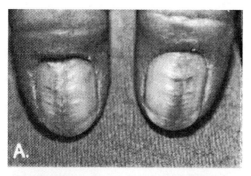

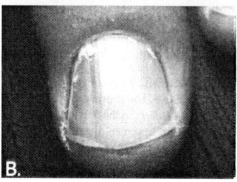

Figure 4.17.4. Irregularity of intact nail plate. (A) Transverse ridging caused by chronic, severe systemic illness. (B) Longitudinal grooving caused by trauma that injured the nail matrix beneath the proximal nail fold.

The appearance of small white dots or patches in the nails (**punctate leukonychia**) is extremely common and is caused by the persistence of small islands of uncornified cells on the lower surface of the nail plate. As many as a dozen or more of these white areas may be present at any given time, and they migrate distally with nail growth, eventually to be lost at the free margin. **Striate leukonychia** is similar but occurs in prominent bands traversing the nail from side to side. **Total leukonychia** involves all of the nails, producing an opaque, porcelain-white appearance (Fig. 4.17.5). These last two forms commonly run in families in an autosomal dominant distribution.

4.17.5. Abnormalities

4.17.5.1. Deformations

There are no deformational abnormalities of the nails as such, but of course the shape of the free edge may be altered by mechanical forces from occupational exposure or manicuring.

4.17.5.2. Disruptions

Trauma that injures or destroys the nail matrix will produce permanent changes in configuration of the nail. Localized loss of matrix will result in a longitudinal zone of thinning and fragility of the nail plate or, if extensive enough, absence of a segment of nail

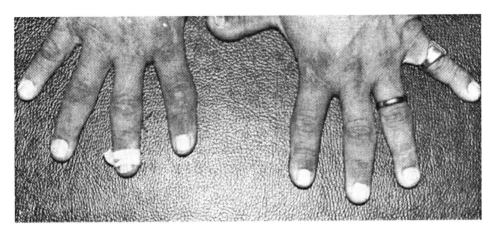

Figure 4.17.5. Leukonychia. Note sparing of thumb nail.

extending the length of the nail bed. Total avulsion of a nail, however, usually is followed by complete regeneration, since most of the matrix remains intact and immediately begins the elaboration of new nail plate material.

4.17.5.3. Dysplasias

Overgrowth of the nails occurs in a few rare dermatologic diseases. The best known genetic cause of **thickened nails** is *pachyonychia congenita,* in which the distal two-thirds of the nail plate is lifted from the nail bed by the accumulation of hard keratinous material beneath it (Fig. 4.17.6A). The nail plate itself also may be thickened and extremely hard, projecting upward at an abrupt angle. Nail changes of this kind may be associated with a number of other systemic abnormalities. Extreme hypertrophy of the nail plate, called

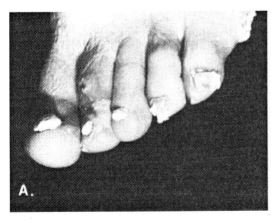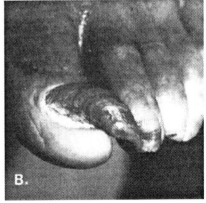

Figure 4.17.6. Overgrowth of nails. (A) Pachyonychia congenita. (B) Onychogryposis. (Photos courtesy of Dr. Walter Burgdorf, Albuquerque, N.M.)

onychogryposis, is manifested by claw- or **horn-shaped nails.** The nails are dull, yellow-brown in color and exceedingly long, with an irregular, furrowed surface (Fig. 4.17.6B). They become twisted or curved backward, assuming bizarre shapes. The first toenails are most commonly affected, but in the inherited forms, fingernails, especially those of the index fingers, may also be involved.

Dystrophic nails occur in many dermatologic and dysmorphic syndromes, including several varieties of ectodermal dysplasia. The nails have an irregular, striated, lusterless surface and are quite fragile (Fig. 4.17.7). Because they break and split easily, they are often very short. Longitudinal splitting may create fissures extending onto the nail bed, and splitting in the plane of the nail plate results in delamination of thin sheets from the distal nail surface.

4.17.5.4. Malformations

As mentioned in Section 4.17.2, the size and configuration of the nails, especially their width, bears a strong relationship to the shape and size of the underlying distal phalanx. **Narrow nails** are often **hyperconvex** as well and usually denote hypoplasia of the distal bony tuft of the phalanx (Figs. 4.17.2B and E and 4.17.8A). Occasionally, this takes the form of **tapered nails** that become progressively narrower and more hyperconvex as they grow distally (Figs. 4.17.2C and 4.17.8B). Unusually **broad nails** of normal length are found over digits with *duplication of the distal phalanx* (Figs. 4.17.9 and 4.20.21D). In hands with total *syndactyly,* there is often a single **nail band** surmounting the dorsal surface of the fused fingertips.

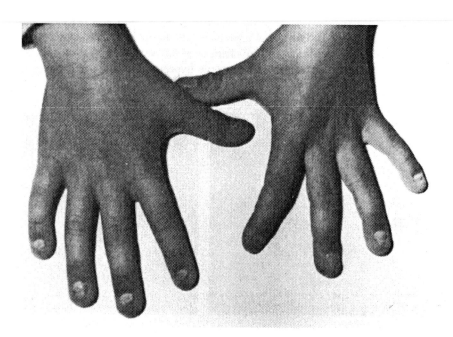

Figure 4.17.7. Generalized nail dystrophy in Clouston ectodermal dysplasia.

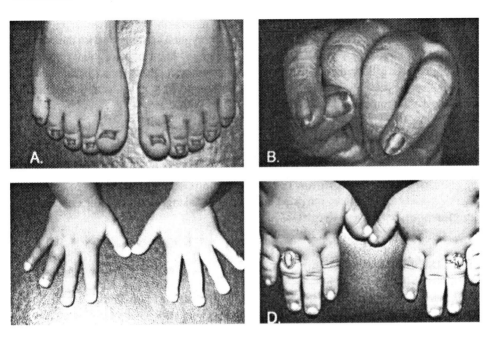

Figure 4.17.8. Minor variants of nail configuration. (A) Short, hyperconvex nails often found with hypoplasia of the distal phalanges. (B) Narrow, tapering nails of normal length. (C) Broad, doubly convex nails. There is no cyanosis of the nail beds or true clubbing. (D) Small nails with normal convexity.

Hypoplasia of the nails may take several forms. **Small nails** are found over underdeveloped distal phalanges. Both length and width are diminished, sometimes leaving only a tiny chip of nail plate arising perpendicular to the surface of the skin (Figs. 4.17.2D, 4.17.8D, and 4.17.10A). In nail-patella syndrome, **partial nail aplasia** occurs, particularly on the thumbs and index fingers. The remaining nail segments are small,

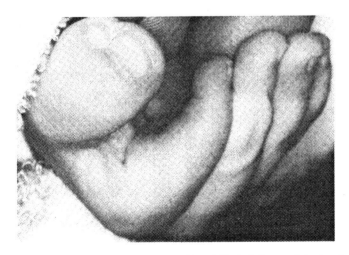

Figure 4.17.9. Broad, fused nails over duplicated distal phalanges of the thumb.

irregular, dull, and friable and are often embedded in the skin, with no free edges. Lateral nail remnants may be separated by a tapering skin pterygium continuous with the proximal nail fold (Fig. 4.17.10B). **Total nail aplasia** is very rare. At birth, some or all fingers bear a rudimentary nail bed, but no nail plate has developed, although an occasional tiny fragment may be present, which soon will be permanently shed. This condition is found in Coffin-Siris syndrome and occasionally in cases of *ectrodactyly*.

4.17.6. Summary

The nail is an extremely simple structure, and its developmental anomalies affect its size and shape within fairly narrow limits. In dysmorphology, examination of the nails is valuable mainly for the clues provided about distal phalangeal size and for indications of some forms of ectodermal dysplasia.

4.18. LIMBS—GENERAL

Anatomical integrity of the limbs is vital in performing many human activities, and therefore any major structural anomalies in this system may be severely handicapping. Furthermore, the lower limbs make a large contribution to statural size, so that many types of disproportionate short stature are produced by aberrant growth of limb bones.

4.18.1. Embryology and Development

Limb development first can be detected at the beginning of gestational week 5, when the *arm buds* appear on the lateral body wall at a level overlapping the lower cervical and the uppermost thoracic somites. A few days later, the *leg buds* will be present, arising in the region of the junction between the lumbar and sacral somites. Development of the lower limbs lags behind that of the upper throughout embryonic life. Both sets of limb buds initially grow in a caudal direction, but by the end of week 5 they have begun to curve ventrally. By this time, the distal ends of the limb buds also have expanded into the

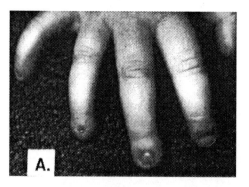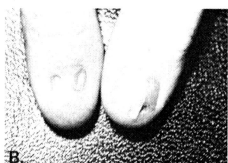

Figure 4.17.10. Nail dysplasia. (A) Tiny, distorted nails over short, bulbous distal phalanges in fetal hydantoin syndrome. (B) Severe medial dysplasia with loss of nail matrix in nail-patella syndrome.

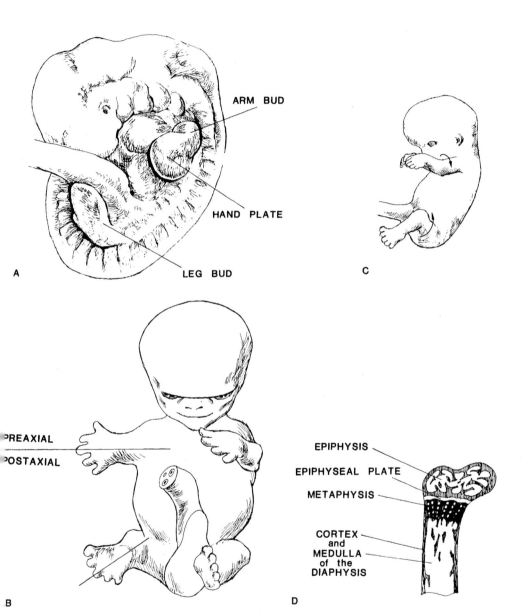

Figure 4.18.1. Embryogenesis of the limb. (A) Embryo at 5 weeks of gestation, showing distinct limb buds and paddle-shaped hand plate. (B) Embryo at gestational week 6, showing normal flexed limb position on the left. The right limbs have been extended to demonstrate the limb axes. [Modified after Langman (1969).] (C) A 7-week old embryo, showing limb rotation to fetal positions. (D) Diagrammatic section of developing long bone to show anatomic divisions.

flat, paddle-shaped *hand* and *foot plates,* and faint indications of segmentation of the upper limb can be seen (Fig. 4.18.1A). These are produced by condensations of mesenchyme that form the *bone primorida,* including the *digital rays* (Fig. 4.20.1A).

During week 6, the limbs lengthen rapidly, such that the developing hands come to lie over the cardiac swelling, near the face. The palmar surfaces of the hands and the soles of the feet are facing each other at this stage, and elbow and knee flexions are present, pointing outward (Fig. 4.18.1B). The primordia of the long bones are clearly outlined and are beginning to undergo chondrification to become miniscule models, in hyaline cartilage, of the future limb bones (Fig. 4.20.1B). The surrounding mesenchyme is also beginning to differentiate into the *limb muscles.*

In gestational week 7, rapid growth continues, and the proximal segments of the limbs rotate around their long axes such that the elbow and knee on each side come to point toward each other (Fig. 4.18.1C). A week later, the limbs appear quite mature, although still disproportionately small and slender in relation to the head and trunk. From this point forward, growth continues at a steady pace, and the development of limb musculature permits increasingly vigorous movement of the arms and legs.

Ossification of the long bones begins by week 12 and continues until final adult stature is achieved at puberty. The central, cylindrical shaft of the bone is called the *diaphysis,* terminating at each end in a *metaphysis.* These, in turn, are separated by cartilaginous epiphyseal plates from the *epiphysis* at each end (Fig. 4.18.1D). Elongation of the bone occurs only at the ends of the diaphysis as new bone is deposited beneath the epiphyseal plate. The bone shaft grows in diameter by the formation of new bone under the *periosteum* on its surface, which exactly keeps pace with the resorption of bone from its inner surface in the *medullary space,* thus maintaining the thickness of the bone *cortex.*

At birth, the arms and legs are still somewhat short in relation to the trunk, but differential growth occurs during childhood, and adult limb length ratios are finally attained by the time of adolescence. The pubertal growth spurt affects the limbs more than the axial skeleton, and a rapid increase in muscle mass also takes place at that time.

4.18.2. Anatomy and Landmarks

The limbs are normally symmetric in length and bulk, tapering slightly from proximal to distal in each segment (*upper arm, lower arm, thigh,* and *leg*), although the smaller *muscle mass* in young children may produce a cylindrical appearance of the arms. The long axis of each segment is generally straight, but some *bowing* of the leg in infants is not unusual (see Section 4.18.4). In the standing position, at rest, the arms hang in such a way that the thumbs point forward and medially, while the patellas and first toes are angled slightly outward from the midplane. If the feet are brought tightly together, the medial surfaces of the thighs, knees, and medial malleoli touch each other. In infants, the fingertips reach the level of the greater trochanters; in older children and adults, they should extend beyond this point (Fig. 4.18.2).

The most useful landmarks in the limbs are the *joints* and some nearby bony prominences, including the *acromion,* the *anterior superior iliac spine,* the *pubic symphysis,* and the *medial malleolus.*

Several special terms are helpful in describing normal and abnormal configuration of the arms and legs. The *axis* of the limbs is determined by embryologic considerations and

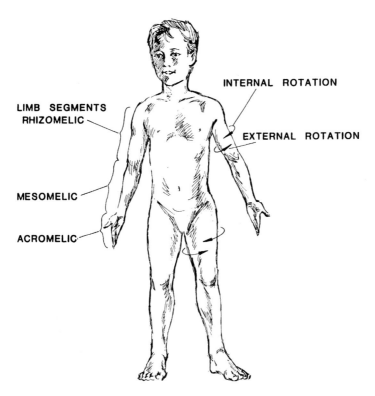

Figure 4.18.2. Frontal view of child in "anatomic position" to show limb subdivisions and axes of rotation.

can best be understood by visualizing a stylized view of the embryo at 7 weeks (Fig. 4.18.1B). The axis of each limb runs down the center of its length to the end of the middle digit. The cranial half of each limb is termed *preaxial;* the caudal half is called *postaxial.* Thus, the thumb and big toe are homologous and lie on the preaxial side of their respective limbs. Specific adjectives also are used to define each of the longitudinal segments of the limbs. *Rhizomelic* refers to the proximal portions (upper arms and thighs), *mesomelic* refers to the central segments (forearms and legs), and *acromelic* refers to the hands and feet (Fig. 4.18.2). Finally, *internal rotation* of a limb involves movements at the joints that turn lateral structures toward the front, whereas *internal torsion* implies an abnormal twisting of a bone on its long axis in the same direction. *External rotation* and *external torsion* are the complementary terms (Fig. 4.18.2).

4.18.3. Examination Techniques

Inspection of the limbs is best carried out with the patient standing, but infants or small children may be examined in the sitting or recumbent position. *Symmetry* of the limbs in length and bulk is first judged by eye. More than about 1 cm of difference in leg length will produce *pelvic tilt,* which is best seen from behind the standing patient. A fingertip placed on the iliac crest on each side helps in determining whether the pelvis is level. Some children compensate for pelvic tilt by habitually bending the knee of the longer leg, so care must be taken that both knees are fully extended during this part of the examination. Infants or children who cannot stand can be evaluated for leg length discrepancy in the supine position. One foot is grasped in each hand, and with the knees straight, the medial malleoli are brought together. The relative positions of the patellas and hips on the two sides provide a rough estimate of leg length equality. A similar maneuver helps detect significant differences in arm length. The child is asked to interlock his fingers and then to extend his arms straight forward, locking the elbows. A discrepancy of 2 cm or more in total arm length will have the effect of swinging the clasped hands away from the midline toward the shorter side. Any suspected differences in limb length detected by these rather crude techniques should be documented by measurement (see below).

Examination for abnormal *torsion* of the leg bones should begin with the patient lying supine, with both hips extended. When the patella is facing straight upward, the first toe should be pointed in the same direction, and an imaginary line drawn from the medial malleolus through the lateral malleolus should slope downward at an angle of about 10°. If the foot points considerably away from the vertical in this position, *tibial torsion* is likely. Testing for *femoral torsion* is carried out in a similar fashion, preferably with the patient standing. Again, the patella and the foot should both point straight forward. If both are directed laterally or medially, femoral torsion or an aberrant angle of the femoral neck should be suspected.

Palpation of the soft tissue of the limbs provides information about the size and consistency of the muscles and the relative amounts of subcutaneous fat. The mid-upper arm and the calf are good places to palpate the muscles, which should be clearly different in texture from overlying fat: firm, but not hard or "woody." Hypoplastic or atrophied muscle bellies feel like narrow bands of firm connective tissue and may be buried within copious deposits of fat that has much less substance and a yielding or "doughy" consistency.

Careful measurements of limb dimensions may be helpful in selected cases. Unfortunately, comparison of such measurements with "normal standards" is of little value because of the wide range of normal variation in body size. More useful is the comparison of dimensions on the two sides of the body or the calculation of ratios relating the size of one structure to another. An example of the latter is the relationship between height and *arm span*. An accurate if slightly strenuous method of determining arm span is to ask the patient to touch the floor at the base of a wall with the fingertips of one hand and then stretch the fingers of the other hand as high up the wall as possible, pressing the chest firmly against the wall (Fig. 4.18.3A). A pencil mark is made at the tips of the upper fingers, and the patient is then asked to stand (barefoot) with the back and heels against the wall under the mark so that span and height can be compared directly (Fig. 4.18.3B). After the age of 6 or 7 years, these two measurements should be approximately equal, and a discrepancy of 4 cm or more is probably of clinical importance.

The *upper/lower segment ratio* is another clinically valuable measurement that is easily obtained. With the patient standing (without shoes), the examiner palpates the upper surface of the pubic bone and anchors the zero mark of a flexible steel tape measure at that point with pressure of a finger. The tape is then extended vertically to the floor, and the distance is recorded as the length of the lower segment. This number is then subtracted

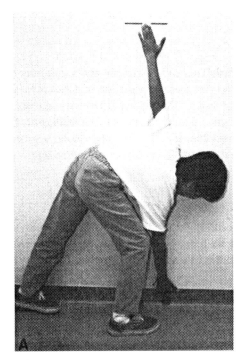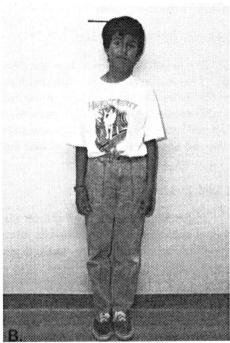

Figure 4.18.3. Estimation of arm span. (A) Patient touches floor with fingertips, reaches up wall as far as possible. (Arms should be more vertical than depicted here.) (B) Patient then stands against wall. Height (without shoes) should be within 1–2 cm of length of arm span.

from the patient's height to obtain the length of the upper segment. Finally, the upper/lower segment ratio is calculated by dividing the upper segment measurement by that of the lower. The normal value of this ratio varies with age, and comparisons should be made with standard curves.

When asymmetry in the size of the limbs is suspected, accurate measurements to compare the two sides provide the best means of clinical confirmation. With the patient supine, *leg length* is measured from the apex of the medial malleolus to the anterior superior iliac spine. A difference of 1 cm between measurements from the two sides is significant. (Measuring between the medial malleoli and the umbilicus is less accurate.) *Arm length* can be measured between the acromion process and the head of the radius at the wrist, with the elbow fully extended. Occasionally, measurement of individual segments of the limb may be useful, and the most convenient additional bony landmarks are the olecranon and the upper margin of the patella. These points may also be used in the comparison of *limb girth* on the two sides, usually to document asymmetric hyperplasia or atrophy of muscle. The tape measure is extended from the bony landmark along the normal limb until it falls over the area of interest, where a mark is made on the skin. The circumference of the normal limb is measured at this point and then compared with a similar measurement taken at the same distance from the landmark on the affected side.

4.18.4. Minor Variants

4.18.4.1. Spectrum Variants

The length of the lower limb is a major contributor to body height and varies over as wide a range. *Femoral length,* particularly, shows considerable variation in different racial groups, being greatest in blacks of sub-Saharan Africa. The normal differences in muscle mass between the sexes involve primarily the limbs, and the amount of subcutaneous fat deposited over the arms and legs is similarly variable. Finally, the upper/lower segment ratio and some other body proportions have a range of variability at any given age.

4.18.4.2. Minor Anomalies

Segmental shortening of a limb may occur as an isolated defect in an otherwise normal individual. The condition is rare, but its most common form is unilateral *rhizomelic shortening* of the arm. Strength and function are secondarily impaired in the more severely affected limbs.

4.18.5. Abnormalities

4.18.5.1. Deformations

Because of their length and position, the limbs, particularly the lower legs, are frequently exposed to deforming stress in utero. This most commonly occurs as **tibial bowing,** seen at birth. One or both tibias curve gently toward the midline, sometimes to the extent that the soles of the feet face each other (Fig. 4.18.4). Rarely, the bowing may be severe enough to produce a skin dimple over the apex of the convexity (see Section 4.15). The fibulas, of course, are also deformed in this condition. **Femoral bowing** is much rarer but is occasionally present in babies born after prolonged breech positioning. Again, the curve is usually gentle and convex laterally. Congenital bowing of the humerus and forearm is almost never seen.

Aberrant intrauterine positioning can also cause torsional deformities. This usually takes the form of *tibial torsion* (either internal or external), but congenital *femoral torsion* is also fairly common.* These deformations both produce **intoeing** or **outtoeing** on the affected side(s), but the site of torsion can be determined by the examination techniques described in Section 4.18.3. Once again, the arms seem to be exempt from this type of deformity. As is the case with all true deformations, these abnormalities tend to improve gradually with time once the deforming stresses have been removed. When the involvement is especially severe, however, permanent orthopedic problems may result, and bracing or surgical correction may be necessary.

---

*It had long been thought that the tendency of some children to sit in the W position, with the knees sharply flexed and the legs drawn back on either side of the thighs, might produce internal femoral torsion during childhood. It now seems most likely that this is simply a position of comfort for children who already have congenital femoral torsion.

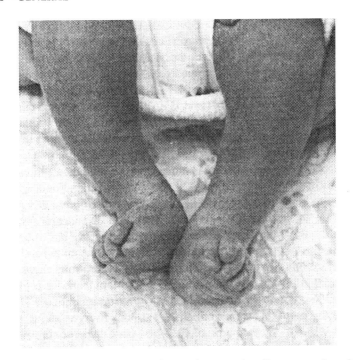

Figure 4.18.4. Tibial bowing caused by intrauterine constraint. Also note overlapped toes.

4.18.5.2. Disruptions

The only significant congenital disruptions of the limbs are those caused by amniotic bands. The severity of damage depends on both the site of attachment of the adherent bands and the depth to which they affect the fetal tissues. Shallow **constricting rings** can encircle a limb at any level and destroy subcutaneous tissue, sometimes producing distal edema (Fig. 4.15.10). Complete **congenital amputation** is most common in the fingers and toes (see Section 4.20.5.2) but may be found in almost any region of the limb. The distal structures are totally lost, and the skin of the stump bears a thin, well-healed scar that lies directly over the end of the severed bone (see Appendix C).

4.18.5.3. Dysplasias

The bulk or texture of the limb muscles may be affected in certain dysplastic disorders. **Diminished muscle mass** is a prominent feature of several congenital syndromes. The muscles may be reduced to narrow bands surrounded by fat deposits. Some of the muscular dystrophies show such changes in their late stages, but in the early phase of Duchenne muscular dystrophy, **bulky, firm muscle** is the rule. Some storage diseases also produce unusually firm muscle consistency.

Skeletal dysplasias of the limbs form a large and varied class of congenital disorders. Although their clinical delineation is important, all require skeletal X-rays examination for definition of the diagnosis. The most common manifestation of these chondrodystrophies is *inadequate bone growth* that may affect the entire limb or only one anatomic division. **Rhizomelic shortening** involves the proximal segment of a limb and may affect all four limbs, as in Conradi-Hunerman syndrome (Fig. 4.18.5A), or only the femurs, as in focal femoral hypolasia syndrome (Fig. 4.18.5B). **Mesomelic shortening** of the forearms is a hallmark of Robinow syndrome (Fig. 4.18.6) and several other dysmorphic entities. Depending on the specific condition in question, such dysplasia again may involve just the upper or lower limbs or all four. **Acromelic shortening** takes place in the bones of the hands and feet (see Section 4.20). The three types of segmental growth deficiency may occur in various combinations, and sometimes all three segments are affected simultaneously but unequally, as is the case in achondroplasia (Fig. 4.18.7).

Some types of chondrodystrophy may produce *localized bone overgrowth,* with or without shortening of the limbs. Of the three structural divisions of long bones, such disorders primarily affect the diaphyses or metaphyses (Fig. 4.18.8). (Almost all of the epiphyseal dysplasias impair endochondral bone growth at the epiphyseal plate and thus impede longitudinal bone growth.) The diaphyseal dysplasias may cause bowing of the bone shaft and a smoothly tapering **diaphyseal enlargement** that widens toward the distal end of the bone. In contrast, *metaphyseal chondrodystrophies* produce sharply outlined *metaphyseal* **enlargement** that is seen or palpated as bony overgrowth just proximal to the epiphysis (Fig. 4.18.8). Another type of localized bone hyperplasia causes **exostoses,** which again are found near the distal ends of the long bones. They are often palpable as discrete, fixed bony spurs over the metaphysis. Large ones often grow into a hook shape, with the free end curving away from the joint.

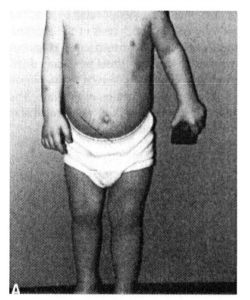
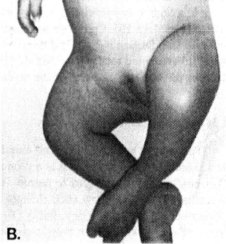

Figure 4.18.5. Rhizomelic limb shortening. (A) Moderate shortening of femurs and humeri. Note fingertips reaching only to level of pubis. (B) Severe rhizomelic shortening in focal femoral hypoplasia.

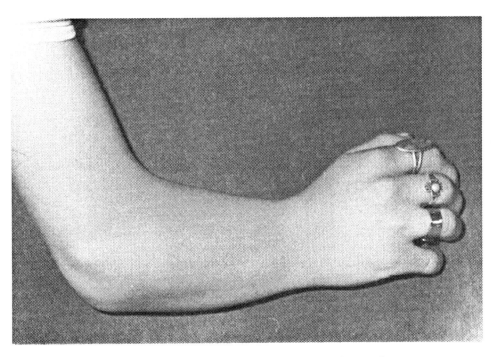

Figure 4.18.6. Mesomelic shortening of the forearm in Robinow syndrome.

A characteristic feature of the osteogenesis imperfecta family of skeletal dysplasias is **bone fragility.** Fractures of the limb bones occur with mild trauma or even as a result of the child's own movements. In some forms, breakage of limb bones is infrequent and heals rapidly; in the more severe types, repeated fractures with callus formation can lead to marked distortion and shortening of the arms and legs. In such cases, incomplete healing may lead to the formation of a **pseudarthrosis,** in which aberrant movement persists between fragments of the shaft of a long bone, producing pain and instability in the limb. Isolated pseudarthroses also can be found in some patients with neurofibromatosis.

4.18.5.4. Malformations

The most important malformations of the limbs involve abnormal development of their bony elements. Skeletal *overgrowth* can produce generalized increase in body size (**macrosomia**) with proportional enlargement of all structures, as in *Weaver syndrome* (Fig. 4.18.9A). A different growth pattern causes the **disproportionately long limbs** in conditions such as Marfan and Stickler syndromes. Trunk length remains about normal (or may be decreased by scoliosis), while the arms and legs grow unusually long but remain quite slender. Clinically, this disproportion often can be detected by noting that the fingertips reach much further down the thigh than usual in the standing position (Fig. 4.18.9B). The abnormally long legs also will diminish the upper/lower segment ratio.

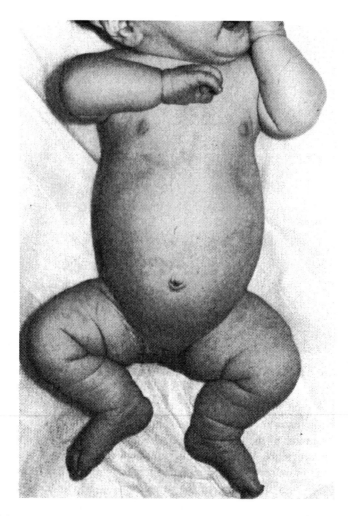

Figure 4.18.7. Shortening of all limb segments (but with most severe effect in proximal segments) in achondroplasia.

Marked **limb asymmetry** sometimes can be caused by *vascular anomalies* that produce localized overcirculation but more commonly is found as an isolated phenomenon. When such asymmetry affects one entire side of the body, the term *hemihypertrophy* is used (Fig. 4.18.9C); "crossed" varieties, in which one arm and the opposite leg are involved, are also seen.

Skeletal deficiencies represent aplasia rather than dysplasia of bone and are also found in a variety of configurations. While some are syndromic, many occur as isolated anomalies (which may, however, affect all four limbs). For convenience, they have been classified by anatomic distribution.

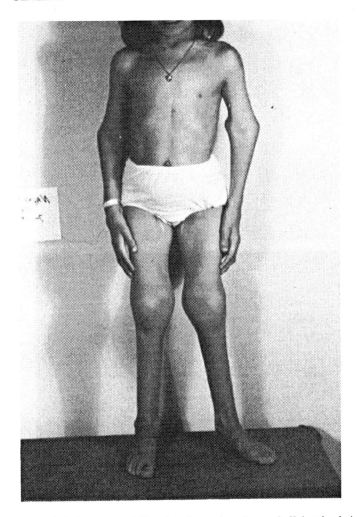

Figure 4.18.8. Enlargement and distortion of metaphyseal zones in Kniest dysplasia.

Longitudinal defects affect the limb on one side of the central axis. Thus, **radial aplasia** with absence of the thumb and forefinger is categorized as *preaxial longitudinal hemimelia of the upper limb* (Fig. 4.20.16B). Similar involvement of the lower limb would produce **tibial aplasia.** The affected limb will be curved toward the side of the deficiency and usually will be somewhat shortened.

In **transverse defects,** the limb is truncated abruptly, as if severed with a knife (Fig. 4.18.10). The limb may terminate at any level, but distal involvement is much more common than proximal. This abnormality strongly resembles a congenital amputation, but on close examination there is usually some degree of hypoplasia of the remaining proximal structures, and the distal stump of the limb is not scarred but commonly bears small

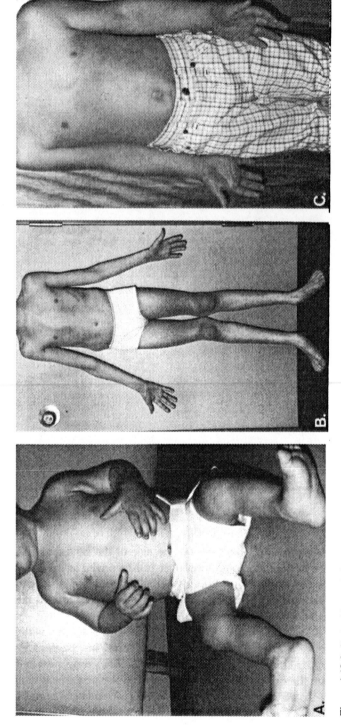

Figure 4.18.9. Skeletal hyperplasia. (A) Generalized skeletal overgrowth in Weaver syndrome. At 9 months, baby has a height age normal for 2.5 years. (B) Elongated, slender limbs in Marfan syndrome. Note that the fingertips almost reach the level of the knees. (C) Lateralized overgrowth of the left arm (hemihypertrophy).

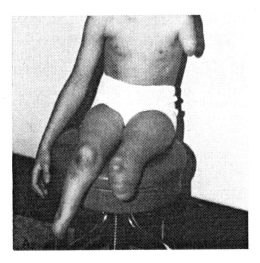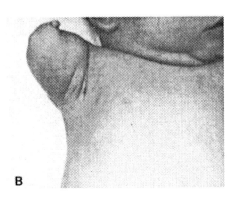

B

Figure 4.18.10. Transverse hemimelia. (A) Multiple-limb involvement in Hanhart syndrome. (B) Unilateral hemimelia of the arm. Note terminal nubbin of tissue representing rudimentary distal limb structures.

nubbins of tissue representing rudimentary digits (Fig. 4.18.10). Failing that, a terminal field of dermal ridges may be found, showing that the distal skin has differentiated toward the type specific to the palmar and plantar zones. Either of these findings proves that the distal structures have not been lost by amputation but have undergone severe hypoplasia.

Intercalary defects are those in which a more proximal portion of a limb fails to develop properly, leaving distal structures relatively intact. An extreme example is **phocomelia,** which involves partial or complete underdevelopment of the rhizomelic and mesomelic limb segments. The structures of the hands and feet may be reduced to a single small digit or may appear virtually normal but arise directly from the trunk, like the flippers of a seal (Greek *phocos*). In less severe cases, portions of the proximal limb may remain, but the functional deficit is still profound (Fig. 4.18.11). In **total amelia,** no limb elements whatever are present. This may represent the most extreme form of an intercalary defect.

Some dysmorphic syndromes show varying combinations of these three types of limb deficit, sometimes combined with bone dysplasias. For example, children with thrombocytopenia-absent radius syndrome have a preaxial longitudinal defect (absence of the radius) but the ulna is also very short, and the thumb and forefinger invariably are intact, as would be expected in an intercalary defect (Fig. 4.18.12). Other combinations of these developmental abnormalities also have been described.

4.18.6. Summary

A wide variety of genetic bone dysplasias affect the length and proportions of the limbs, while intrinsic developmental hypoplasias and aplasias of bone cause specific structural deficits that may be seen in isolation or as part of various dysmorphic syndromes.

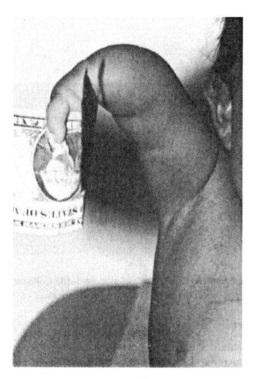

Figure 4.18.11. Phocomelia. In this child, the humerus is only mildly shortened, but the forearm is completely absent and the thumb and forefinger also are missing.

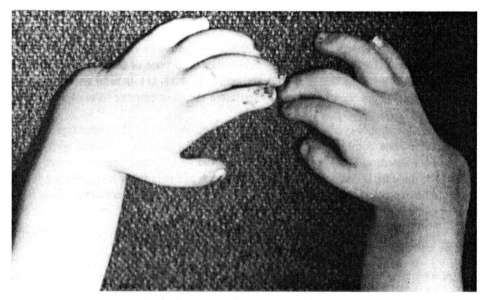

Figure 4.18.12. Radial hypoplasia with severe radial deviation of the hands but with intact thumbs in thrombocytopenia-absent radius syndrome.

4.19. LIMBS—JOINTS

The limbs are provided with a variety of joints to permit motor activity for locomotion and prehension. Limbs with limited joint movement show varying degrees of functional impairment, while hyperelastic joints may be unstable and prone to trauma. Both types of abnormality may be clues to underlying dysplastic or dysmorphic disorders.

4.19.1. Embryology and Development

The first indication of joint development in the limbs is seen at about the middle of gestational week 6, when the mesenchyme in the center of the developing limb begins to condense to form the *long bone primordia.* These regions undergo rapid conversion to cartilage, creating tiny models of the bone to come (see Section 4.18.1). At the end of week 6, selective cell death begins to take place in the zones lying between the ends of these cartilaginous bars, forming lacunae in the loose mesenchymal tissue (Fig. 4.19.1A). These lacunae soon coalesce to form the *joint cavity,* while the peripheral mesenchyme, enclosed by the *perichondrium,* begins to condense to form the *articular cartilages,* as well as the supporting *capsule* and *ligaments* of the joint (Fig. 4.19.1B). Successful development apparently requires repeated movement of the joint, which seems to help shape the articular cartilages and properly stretch the joint ligaments and capsule.

4.19.2. Anatomy and Landmarks

The joints of the limbs are traditionally classified by the type of motion that they accommodate. *Hinge joints,* such as the knee, permit flexion and extension in one plane. *Ball and socket joints* (shoulder and hip) allow movement of a limb through a large range of positions in three dimensions. *Compound joints* (wrist and ankle) permit at least limited

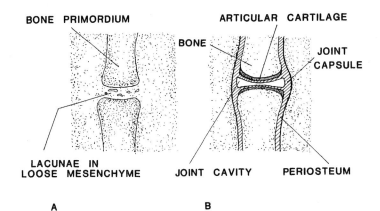

Figure 4.19.1. Joint embryogenesis. (A) Diagram of developing joint at about 6 weeks of gestation. Lacunae are beginning to form in the loose connective tissue between the ends of the primitive long bones. (B) At 8 weeks, joint formation is almost complete, and the surrounding and supporting connective tissues have also become differentiated.

motion in two major planes. The elbow is a special case, having the characteristics of a hinge joint but allowing rotary motion of the forearm.

The connective tissue of the ligaments and capsule provides support and stability for the joint, but it is the *tendons* which pass across it that translate muscle contraction into joint motion. In some tendons, cartilage and then bone develop at sites of particular stress. These specialized intratendinous *sesamoid bones* provide a sturdy bearing surface for tendon travel, and their articulation with the underlying joint helps prevent sideways motion of the tendon. The *patella* and the pisiform bone of the wrist are the largest of the sesamoid bones in humans.

The limits of excursion of a joint's movement are determined by the contours of the articular cartilages and by the elasticity of the joint capsule and ligaments. The approximate normal range of motion for each of the major limb joints is outlined in Table 4.19.1.

Table 4.19.1. Ranges of Joint Movements[a]

Joint	Rotation (in degrees from neutral position)						
	Flex	Ext	Abd	Add	Int	Ext	Other
Neck	45	45	NA	NA	60	60	Lateral flexion = 45
Shoulder							
Without scapular motion	90	30	80	0	90	80	
With scapular motion	180	50	180	0	90	80	
Elbow	150	0	NA	NA	90	80	
Wrist	80	70	20	30	NA	NA	
Thumb							
C-M	15	20	75	0	90	NA	
M-P	Var	0	NA	NA	NA	NA	
DIP	90	NA	NA	NA	NA	NA	
Fingers							
M-P	90	Var	15	15	NA	NA	
PIP	100	0	NA	NA	NA	NA	
DIP	90	0	NA	NA	NA	NA	
Spinal column	80	25	NA	NA	20	20	Lateral flexion = 35
Hip	120	0	45	30	40	40	Abduction in flexion = 70
Knee	130	0	NA	NA	NA	NA	
Ankle	50	20	NA	NA	NA	NA	
Foot							
Subtalar	NA	NA	5	5	NA	NA	
Midtarsal	NA	NA	NA	NA	10	20	
First toe							
M-P	Var	90	5	5	NA	NA	
DIP	90	0	NA	NA	NA	NA	
Toes 2–5							
M-P	40	90	NA	NA	NA	NA	
PIP	35	0	NA	NA	NA	NA	
DIP	Var	60	NA	NA	NA	NA	

[a]Each value represents the average limit of passive joint excursion, with 0° being the neutral or "anatomic" position. Most ranges are wider in young children. Flex, Flexion (plantar flexion of foot); Ext, extension (dorsiflexion of foot); Abd, abduction; Add, adduction; Int, internal rotation (pronation of forearm, eversion of foot); Ext, external rotation (supination of forearm, inversion of foot); C-M, carpometacarpal joint; M-P, metacarpophalangeal joint; PIP, proximal interphalangeal joint; DIP, distal interphalangeal joint; NA, no normal joint motion in this plane; Var, variable.

A few special descriptive terms are useful in discussing joint abnormalities. In the usual "anatomic position" (Fig. 4.18.2), the joints are in *neutral position*. If the portion of a limb distal to a joint deviates laterally from neutral, it is said to be in a *valgus* position; medial deviation is *varus*. A mild degree of valgus deviation at the elbow is normal, and this *carrying angle* is usually larger in females (Fig. 4.19.2A). *Supination* of the forearm is the process of turning the palm upward, while *pronation* turns the palm down. Similarly, *inversion* of the foot at the ankle turns the sole toward the midline, and *eversion* lifts the lateral edge of the foot. *Dorsiflexion* of the foot brings the toes closer to the shin, while *plantar flexion* puts the foot in a "tiptoe" position.

4.19.3. Examination Techniques

Initial inspection of the joints is carried out during examination of the limbs by noting their alignment and position at rest. Significant *joint enlargement* can also be observable at this time unless the patient is excessively obese. In infants, the posterior thighs should be examined for any unusual or *accessory transverse skin creases* that could signal *congenital dislocation of the hip*. In older children, the presence of an abnormal carrying angle usually is evident on gross inspection and may be confirmed by measurement (see below). If the patient has a low plantar arch, it is helpful to examine the standing foot from behind. The posterior surface of the heel and the Achilles tendon normally form one continuous vertical line (Fig. 4.19.3A). If the calcaneus is tipped away from the vertical, this line will deviate medially or laterally (Fig. 4.19.3B).

Direct palpation of joints occasionally may be useful if they seem enlarged or locally thickened. In such cases, it is important to determine whether the apparent enlargement is caused by overgrowth of bone adjacent to the joint, by local thickening of the connective tissue, or by fluid within the joint. These are easily discriminated by their differences in consistency. Palpation may also elicit *tenderness* over joints, which usually indicates acute inflammation.

The clinical information most helpful for dysmorphic diagnosis of joint abnormalities comes from determining the *range of motion*. Rotation and flexion/extension at the elbow can be evaluated easily by holding the joint lightly from behind to steady it while it is passively extended and supinated and then flexed and pronated. Because rotation of the humerus at the shoulder can partly compensate for limited forearm supination, the patient then should be examined with the upper arm held against the lateral rib cage and the forearm pointing horizontally forward. In this position, full pronation of the forearm should result in the palm facing downward, parallel to the floor. Full supination rotates the forearm almost 180°, so that the plane of the hand is only 10–20° short of being horizontal again, but this time palm up. The two arms should be compared for symmetry of movement.

The range of motion in the hips should be checked routinely in infants. The *Ortolani maneuver* is performed with the baby supine and preferably not wearing diapers. The examiner stands at the foot of the crib or examining table and grasps the baby's flexed knees firmly, with the thumbs on the medial surface, the fingers on the lateral thigh, and the palms against the front of the knees. Outward pressure is applied with the thumbs, balanced by firm inward pressure with the fingers, and maintained while the hips are fully abducted. A positive *Ortolani sign* is the palpable "clunk" of the posteriorly displaced

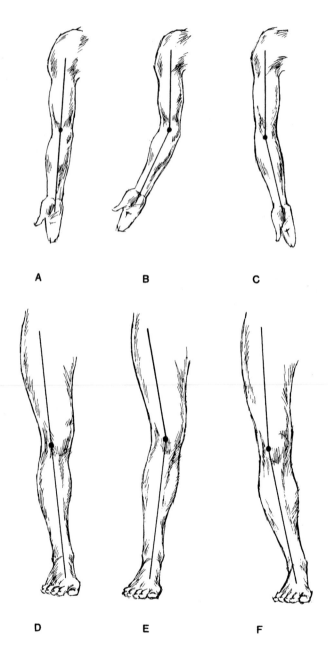

Figure 4.19.2. Positional anomalies of large joints. (A) Frontal view of normal arm. (B) Increased carrying angle at the elbow (cubitus valgus). (C) Negative carrying angle (cutibus varus). (D) Frontal view of normal leg, showing approximately straight weight-bearing angle between hip and ankle. (E) Genu valgum. (F) Genu varum.

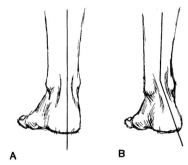

Figure 4.19.3. Posterior view of foot and ankle. (A) Normal conformation of posterior foot. The lower leg, Achilles tendon, and calcaneus lie in a straight line. (B) Valgus position of calcaneus. The posterior heel deviates laterally.

femoral head reseating itself in the acetabulum. Small "clicks" are of no concern, but marked *asymmetry of abduction* is decidedly suspicious. This or a positive Ortolani sign should prompt immediate X-ray evaluation of the hips, and further manipulation of the joint should be avoided to prevent injury to the acetabular lip.

Examination of the elbows, hips, and small joints of the hands (discussed in Section 4.20) will usually serve to detect the most important *isolated* joint abnormalities seen in dysmorphic disorders. *Generalized* joint abnormalities usually become apparent during the assessment of these same joints, and seldom is it necessary actually to measure range of motion for the purpose of dysmorphologic diagnosis (see Table 4.19.1 and Appendix A).

4.19.4. Minor Variants

4.19.4.1. Spectrum Variants

Joint function, as estimated by position at rest and range of motion, shows a relatively narrow range of normal variation. Members of some families may show unusual *loose jointedness,* with mild hyperextensibility in the elbows, knees, and small joints of the hand. An even milder manifestation of ligamentous laxity is **flexible flat foot,** in which the longitudinal arch is flattened with weight bearing but remains asymptomatic and has no detectable bony abnormalities. In the arm, the carrying angle at the elbow is normally larger in females (5–15°) than in males (0–5°) (Fig. 4.19.2A and B).

4.19.4.2. Minor Anomalies

Mild *genu varum* frequently creates slight **bowleg** in infants and toddlers, often accentuated by some actual bowing and *internal rotation* of the tibias. **Knock-knee** is less common but may result from a mild degree of *genu valgum* during midchildhood.

4.19.5. Abnormalities

4.19.5.1. Deformations

Prolonged mechanical stress produced by intrauterine constraint frequently causes joint deformities. Mild to moderate degrees of distortion are found quite frequently in the

feet (see Section 4.19.5.3) and may involve multiple joints if the fetus has been immo-
bilized for a month or more in late gestation. In most instances, once the constraining
forces are removed, motion at affected joints is gradually restored by normal muscle pull,
and treatment is seldom necessary. A major exception occurs in the case of congenital
dislocation of the hip, whose pathogenesis, at least in part, depends on deforming forces
acting directly on the hip joint. The femoral head is displaced posteriorly and inferiorly
and may be partly or totally outside the acetabulum. Prompt diagnosis of this anomaly is
important and is based on clinical signs, with radiologic confirmation (see Section
4.19.3).

Rarely, extreme intrauterine compression over an extended period of time can produce such severe distortion in multiple joints that supporting ligaments become contracted
and opposing tendons stretch. The muscles acting across these joints may atrophy, creating a clinical picture indistinguishable from the intrinsic forms of arthrogryposis congenita
described in Section 4.19.5.4. Only nerve conduction studies, electromyography, or
muscle biopsy can discriminate between malformational and deformational forms of
arthrogryposis, and the requirements for prolonged physical therapy and surgical intervention are the same in both types. Nevertheless, determination of the pathogenesis (when
possible) is of great value for prognosis and recurrence risk counseling.

4.19.5.2. Disruptions

There seem to be no disruptive abnormalities that affect primarily the joints of the
limbs in prenatal life. Several forms of acquired *arthritis* may occur in childhood, however, some of which can produce a clinical picture reminiscent of certain bone dysplasias.
X-rays, rheumatologic evaluation, and special laboratory studies may be needed to dis-

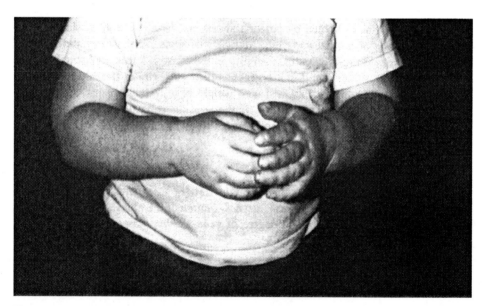

Figure 4.19.4. Joint thickening and limited range of motion in the hands of a boy with mucopolysaccharidosis.

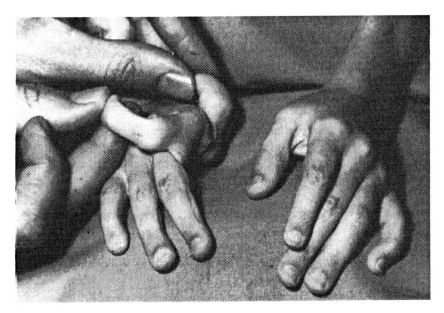

Figure 4.19.5. Extreme hyperextensibility of small joints in one form of Ehlers-Danlos syndrome (also see Fig. 4.20.5).

criminate these disorders. Furthermore, *traumatic arthritis* may occur in some genetic disorders with severe joint laxity as a feature (see Section 4.19.5.4).

4.19.5.3. Dysplasias

Generalized abnormalities of limb joints usually denote the presence of a systemic disease or a dysplastic syndrome. **Joint enlargement** in multiple sites may take place in inflammatory arthritis but also occurs in a number of dysmorphic conditions. In some of these, such as the mucopolysaccharidoses, the thickening is in the soft tissues around the joint (Fig. 4.19.4). Other disorders cause actual hyperplasia of periarticular bone (Fig. 4.18.8), and the difference becomes apparent upon palpating the joints. For diagnostic purposes, it is important to discriminate between these two types of joint enlargement, as well as between them and the *joint effusion* of acute or chronic arthritis.

Varying degrees of *limited joint movement* may be generalized or involve only a few sites. In some instances, the joints may be affected by actual soft tissue contractures, usually holding the limb in a slightly flexed posture; in others, movement may be limited in all directions by thickening of the joint capsule.

Widespread and severe *ligamentous laxity* produces **joint hypermobility** in disorders such as the various types of Ehlers-Danlos syndrome. The joints can be moved far beyond their normal range (Fig. 4.19.5), and their stability may be impaired to the extent that standing and walking become difficult. Repeated excursions of the joints beyond the normal range of motion will eventually lead to traumatic arthritis. **Multiple joint dislocations** are found in Larsen syndrome and a few other conditions. The affected joints are somewhat enlarged, with an abnormal range of motion, and there is aberrant positioning of the limb distally (Fig. 4.19.6). Congenital anterior *subluxation of the knee,* otherwise an extremely rare abnormality, strongly suggests the presence of such a syndrome. Again, traumatic arthritis in later life is a frequent complication of these disorders.

4.19.5.4. Malformations

Local changes in joint configuration or function may represent isolated malformations or be part of a syndrome pattern. For instance, several dysmorphic conditions have as a feature **limited forearm supination.** The plane of the hand often can be brought only to 90° or less from the horizontal (see Section 4.19.3 for examination techniques). Rota-

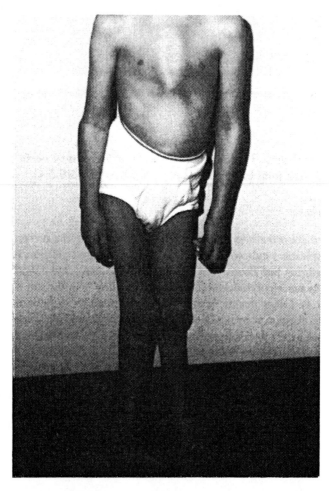

Figure 4.19.6. Genu valgum and thickening of periarticular tissue in Larsen syndrome. Note also flexion contractures at hips and pectus carinatum.

tional abnormalities of the elbow are often accompanied by **incomplete elbow extension,** but *flexion* at the elbow is seldom impaired. Elbow joint abnormality of this kind may be unilateral or asymmetric in severity. In the knees, moderate to severe degrees of **genu varum** are usually bilateral, and the legs seem badly bowed. Actual bowing of the femur and lower leg may contribute to this appearance, but in most cases, hypoplasia of the medial femoral condyle is responsible for the largest part of the abnormal leg configuration. Severe **genu valgum** is less often seen in isolation but may be part of conditions affecting multiple joints (see below). **Genu recurvatum** or *back knee* may occur in some neurologic disorders and also is seen in syndromes with generalized joint laxity.

Widespread **joint contractures** are the hallmark of a heterogeneous group of conditions loosely termed arthrogryposis multiplex congenita. The limbs are partially or completely fixed in position and may be held in attitudes of flexion or extension (Fig. 4.19.7). A *diminished muscle mass* is often noted, and the joints are fusiform or tapered. Some forms of severe contracture are accompanied (or produced) by **joint webbing.** A strong connective tissue band covered with normal skin bridges the flexor aspect of the joint like a bowstring, preventing full extension (Fig. 4.19.8). In multiple pterygium syndrome, such webbing may involve the neck and the groin as well as more peripheral areas.

4.19.6. Summary

Many dysplastic disorders tend to produce abnormalities of joint function, whereas structural defects are more likely to cause aberrant joint position.

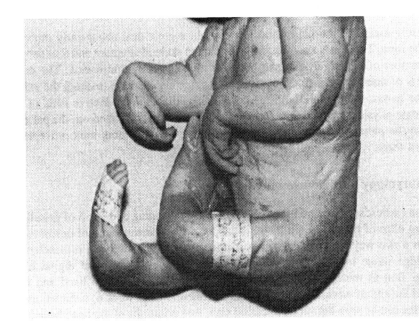

Figure 4.19.7. Widespread severe joint fixation in arthrogryposis multiplex congenita.

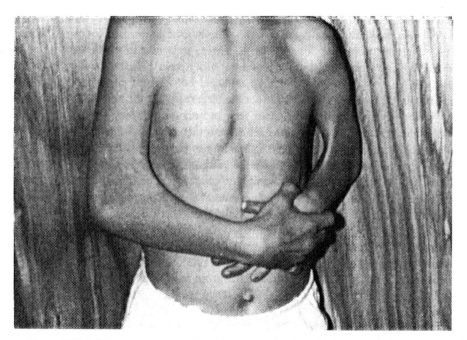

Figure 4.19.8. Elbow contractures and webbing across joints in multiple pterygium syndrome.

4.20. HANDS AND FEET

The configuration of the hands and feet reveals a great deal about early embryo-genesis of the limb. The hands are especially intricate in skeletal structure and thus subject to a large number of distinct dysmorphic changes of diagnostic significance. The progressive effects of many dysplastic disorders also become evident here, making the examination of the hands, along with the face and the skin, the most productive parts of the dysmorphologic physical examination. Readers of palmistry notwithstanding, the patterns of creases on the palms reveal only the past, reflecting the continuing joint movements that produced them.

4.20.1. Embryology and Development

From the earliest stages of limb development at the beginning of week 5 of gestation, the advancing edge of the finlike limb bud is capped with a narrow band of *apical ridge ectoderm.* In a two-way biochemical "conversation" with the underlying mesenchyme, the apical ridge tissue induces general limb growth and the formation of digital rays. These appear first as mesenchymal condensations in the paddle-shaped hand and foot plates toward the end of week 5 (Fig. 4.20.1A). By the middle of week 6, indentations of the apical ridge can be seen between the digital rays, and primordia of the hand bones can be seen (Fig. 4.20.1B). The notches in the edges of the hand plate deepen rapidly through localized *cell death,* and by the end of week 7, cartilaginous models of the *phalanges,*

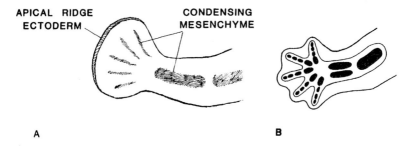

APICAL RIDGE
ECTODERM

CONDENSING
MESENCHYME

A

B

Figure 4.20.1. Embryogenesis of the hand. (A) Distal limb development at 5.5 weeks of gestation. The five digital rays are represented by mesenchymal condensations. (B) By 6 weeks, the digital rays are segmenting into metacarpals and phalanges. Regression of interdigital tissues is beginning.

metacarpals, and most of the *carpal bones* are present. As usual, maturation of the lower limb lags behind that of the upper.

Continued growth and deepening of the interdigital clefts produces a remarkably mature appearance of the hand by the end of gestational week 8 (Fig. 4.20.2). Large pads of soft tissue are appearing on the palms and soles and on the tips of the fingers and toes. Their contours will determine the configuration of the dermatoglyphic patterns (see Appendix B). With the growth and functional maturation of the limb muscles, joint movement in the hands probably begins around week 12, initiating the formation of patterns of *flexion creases* on the skin of the palms and fingers, which can be seen by week 20.

Although the hands and feet are embryologically homologous, their component structures develop quite different proportions after the limb bud stage. The fingers becoming elongate in relation to the metacarpal bones, while the toes remain short, so that the length of the foot is determined primarily by the metatarsals. During postnatal growth the hands and feet retain these relationships in size.

4.20.2. Anatomy and Landmarks

4.20.2.1. Hands

The five digital rays are represented by the *metacarpal bones* and the *digits.* The central axis of the hand courses through the *middle* (*third* or *long*) finger and *third*

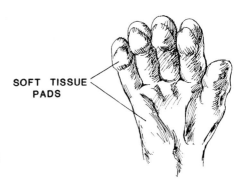

SOFT TISSUE
PADS

Figure 4.20.2. Fetal hand at about week 9 of gestation. Prominent soft tissue pads surmount the fingertips and produce the contours of the palm.

metacarpal. On the *preaxial (radial)* side of the hand are the *thumb* and *index (second)* finger, and on the *postaxial (ulnar)* side lie the *ring (fourth)* and *little (fifth)* fingers (Fig. 4.18.1B). The adjective *volar* refers to the palmar surface of the hand and the sole of the foot.

The hand is about twice as long as it is wide, and the palm has a roughly rectangular outline. The thumb has two phalanges, and the *first metacarpal* extends from the *thumb web* to the level of the wrist joint. An elliptical muscle mass, the *thenar eminence,* lies over the first metacarpal, extending onto the palm to about the midline. A smaller muscle mass, the *hypothenar eminence,* extends up the postaxial side of the palm (Fig. 4.20.3).

The fingers are cylindrical or slightly tapered, and each articulates with its metacarpal at the *metacarpophalangeal (M-P) joint.* The *proximal, middle,* and *distal phalanges* articulate with each other at the *proximal* and *distal interphalangeal joints* (respectively abbreviated PIP and DIP). The thumb has but a single interphalangeal joint. The interphalangeal joints are true hinge joints and normally permit about 90° of flexion. The M-P joints of the fingers, which also flex to 90°, have a small range of lateral motion as well when extended. Each of the M-P joints has a plane of flexion slightly different from that of its neighbors. Thus, when a flat-fingered fist is formed, the axes of the fingers are not quite parallel; the fingertips all point to a spot between the radius and ulna on the distal forearm. Flexion at the M-P joint of the thumb usually is limited to about 20°, but in some individuals up to 90° of flexion is possible. The articulation of the first metacarpal with the trapezium of the wrist can be moved through a broad cone of rotation, facilitating the *opposition* of the thumb.

The ring finger is almost as long as the middle finger, the index is somewhat shorter, and the tip of the little finger just reaches the DIP joint of the ring finger. The *interosseous*

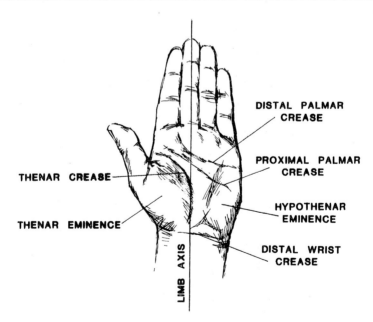

Figure 4.20.3. Superficial anatomy and landmarks of the hand.

muscles contribute to the contours of the dorsum of the hand, with the muscle mass lying between the thumb and index fingers producing a noticeable bulge. The small *skin webs* between the bases of the fingers normally extend distally less than half the length of the first phalanges. When the fingers are widely separated, these form a smooth arc.

The soft tissues of the volar surface of the hand respond to joint movement by the formation of flexion creases. Those lying across the DIP joints are usually single, whereas several roughly parallel creases lie over the PIP joints and the junctions of the fingers with the palms. *Palm creases* form in response to flexion at the M-P joints and opposition of the thumb. Although many normal variants exist, three deep creases are usually seen: the *thenar crease* circles the base of the thenar eminence, extending distally to exit between the thumb and index finger. The *distal palmar crease* traverses the palm beneath the last three fingers, beginning at the ulnar edge of the palm and curving distally to exit between the index and middle fingers. The *proximal palmar crease* may be less well defined, beginning over the hypothenar eminence and extending parallel to the distal crease to exit near or fuse with the distal portion of the thenar crease (Fig. 4.20.3). The *distal wrist crease* defines the proximal limit of the palm. A number of fine creases, many oriented longitudinally, have a variable distribution.

Dermatoglyphic patterns are discussed in Appendix B.

4.20.2.2. Feet

As in the hand, the axis of the foot runs down the length of the central digital ray. In the *neutral position,* the foot forms a 90° angle with the leg, and the axis of the foot is directed straight forward, in the same direction the patella faces. Seen from above, the distal third (*forefoot*) is widest over the *metatarsal heads* at the base of the toes. The medial (*preaxial* or *tibial*) border is nearly straight from the heel to the tip of the *first* (*great*) toe, while the lateral (*postaxial* or *ulnar*) plantar margin may be slightly convex. Viewed from the side, the foot is wedge shaped. In the standing position, the medial third of the sole is raised in the *longitudinal* (*plantar*) *arch* between the major weight-bearing areas of the metatarsal heads and the *calcaneus* (Fig. 4.20.4). In infants, the foot is thicker in relation to its length and width, and the arch is poorly developed.

The toes, which are simply numbered *first* through *fifth* from medial to lateral, normally are graduated in length in the same direction (the "plebian" foot). A very common variation, however, has a second toe longer than the first (the "patrician" foot). The toes have a variable range of motion, although in some cases 90° of flexion and extension can be obtained at the M-P joints. Two distinct flexion creases may be found on the volar surface of the toes except the fifth, which commonly bears just one. Because of its relative immobility, the sole of the foot normally has only a few poorly defined flexion creases.

4.20.3. Examination Techniques

Inspection of the hands and feet provides information concerning their general proportions, the positions and relative length of the digits, and the contours of the intrinsic muscles.

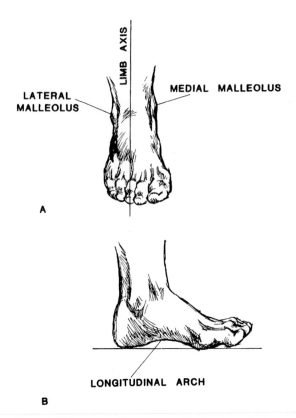

Figure 4.20.4. Superficial anatomy and landmarks of the foot.

4.20.3.1. Inspection of the Hands

Special attention should be paid to the palmar and digital crease lines, which provide valuable clues concerning joint location and function. The patient should be asked to make a fist with each hand so that adequacy of finger flexion and the relative length of the metacarpals can be assessed. Mild skin *syndactyly* often can be detected by flexing the M-P joints and spreading the fingers slightly to determine how far the interdigital webs extend down the first phalanges. Placing the hands together, palm to palm and with the distal wrist creases aligned, permits determination of hand symmetry and also accentuates mild degrees of bilateral flexion contractures of the fingers.

4.20.3.2. Inspection of the Feet

With the patient standing, the height of the plantar arch can be judged, and unusual intoeing or other positional abnormalities can be seen.

Palpation of the structures of the distal limbs is particularly helpful in detecting joint abnormalities.

4.20.3.3. Palpation of the Hands and Wrists

Each finger should be extended passively to its full extent; anything short of a full 180° angle at any joint signifies joint contracture or *camptodactyly*. With the palm held flat against the examining table, the M-P joints are gently hyperextended. In infants and young children, the angle of the first phalanx with the plane of the hand may be 60° or a bit more; older children and adults can usually extend less than 45°. Passive extension to 90° or beyond signifies *joint laxity*. No hyperextension normally is present in the M-P joints of the thumbs. Some younger children have sufficient laxity at the wrist that the thumb can be brought down to touch the anterior surface of the forearm. Passive movement of the thumb backward usually is more limited, however, and extreme hyperextension at the first carpometacarpal joint, so that the nail touches the dorsal forearm, is a definite sign of joint hypermobility (Fig. 4.20.5).

4.20.3.4. Palpation of the Feet and Ankles

With the patient supine or seated, the range of motion of the foot at the ankle is tested. Plantar flexion to 45° is normal, and dorsiflexion is usually about 20°, although it may be much greater in newborn infants. Internal rotation of the calcaneus may approach 30°, whereas external rotation is minimal. If any apparent positional abnormality is noted with the foot at rest, an effort should be made to bring the foot back to the neutral position. The heel is grasped firmly with one hand and the forefoot is manipulated with the other. A *flexible* deformity can be restored to neutral position; a *fixed* abnormality cannot.

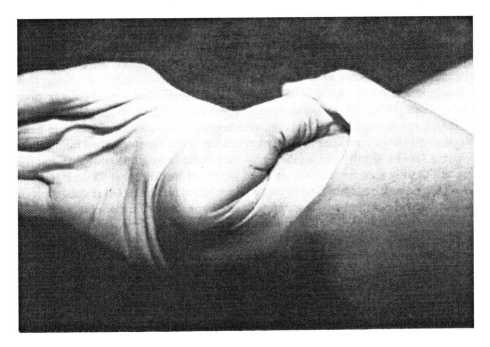

Figure 4.20.5. Extreme joint laxity in Ehlers-Danlos syndrome type I (also see Fig. 4.19.5).

Measurement of the hands is useful if abnormalities of finger length are suspected. *Palm length* is measured from the distal wrist crease to the flexion crease at the base of the middle finger. The distance from the latter point to the tip of the middle finger is the *midfinger length*. Both the absolute and relative values of these measurements should be compared with charts of normals for age. *Foot length* may be determined with the patient supine by resting the heel on the examining table and measuring from that point to the tip of the first toe. (Standing foot length is somewhat greater.)

4.20.4. Minor Variants

4.20.4.1. Spectrum Variants

Joint mobility varies over a fairly broad range in normal individuals and families, from "stiff-jointedness" at one end to **benign familial hypermobility** at the other. Minor degrees of joint limitation usually are not brought to medical attention, but children with unusually "loose" joints may be sent to dysmorphology clinics because of suspicion of Ehlers-Danlos syndrome or some other connective tissue disorder. Joint hypermobility in such instances is especially notable in the small joints of the hands, where the fingers may be extended (dorsiflexed) to an unusal extent. There are no accompanying skin abnormalities, and the large joints of the limbs show little or no hypermobility. Another common manifestation of benign joint laxity is **pes planus** (*flat foot*), in which the longitudinal arch of the foot is low or entirely absent. Flexible flat foot is also found as an isolated feature in people with no remarkable joint extensibility elsewhere. In the majority of cases, this condition is asymptomatic, and no bony abnormalities of the foot can be found. Instead, an unusual degree of laxity of the supporting ligaments permits sagging of the plantar arch at the joints between the metatarsal and tarsal bones.

Palmar crease patterns show a great deal of normal variation that probably reflects mild differences in joint placement in the underlying bones. In fact, there are no pathognomonic crease patterns at all. Children are sometimes suspected of having Down syndrome solely on the basis of the presence of a **single transverse palmar crease** (*simian crease*) (Fig. 4.20.6A). This variant is seen unilaterally in about 4% of the normal population and bilaterally in about 1%. (Furthermore, it is present in less than half of children with Down syndrome.) Its only implication is that the second and third metacarpal bones may be slightly shorter than usual and closer in length to the fourth and fifth. This will slightly alter the relative planes of flexion of the fingers at the M-P joints and require only a single palmar flexion crease to accommodate them. Other common variations include **bridging creases** connecting or extending the three major creases, a **Sydney line,** which is an extension of the proximal transverse crease to reach the ulnar border of the hand, and the **hockeystick crease,** in which the distal transverse crease runs quite horizontally across the postaxial palm and then abruptly angles distally to exit between the index and middle fingers (Fig. 4.20.6B–D).

On the sole, *plantar crease patterns* are less well defined. A **longitudinal plantar crease** may be found in newborns after the foot has undergone prolonged transverse compression in utero. Similar creases that persist and deepen are a feature of a few syndromes (Fig. 4.20.7).

For diagnostic purposes, the most important crease anomaly is **absence of flexion**

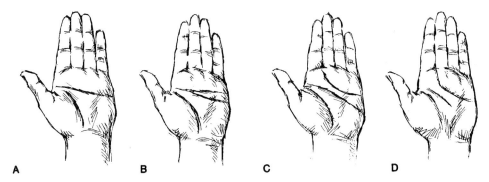

A   B   C   D

Figure 4.20.6. Normal variation in palmar crease patterns. (A) Single transverse distal palmar crease. (B) Fused distal and proximal transverse creases. (C) Sydney line (extension of the proximal transverse crease to the extreme medial edge of the palm. (D) Abrupt angulation of the distal transverse crease, exiting between the index and middle fingers (hockeystick crease).

creases in zones where they are normally present. This invariably signifies inadequate movement of the underlying joint(s).

4.20.4.2. Minor Malformations

A number of minor structural variants of the hands and feet occur sporadically in some populations or in an irregular autosomal dominant familial distribution.

Hands. **Clinodactyly** is the curving of a finger to one side, usually toward the mid-

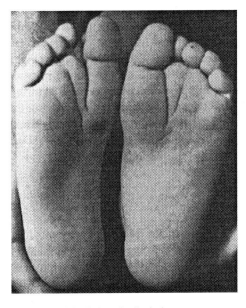

Figure 4.20.7. Longitudinal plantar creases.

line, in the plane of the palm. Involvement of the fifth finger is most common and is caused by varying degrees of hypoplasia of the middle phalanx, which changes the planes of joint movement in the finger (Fig. 4.20.8A). Mild clinodactyly is most easily detected by examination of the flexion creases, which will slope toward each other rather than being parallel. Markedly **tapered fingers** are seen in some obese individuals but may also indicate mild hypoplasia of the middle and distal phalanges (Fig. 4.20.8B). A form of *polydactyly* common in blacks is a small **accessory digit** (*postminimus*) arising on the ulnar aspect of the first phalanx of the fifth finger. Unilateral or bilateral, these extra digits sometimes may be fairly well formed, with one or more rudimentary phalanges (Fig. 4.20.8D). More often, they take the form of a small nubbin or a pedunculated mass, joined to the fifth finger by a narrow stalk. A disproportionately short and broad distal phalanx of the thumb produces what has been called potter's thumb, apparently in reference to supposed wearing down of the digit by constant application to clay on a potter's wheel (Fig. 4.20.8C). This anomaly is commonly seen as a familial feature. (See Section 4.17.2.)

A **short fourth metacarpal** causes the ring finger to seem unusually short, appearing equal in length to the index or even the fifth finger (Fig. 4.20.9A). The actual cause for this appearance can be demonstrated by clenching the fist, when the normal prominence of the fourth knuckle will be absent (the *knuckle-knuckle-dimple-knuckle sign*) (Fig. 4.20.9B). Moderate degrees of **cutaneous syndactyly** also may be best appreciated from a dorsal view of the hand, with the M-P joints flexed. The interdigital skin webs will be seen to extend distally, almost to the level of the PIP joints (Fig. 4.20.10A). On the palm, the distance between the distal transverse crease and the margin of the skin web will be increased (Fig. 4.20.10B).

Feet. Several minor anomalies of the feet are homologous to those of the hand. Clinodactyly of the toes is quite common, probably because their phalanges are so short. Postaxial polydactyly of the foot is fairly common, and the accessory digits have much the same form and relative position as those found on the hands. A short, **broad distal hallux** may occur with or without similar involvement of the thumbs (Fig. 4.20.11A). A **short fourth metatarsal** causes apparent irregularity of toe length (Fig. 4.20.11B) and may also produce **overriding toes,** although these may be found in otherwise normal feet (Fig. 4.20.11C). Dorsiflexed **hammertoes** rarely may be seen at birth, more frequently developing in adult life because of relative shortening of the extensor tendons. **Toe syndactyly,** usually involving the second and third digits, is quite common and in its most pronounced form may extend almost to the tips of the toes (Fig. 4.20.11D).

4.20.5. Abnormalities

4.20.5.1. Deformations

Deformational abnormalities of the hands are very rare, probably because of their relatively protected intrauterine position. In contrast, the legs and feet may be subjected to considerable mechanical stress during the last weeks in utero, especially if the baby is in the breech or other aberrant position. The usual response to this stress is some form of *clubfoot*. If the constraint has been mild or relatively brief, the deformity usually is flexible in that the foot can be manipulated back into neutral position. A fixed deformity

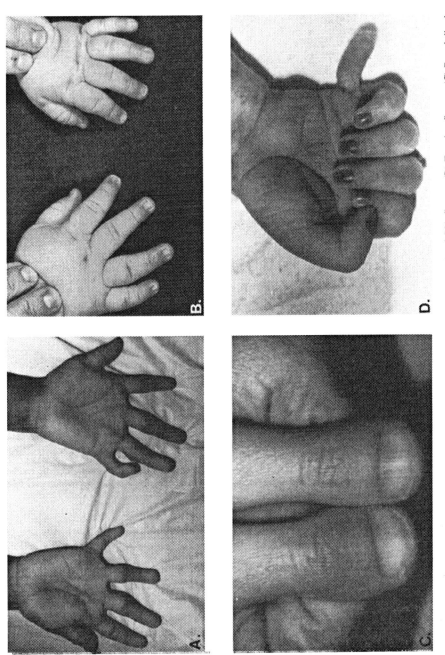

Figure 4.20.8. Minor anomalies of hand development. (A) Clinodactyly and camptodactyly of fifth fingers. (B) Tapering fingers. (C) Broad distal phalanges of the thumbs, with wide, relatively short nails (racquet nails). (D) Postaxial polydactyly.

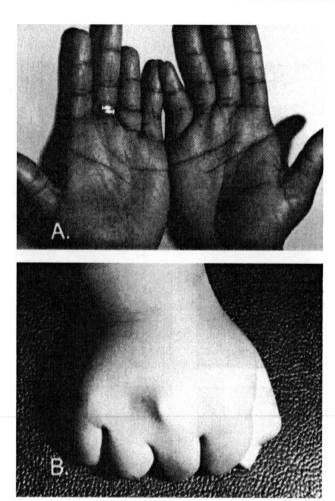

Figure 4.20.9. Isolated shortening of fourth metacarpal. (A) Palmar view showing left fourth fingertip reaching only to distal flexion crease of middle finger. (B) Dorsal view in another patient showing depression over fourth M-P joint (knuckle-knuckle-dimple-knuckle sign).

implies either severe and prolonged immobilization, with contractures of the ligaments and capsules of joints or, more ominously, an *intrinsic* skeletal anomaly. This type is resistant to conservative treatment, and serial casting or surgical correction is more often required. Positional foot abnormalities also may be caused by hypoplasia, weakness, or denervation of the muscles that act on the foot. In this case, the abnormal position will eventually become fixed if the muscular imbalance is prolonged.

In **talipes calcaneovalgus,** the foot is dorsiflexed onto the fibular side of the ankle and everted, with the sole facing anterolaterally. As implied by the name, the calcaneus

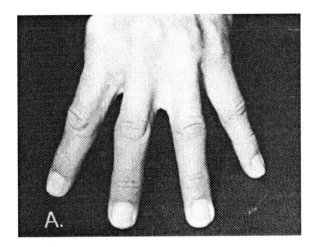

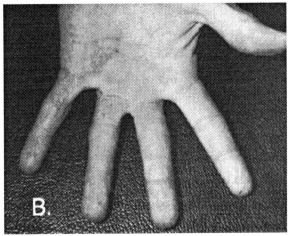

Figure 4.20.10. Mild cutaneous syndactyly. (A) Dorsal view with fingers partly flexed. The skin web between the middle and ring fingers lies at more than two-thirds of the distance from the M-P to the PIP joints. (B) Palmar view of the same hand. Note increased distance between transverse palmar crease and margin of interdigital web.

also is deviated laterally (see Fig. 4.19.3B). A deep skin crease is often present in the plane of abnormal flexion, and subcutaneous tissue is diminished over the anterolateral region of the foot (Fig. 4.20.12A). This anomaly is common in babies born in the breech position, especially if the knees were flexed in utero, and it usually responds to repeated postnatal manipulation. With **metatarsus adductus,** the forefoot is turned medially so that the lateral border of the sole is quite convex. The heel is in neutral position, and the foot can be dorsiflexed normally. If intrauterine constraint has been prolonged, a deep plantar crease will be seen on the medial sole (Fig. 4.20.12B). **Talipes equinovarus** causes the foot to be sharply plantar flexed and inverted, so that the sole is turned toward the median plane. The calcaneus is in varus position, and some degree of metatarsus adductus is almost always present. The skin and subcutaneous tissues over the lateral part of the foot may be thin, and dorsiflexion is minimal or absent (Fig. 4.20.12C). This foot

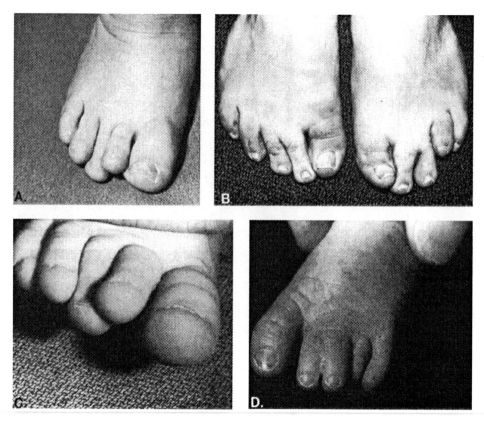

Figure 4.20.11. Minor toe anomalies. (A) Dorsally positioned second toe overlapping the third. (B) Isolated short fourth metatarsal. The fourth toe appears "inset" into the foot. (C) Hypoplastic toe nails. (D) Skin syndactyly of second and third toes.

position is frequently fixed and is caused by a malformational abnormality in almost half of the cases. Casting or surgery is frequently required.

4.20.5.2. Disruptions

Probably because of their distal position and mobility, the hands and feet (and especially the digits) are the commonest sites of damage from amniotic bands. The mechanisms causing this injury remain obscure, but the resulting lesions range from shallow *constricting rings* to those that are deep enough to occlude lymphatic circulation, producing distal edema. Even more severe compression can apparently disrupt tissue down to the periosteum, with eventual loss of the distal avascular portion, a congenital amputation (Fig. 4.20.13A). At birth, the amputation site will be scarred, and sometimes bands of fibrous tissue still will be attached to the injured area. The damage is usually asymmetric with digits affected at different levels. Occasionally, several digits will be bound together at the tips by scar tissue, producing a form of pseudosyndactyly (Fig. 4.20.13B).

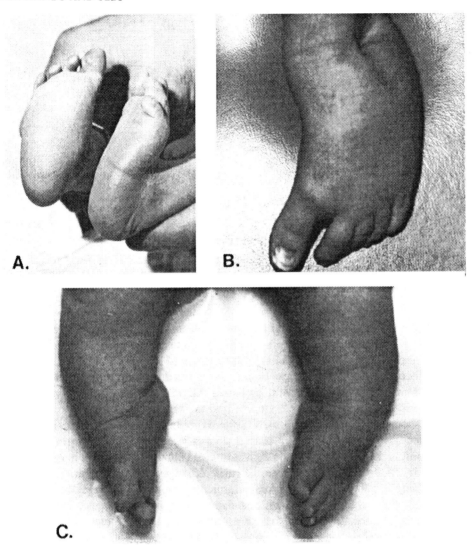

Figure 4.20.12. Positional foot abnormalities. (A) Plantar view of calcaneovalgus feet. Note dorsiflexion and lateral deviation of calcaneus on left. (B) Metatarsus adductus. The forefoot is "windswept" medially. (C) Severe equinovarus foot position in a baby with epiphyseal dysostosis. Note "tiptoe" position with soles nearly facing each other.

4.20.5.3. Dysplasias

The soft tissues of the hands, especially around the joints, are sites of deposition of storage substances in several metabolic diseases, which cause *skin thickening* and **limitation of joint movement** (Fig. 4.19.4). These diseases also produce **phalangeal broadening,** which sometimes can be palpated but is much more evident in hand radiographs.

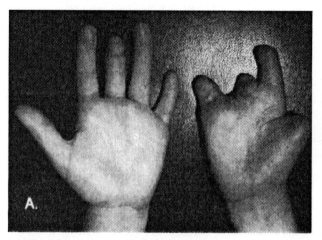 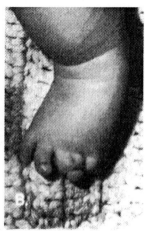

Figure 4.20.13. Digital amputations from amniotic bands. (A) Multiple finger amputations. The dermatoglyphic patterns were interrupted at the terminus of involved fingers. (B) Pseudosyndactyly and constriction ring formation involving the third and fourth toes.

Bone changes in the hands and feet are also features of some of the chondrodystrophies, usually resulting in shortening of the long bones (acromelic shortening.) Short fourth metacarpals and metatarsals have been mentioned as minor anomalies, but shortening may occur in any or all of these bones. **Short third, fourth, and fifth metacarpals** may be found in several disorders, including Albright hereditary osteodystrophy and nevoid basal cell nevus syndrome. Generalized **metacarpal hypoplasia** produces a noticeably short palm, while overall **metatarsal hypoplasia** gives the foot a similar short, stubby appearance. A **proximally placed thumb** is caused by *hypoplasia of the first metacarpal,* and the long axis of the digit is oriented almost horizontally in relation to the palm (Fig. 4.20.14B). Hypoplasia of the phalanges produces various forms of **brachydactyly.** Shortening of the proximal, middle, and distal phalanges occurs in different combinations in each type, often associated with clinodactyly, and may affect one, several, or all of the fingers and toes (Fig. 4.20.14C). Finally, generalized mild hypoplasia of all of the long bones produces **small hands and feet,** with no evident disproportion in finger length in relation to the palms. Measurements usually are necessary to confirm a clinical impression in this regard.

Dysplastic conditions that affect primarily the skin and nails have been discussed in Sections 4.15 and 4.17.

4.20.5.4. Malformations

Of the many intrinsic malformations of the hands and feet, several affect primarily the joints. The clinical features of the three major types of deformational *talipes* (clubfoot) were discussed in Section 4.20.5.1. Malformational talipes may be identical in appearance but is caused by abnormal development of the bones of the foot. These anomalies are often syndromic, forming part of a larger pattern that may include abnormal bone formation or muscle function in many areas of the body. In the hands, deformations are

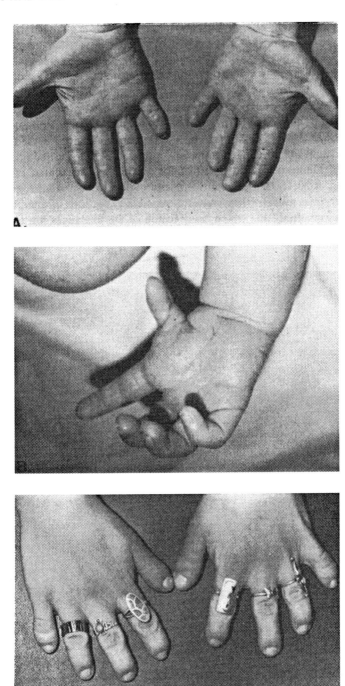

Figure 4.20.14. Finger malformations. (A) Symphalangism. The DIP joints of the third, fourth, and fifth fingers are fixed. Note absence of distal flexion creases. (B) "Hitchhiker's thumb," retroflexed with hypoplasia of the thenar musculature. (C) Acromelic shortening (brachydactyly) in Robinow syndrome.

rare, and therefore the presence of joint anomalies usually has more diagnostic specificity. A good example is found in **camptodactyly**, in which the proximal interphalangeal joints are held in a partially flexed position, sometimes with thickened connective tissue on the volar surface (Fig. 4.20.15A). The fifth finger is most commonly affected, but others may be involved as well, usually bilaterally and symmetrically. **Clasped thumbs** are held in a flexed and adducted position across the palm and cannot be abducted or extended. This anomaly should be differentiated from the *cortical thumbs* seen in normal infants until about 3 months of age and in children with severe brain damage. In the latter condition, the thumb is freely mobile but is habitually positioned over the palm, grasped by the flexed fingers. **Ulnar deviation** of all of the fingers is a feature of Freeman-Sheldon syndrome (Fig. 4.20.15B). Occasionally, **incomplete flexion** is found, especially in the M-P joints. No joint movement whatever is possible at the sites of interphalangeal joints affected by **symphalangism,** where bony fusion of the phalanges has taken place. The absence of flexion creases is an excellent clue to the presence of this anomaly (Fig. 4.20.14A).

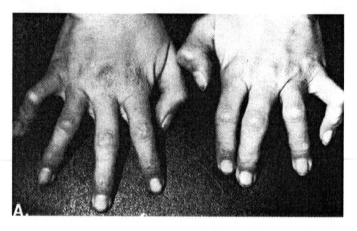

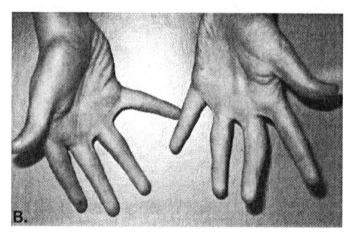

Figure 4.20.15. Positional abnormalities of fingers. (A) Camptodactyly. Flexion contractures most severely affect the PIP joints. (B) Mild ulnar deviation of the fingers in Freeman-Sheldon syndrome.

Various types of localized *skeletal aplasia* or hypoplasia may affect the bones of the hands and feet, either in isolation or as part of a larger pattern of bony abnormality involving the limbs. They may be discussed most conveniently when categorized by the anatomic distribution of deficiency, as has been done earlier with the limbs in general.

Longitudinal skeletal defects may be limited to the digital rays or involve the more proximal limb structures as well. Most of these probably have their embryologic basis in abnormal development of the apical ridge ectoderm, which plays a role both in early growth of the limb and definition of its skeletal elements. For example, inadequate induction of growth and differentiation on the preaxial side of the upper limb can produce various degrees of isolated **thumb hypoplasia,** ranging from a relatively long **triphalangeal thumb** that lies in the same plane as the fingers (Fig. 4.20.16A) to a small, pedunculated rudimentary digit (Fig. 4.20.16B). The muscle mass making up the thenar eminence is also diminished in size or absent in these cases. More extensive involvement of the preaxial side of the upper limb may result in total absence of the first and second digital rays, with severe **radial hypoplasia** (Fig. 4.20.17A). Homologous deficiencies occur in the foot and leg with *tibial hypoplasia.* Similar but rarer are abnormalities of the postaxial side of the limb, affecting the fifth and fourth digital rays (Fig. 4.20.17B and C). The central digital rays are not immune from longitudinal bone deficits, which produce **ectrodactyly** (*split hand/split foot or lobster-claw deformity*). The severity of this malformation varies considerably, not only among affected individuals but even between different limbs in the same person. In the hand, the typical abnormality consists of absence of the third digital ray, with a deep triangular cleft extending to the level of the carpal bones (Fig. 4.20.18A). Fingers bordering the cleft may show clinodactyly, camptodactyly, or syndactyly and are sometimes hypoplastic or completely missing. Defects of a similar type but varying widely in severity may be found in the other limbs. Rarely, two types of longitudinal skeletal defects may occur in the same limb, resulting in **monodactyly,** in which only a single digit (usually the third) is preserved (Fig. 4.20.18B).

Terminal transverse skeletal deficiencies take the form of hypoplasia or aplasia of all structures distal to a particular level on the limb, usually with preservation of the more

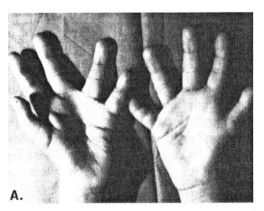
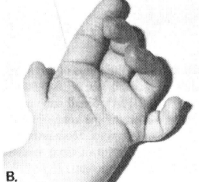

Figure 4.20.16. Digital ray hypoplasia. (A) Mild radial and ulnar hypoplasia with underdevelopment of the thenar and hypothenar muscle masses, producing a triangular palm. Note fingerlike appearance of triphalangeal thumbs. (B) More severe radial hypoplasia with rudimentary, immobile thumb.

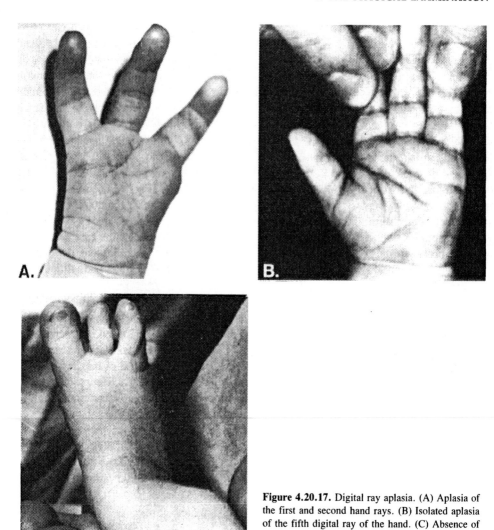

Figure 4.20.17. Digital ray aplasia. (A) Aplasia of the first and second hand rays. (B) Isolated aplasia of the fifth digital ray of the hand. (C) Absence of fourth and fifth rays of the foot.

proximal parts. Variations of this kind of truncation include absence of phalanges (**aphalangia**) (Fig. 4.20.19), digits (**adactylia**), or the entire hand or foot (**acheiria** or **apodia**) (see Fig. 4.18.10A). Small nubbins representing rudimentary digits usually remain over the distal surface of the zone of aplasia, distinguishing these abnormalities from actual congenital amputations. More proximal portions of the limb may be normal or diminished in size. The majority of these terminal transverse deficiencies probably represent true intercalary skeletal defects.

Duplication of digits occurs when one or more extra digital rays are formed during the embryonic period or when excess mesenchymal tissue results in bifurcation of a bone primordium. **Postaxial polydactyly** may take forms ranging from a small postminimus (see Section 4.20.4.2) to a well-developed extra finger or toe, articulating with an ac-

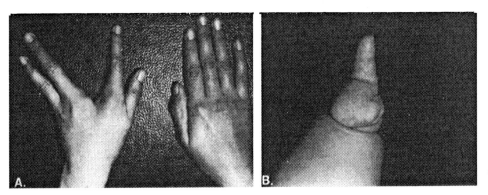

Figure 4.20.18. Forms of ectrodactyly. (A) Unilateral aplasia of the central digital ray (lobster-claw defect). (B) Ectrodactyly involving all but the fourth digital ray, resulting in monodactyly.

cessory metacarpal or metatarsal (Fig. 4.20.20A). **Preaxial polydactyly** is less common but has the same range of severity, with the accessory tissue usually arising from the midportion of the first toe or thumb (Fig. 4.20.20B). Most polydactyly involves only a single extra digit per limb, but rare examples of **multiple polydactyly** occur, producing duplication of two or more digital rays in the same hand or foot (Fig. 4.20.20C). This

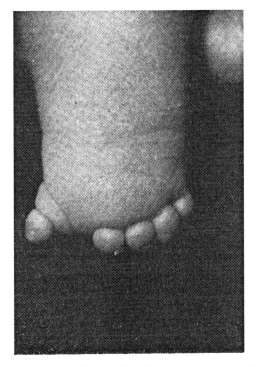

Figure 4.20.19. Distal transverse hemimelia of the foot. The toes are represented by small nubbins containing only a single small rounded remnant of bone.

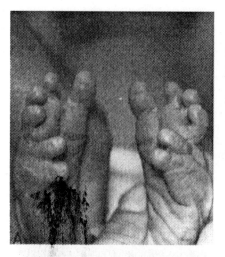
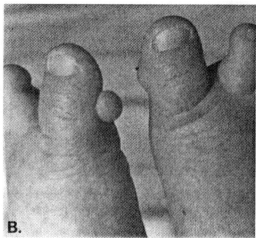
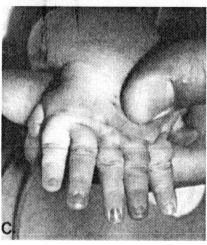

Figure 4.20.20. Forms of polydactyly. (A) Bilateral postaxial polydactyly of the feet. The sixth toes are well formed. (B) Preaxial polydactyly of the feet. The pedunculated supernumerary digit on the left first toe is reflected by only a medial bulge on the right. (C) Preaxial and postaxial polydactyly on the same limb.

form is more likely than the others to be associated with additional structural anomalies as part of a dysmorphic syndrome.

Syndactyly is the fusion of one or more digits into a single mass. The commonest form is **cutaneous syndactyly**, which in its milder expressions is a minor anomaly (see Section 4.20.4.2). With more severe involvement, the digits are joined to the level of the DIP joints or beyond and may share a common nail (Fig. 4.20.21A). In the hands, the longer of the involved fingers is often held in a flexed position to accommodate to the length of the shorter, and the flexion creases reflect the mutual movement of the combined fingers. Cutaneous syndactyly is probably caused by inadequacy of the programmed cell death that normally occurs in the tissues between the digital rays from about the weeks 6–8 of embryonic life. In contrast, the synostosis found in **osseous syndactyly** may result from excessive cell death at this stage, leading to close apposition of the digital blastema

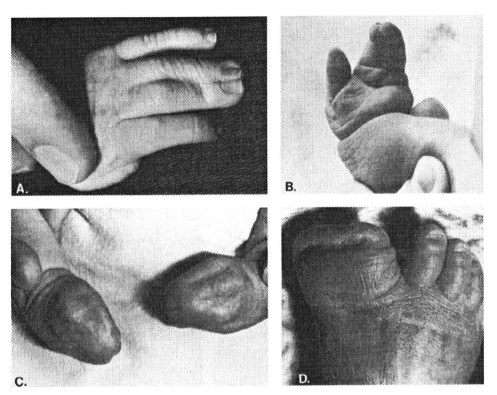

Figure 4.20.21. Forms of syndactyly. (A) Complete cutaneous syndactyly between the middle and ring fingers. (B) Syndactyly combined with aplasia of the ulnar digital rays. (C) Total syndactyly involving the full length of all fingers (mitten syndactyly) in Apert syndrome. (D) Polysyndactyly of the first toe.

and their eventual coalesence. In this type of syndactyly, bony fusion exists between some of the phalanges of adjacent digits, forming an abnormally broad, tapered finger or toe (Fig. 4.20.21B). In several genetic syndromes, complete syndactyly with synostosis involving all the fingers and toes is a common feature. The hands are cupped and mittenlike, with a single undulating, band-shaped nail, and the feet are similarly affected (Fig. 4.20.21C). The thumbs may be free but very short and broad, with ulnar deviation of the distal phalanx. In some of these conditions, supernumerary digital rays also form, giving rise to **polysyndactyly** (Fig. 4.20.21D).

One final category of malformation of the hands and feet consists of *localized overgrowth* of the digits. This may entail isolated enlargement of a random finger or toe (**macrodactyly**) or a generalized elongation of the digits (**arachnodactyly**) as is often seen in Marfan syndrome (Fig. 4.20.22A). In some dysmorphologic disorders, a distinctive overgrowth anomaly may be particularly helpful in diagnosis. Examples include the **broad thumb** and first toes of Rubinstein-Taybi syndrome (Fig. 4.20.22B) or the **bulbous toes,** irregular in length and spacing (which some observers have likened to the foot of a tree frog) in otopalatodigital dysplasia (Fig. 4.20.22C).

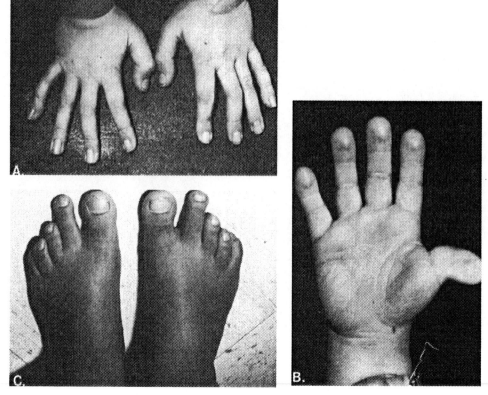

Figure 4.20.22. Variations of digital configuration. (A) Arachnodactyly. The fingers are long, tubular, and relatively slender. (B) Broad thumb in Rubinstein-Taybi syndrome. (C) Disharmony of toe length, with bulbous distal phalanges in otopalatodigital syndrome.

4.20.6. Summary

The distalmost portions of the limbs undergo a form of embryonic development in which aberrations during a very limited time period produce distinctive and striking malformations. Many signs of dysplastic disorders also appear in the hands, and palmar crease patterns provide a helpful record of joint movements.

4.21. NEUROLOGIC AND BEHAVIORAL ABNORMALITIES

Many dysmorphic syndromes have neurologic components beyond that of global mental deficit, and some also show consistent behavioral characteristics that may be helpful in diagnosis. Since these functional abnormalities often can be detected during the clinical examination, they are included in this chapter.

4.21.1. Neurologic Abnormalities

4.21.1.1. Gross Motor Dysfunction

Hypertonicity of a mild to moderate degree, primarily affecting the flexor muscle groups, is found in normal infants until about 4 months of age. After this time, however, persistence of increased muscle tone strongly suggests upper motor neuron abnormality. Associated **hyperreflexia** may also be found in such cases. Babies with increased tone may display unusually rapid attainment of gross motor milestones during early months, rolling over and even sitting earlier than expected. These precocious accomplishments are based on spasticity of major muscle groups and are not accompanied by corresponding advances in fine motor or social skills, which instead are likely to be significantly delayed. **Cortical thumbs** are a manifestation of hypertonicity when they persist beyond the first 3–4 months. The thumbs are held adducted and flexed across the palms, with the fingers clenched tightly over them. Passive motion of the thumbs and fingers is resisted by increased flexor tone, but there are no joint anomalies that limit movement. Severe cortical irritation or damage may produce extreme hypertonicity of the paraspinal musculature, resulting in **opisthotonos.** The neck is hyperextended, and the spine is arched into an extreme lordotic curve.

Decreased muscle tone, or **hypotonia,** is another important neurologic sign and is more frequently of diagnostic significance in dysmorphic conditions than is hypertonicity. Lack of normal flexor hypertonus in early infancy produces the picture of a "floppy baby." Such a child will hang limply when supported in a prone position and seem to slip through the examiner's hands when held upright under the arms. Later in infancy, hypotonia may be manifest in delayed gross motor milestones, especially in attaining head support and sitting. In older children, hypotonia produces a slumped sitting posture, late walking, and an abnormal gait.

Neonatal hypotonia often is an early sign of brain damage that will progress to spasticity and typical cerebral palsy by the end of the first year. Alternatively, diminished muscle tone may be one manifestation of an underlying genetic disease or dysmorphic syndrome, in which case it may persist into childhood or adult life. In some of these conditions, *prenatal hypotonia* is a feature, and diminished fetal movement will have been noted by the mother. A helpful confirmatory sign is the presence of persistent secondary alveolar ridges in the newborn period (see Section 4.8). The detection of significant hypotonia in infancy justifies prompt neurologic consultation and often requires extensive special testing to determine the correct diagnosis. Electromyography, nerve conduction studies, and magnetic resonance imaging or computerized tomography may be called into play for evaluation of the hypotonic newborn.

Muscle weakness is not the same as diminished muscular tone, but the two may be hard to discriminate in infancy. As a general rule, true hypotonia produces abnormalities of posture and inadequate resistance to passive manipulation of the limbs, whereas weakness leads to abnormal movement. At later ages, accurate testing of muscle strength by resistive maneuvers may be possible. Weakness of the levator palpebri superioris muscles produces ptosis, often associated with straight eyelashes (see Section 4.4). Generalized weakness of facial muscles becomes evident by the loss of normal facial expression. An

expressionless face with virtually no muscle movement may represent profound neurologic disease or localized dysfunction of certain nerve pathways, as in Moebius sequence (Fig. 4.21.1A). **Asymmetrical facial movement** or tone also suggests a neurologic impairment, and it is important to differentiate between the central and peripheral types (Fig. 4.21.1B).

A **drooping face** may also indicate a neurologic disorder producing poor muscle tone, but a similar appearance can be caused by a deficiency of skin connective tissue as in cutis laxa (Fig. 4.21.1C). In this condition, of course, the muscles of facial expression are normal, but their effects may be masked by redundant overlying skin. In most of the types of generalized muscular weakness, diminished muscle mass is a feature; in a few of the genetic muscular dystrophies, hypertrophy of affected muscles is the rule, and the consistency of the muscles gradually becomes firm or "woody" to palpation.

Movement disorders such as **ataxia** and **tremor** are found as features of some syndrome diagnoses. In older children, these can be evaluated by standard neurologic examination techniques, but in the infant and toddler, they may be hard to differentiate from normal immaturity of coordination or "jitteriness."

Seizures may produce a broad range of clinical manifestations, and confirmation by

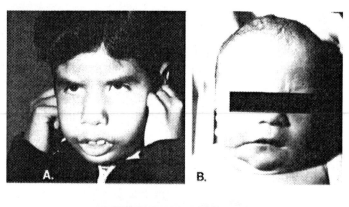

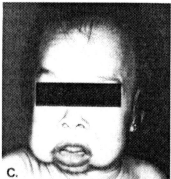

Figure 4.21.1. Expressionless facies. (A) Immobile face in Moebius syndrome. (B) Unilateral loss of facial expression caused by seventh cranial nerve palsy. (C) Face in cutis laxa. Movements of the muscles of facial expression are poorly evident because of loose, redundant facial skin. (Photograph courtesy of Dr. M. Tottori, Honolulu, Hawaii.)

electroencephalography and neurologic consultation should always be sought if a seizure disorder is suspected. In some dysmorphic conditions such as tuberous sclerosis, worsening or intractable seizures may be the first sign to bring the child to medical attention.

Generalized incoordination or **clumsiness** is a feature of a number of dysmorphic disorders and is often associated with conditions in which there is unusually rapid growth, such as Sotos syndrome and Weaver syndrome. Clumsiness usually becomes a problem only after the child has begun to walk, when he begins to run into objects, drop things, and fall frequently. When this tendency is part of a syndrome diagnosis, gradual improvement often takes place over several years, and the problem is usually minimal by teen age. If other neurologic causes are present, however, the clumsiness may become progressive until the child's motor functions are virtually at a standstill.

4.21.1.2. Fine Motor Disturbances

Just as in the case of gross motor dysfunction, abnormalities of fine motor control usually signal a primary neurologic problem, but a few specific fine motor signs may be helpful in the diagnosis of dysmorphic disorders.

Strabismus refers to any deviation of the optic axis of the eyes from parallel in any direction of gaze. *Convergent strabismus* (**esotropia**) and *divergent strabismus* (**exotropia**) are illustrated diagramatically in Fig. 4.21.2. In these conditions, the angle between the optic axes of the two eyes remains roughly the same when the child is looking in any direction. If one eye is consistently used for fixation and the other remains deviated, the deviating eye is designated *eso-* or *exotropic*. If either eye can be used for fixation, the term **alternating eso-** or **exotropia** is applied. There is a high risk of developing amblyopia or *perceptual blindness* in a consistently tropic eye. For unknown reasons, esotropia seems to be more common in children, whereas exotropia prevails in adults.

Another form of strabismus occurs when the gaze is conjugate in some fields of view, but nonconjugate in others. The tendency to "carry" one eye medially or laterally is appropriately called **esophoria** or **exophoria,** respectively. Sometimes these errors of visual tracking are associated with abnormal orbital configuration; *alternating esophoria* is frequently found in children with moderate degrees of hypertelorism, for example. The equivalent term when the gaze in one eye is carried too far upward or downward is **hyperphoria** or **hypophoria,** respectively. These abnormalities are common in children

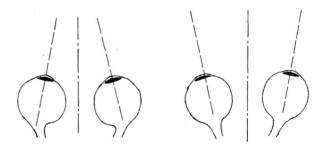

Figure 4.21.2. Diagrams of nonparallel optic axes in strabismus. (A) Convergent strabismus (esotropia). (B) Divergent strabismus (exotropia).   **A**   **B**

with *orbital asymmetry.* An unusual form of strabismus is occasionally seen in individuals with lesions of the central nervous system in the region of the pineal body. The eyes are conjugate in forward gaze but converge when the patient looks up, producing an inverted-V-shaped esophoria. The cause of this phenomenon is unknown.

Nystagmus is a rapid to-and-fro motion of the eyes that has several variations. *Horizontal nystagmus,* the most common, may occur at rest or only during eye movements. Some individuals with constant horizontal nystagmus have perfectly normal visual acuity, whereas others are severely handicapped by this disorder. *Vertical nystagmus* is quite uncommon, as is *pendular nystagmus,* in which the eyes move in a swinging side-to-side fashion. Some of these aberrant eye movements have distinct neurologic significance and, when discovered, justify consultation with a pediatric neurologist or neuro-ophthalmologist.

Dysphagia implies poor coordination of the muscles of the tongue and pharynx and is a feature of such conditions as Smith-Lemli-Opitz syndrome. Affected children may experience aspiration of feedings in infancy and have great difficulty with chewing and swallowing solid foods at later ages. The disability may be so severe as to necessitate placement of a feeding gastrostomy.

4.21.1.3. Autonomic Dysfunctions

The common childhood problems of **constipation** and **diarrhea** usually are transient and self-limiting but can appear in severe and chronic forms in some syndrome diagnoses. Long-standing constipation, such as is found in Opitz-Kaveggia syndrome, responds poorly to the usual laxative regimens and produces a troublesome management problem. On the other hand, severe and unrelenting diarrhea actually may threaten survival and demands immediate intervention. This functional bowel problem may indicate an underlying anomaly such as cystic fibrosis or intestinal lymphangiectasia and is also the hallmark of several metabolic diseases of genetic origin.

An uncommon finding in infants with poor autonomic control of vascular tone is **harlequin discoloration.** The skin capillaries on one side of the body become engorged with blood, while the other side is relatively blanched. There is a sharp demarcation exactly at the midline, and the contrast between the appearance of the two sides of the body is striking. This phenomenon usually occurs when the baby is propped into a position in which she is lying on her side, and the dependent side is the engorged one. If the position in the crib is reversed, the other side will become purple. This condition is almost always benign and self-limiting and only on rare occasions does it signify an underlying neurologic problem.

Some families show an unusual tendency toward **dermatographism** in response to mild trauma. This phenomenon can be elicited by lightly stroking the skin over the back with a fingernail or the edge of a tongue depressor. An immediate flare or reddening of the stroked skin will be seen, followed in a few minutes by a pronounced wheal in the same region, which may persist for an hour or more. This extreme response to minimal trauma seems to be urticarial in nature, probably based on unusual sensitivity of cutaneous mast cells, and is a feature of urticaria pigmentosa. A somewhat similar reaction is seen in instances of severe cortical irritation, such as the early stages of meningitis, when similar stroking of the skin produces bright red lines indicating capillary engorgement but without subsequent wheal formation. This **tache cerebrale** is an ominous sign and, if seen in the absence of an infectious cause, has grave prognostic significance for brain dysfunction.

4.21.2. Behavioral Abnormalities

Many aspects of children's behavior do not lend themselves well to deductive analysis but instead depend on a general impression perceived by the examiner. However, the clinical setting may inhibit some types of behavior and emphasize others, and the brief opportunity for interaction during the usual clinical examination may not provide an accurate picture of a child's usual activity patterns. For this reason, the observations during the exam should be supplemented by specific inquiries directed toward the parents or caretakers about the child's normal behavior at home.

Many children with mild degrees of brain dysfunction demonstrate **hyperactivity.** Tomes have been written on this subject, but for purposes of the dysmorphologic examination, simple observation of the child's ability to sit still, together with a few questions to the parents, should suffice. ("Is Tommy a quiet boy or a busy boy?" "How long can Brenda sit quietly playing with a toy?") Some children with true hyperkinetic activity will seem "driven" by events in their environment and unable to shut out even the most minor outside distractions. More rarely, a child might seem to have some sort of internal timer, set on short cycle. They flit from one activity to another with no apparent external stimulus. Frequently seen in children with fetal alcohol syndrome, this type of activity has been appropriately described as **butterfly behavior.**

The opposite end of the spectrum of spontaneous childhood activity is seen in some patients with certain metabolic disorders that produce **torpid behavior.** These children move slowly, speak slowly, and often seem to think slowly as well. Obvious examples are found in hypothyroidism and the mucopolysaccharidoses, but children with some neurologic conditions such as myotonic dystrophy may also demonstrate slow movements and general hypoactivity.

A few unusual **habit patterns** may provide clues to the existence of an underlying genetic or dysmorphic diagnosis. Children with severe mental deficit from any cause may indulge in a number of stereotyped self-stimulatory activities such as head banging, masturbation, chronic biting of the hands or fingers, and grinding of the teeth (bruxism). Psychiatrically disturbed children may show trichotillomania, plucking or rubbing the hair from areas of the scalp to produce an appearance similar to that of alopecia areata. More specific and diagnostically helpful habit patterns include **blindisms** (the tendency of children with severe visual loss to rub or pat their eyes, probably to produce scotomas as a type of visual self-stimulation) and the **inappropriate laughter** of children with certain hypothalamic lesions and conditions such as Angelmann syndrome. Girls with Rett syndrome show characteristic **hand-wringing** motions almost continuously during waking hours, while boys with Lesch-Nyhan syndrome seem to have a compulsion toward **self-mutilation** such that they repeatedly bite their lips, tongue, and fingers, often causing severe injuries and loss of tissue.

Voice characteristics make up one other aspect of behavior that may have diagnostic importance. Unusually low vocal pitch may be caused by connective tissue disorders such as cutis laxa, while a persisting treble voice may be the result of laryngeal malformation or growth failure, as in panhypopituitarism. A high-pitched **mewing cry** is one of the hallmarks of the appropriately named cri-du-chat syndrome. Heard primarily during the newborn period, the sound most commonly has been likened to that of a kitten or a distant seagull—weak and high, with a rapidly falling pitch. In contrast, a **hoarse voice** will be present in some children with thickening of the vocal cords caused by edema or deposition of abnormal metabolic products. Complete **aphonia** rarely may be produced by laryngeal clefts.

5

Arriving at a Dysmorphologic Diagnosis

*Like all other arts, the Science of Deduction
and Analysis is one which can only be acquired
by long and patient study, nor is life long
enough to allow any mortal to attain the highest
perfection in it.*
—"The Sign of Four"

5.1. INTRODUCTION

Chapters 3 and 4 outlined techniques of gathering information from the history and physical examination. This chapter addresses the process of sifting, evaluating, and synthesizing these clues in order to reach a final diagnosis. Although much has been written on this topic, most writers emphasize "the scientific method" and hypothesis testing. These theoretical models certainly have value in behavioral research and medical education but often bear only a faint resemblance to the actual techniques used by students, practitioners, and specialists in their day-to-day work.

There may be as many diagnostic styles as there are diagnosticians, and no one can or should adhere slavishly to a single approach for every clinical situation. From the broad spectrum of possible strategies, however, a few seem to emerge as archetypes. At the risk of oversimplification, I will briefly consider the strengths and weaknesses of three of these as a basis for discussion of an appropriate approach to diagnosis of the child with birth defects.

5.2. COMMON STRATEGIES IN THE PROCESS OF DIAGNOSIS

5.2.1. The Scotland Yard Model

*I have been down to see friend Lestrade at the
Yard. There may be an occasional want of
imaginative intuition down there, but they lead
the world for thoroughness and method.*
—"The Three Garridebs"

In medical training, instruction in the art of diagnosis may take several forms, but emphasis usually is placed on what might be called the classic, linear/recursive, or Scotland Yard technique. This procedure involves a number of clearly defined sequential

259

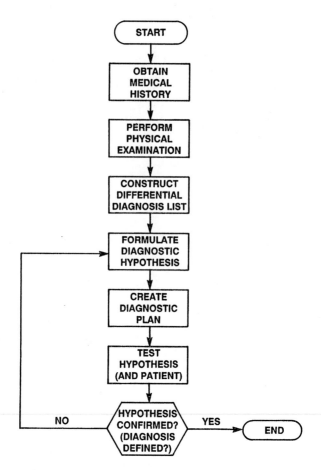

Figure 5.1. Diagnostic strategies: The Scotland Yard model.

steps (Fig. 5.1). The medical history, social history, and review of systems are obtained and recorded in a set format, and the physical examination also is performed according to a fixed protocol. Consistent with the scientific method, all this theoretically takes place before any diagnostic conclusions are entertained. Next, a differential diagnosis list is created, and then a diagnostic plan is formulated to determine which of these possibilities best accounts for the patient's problems. Discrimination among the various possible diagnoses is accomplished by laboratory testing, by X-ray and other imaging techniques, and sometimes by trials of therapy. Beginning with the most likely, each diagnostic hypothesis is examined, and if it cannot be substantiated, it is discarded and another is put forward, to be tested in turn. A final diagnosis is achieved when all of the competing candidates can be eliminated.

Like the mills of the gods, this "by-the-book" approach grinds slow but exceeding fine. The process demands and rewards thoroughness, and for this reason it is time consuming and relatively inefficient and may be quite expensive, since it often entails hospitalization of the patient. If the data-gathering phase (history and physical examination) is performed as a rote drill, there is a danger that important information will be overlooked or ignored. This approach also encourages extensive and sometimes random or "shotgun" testing, which may come to be regarded as part of the data-gathering phase rather than as an aid in discriminating among competing diagnostic possibilities. The value of the technique hinges on the completeness and pertinence of the differential diagnosis list, the assembly of which is the only really creative part of the exercise and the greatest challenge to the neophyte. With enough persistence, however, the achievement of an accurate diagnosis is almost assured. Furthermore, this technique is easy to teach and evaluate, and it can be used in the earliest stages of medical training, since clinical experience plays only a minor role in its use. For these reasons, the Scotland Yard model remains the standard for teaching clinical diagnosis in most training programs.

5.2.2. The Doctor Watson Model

Excellent, Watson! Compound of the Busy Bee
and Excelsior.
— "The Creeping Man"

Experienced clinicians often seem to use a process of diagnostic reasoning that is at once more complex, more idiosyncratic, and less formal than the theoretical ideal. This process bears more resemblance to solving a puzzle than to following a computer algorithm. It usually abbreviates and blends many of the separate steps of the classic model (Fig. 5.2) and involves a large component of pattern recognition based on prior experience (the "Aha! response"). The method is both efficient and practical in most clinical situations.

An initial diagnostic hunch is formulated almost as soon as the patient's symptoms

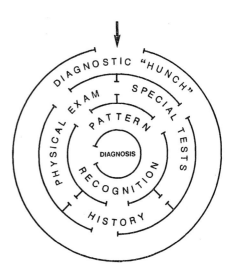

Figure 5.2. Diagnostic strategies: The Doctor Watson model.

are presented, and the ensuing history taking and physical examination may be quite limited in scope, directed toward confirmation of this notion. Dozens of elements, such as the age and sex of the patient, duration of the illness, characteristic physical signs, and "what's going around this season" are factored into the diagnostic equation, rapidly and often unconsciously. If the first clinical impression is not supported by the results of the initial history and physical findings, a new diagnostic guess is made, and the net is cast more broadly to seek further information that might confirm the new hypothesis.

In this model, diagnosis is accomplished largely by recognition of known disease entities, and the success of the technique depends to a large extent on the accumulated clinical experience and the knowledge base of the physician. Happily, physicians soon become both proficient and careful in using this new strategy, and since the more common maladies are seen most often, their recognition is continually reinforced. The process is efficient in the use of time for both patient and diagnostician, and the resulting diagnosis has a high degree of probability in practical terms. The greatest pitfall in this method, however, lies in the danger of misdiagnosis of conditions with which the practitioner is not familiar, and thus the Dr. Watson model frequently falls short in the diagnosis of rare disorders.

5.2.3. The Sherlock Holmes Model

> *You know my method. It is founded upon the*
> *observance of trifles.*
> —"The Boscombe Valley Mystery"

The diagnostic strategy of the Sherlock Holmes model combines the worst features of the first two, but in so doing it achieves the greatest usefulness in the diagnosis of rare medical conditions. As in the Scotland Yard model, the process begins with a detailed and complete medical history and a meticulous physical examination (Fig. 5.3). On the basis of this information, a few pivotal features are selected, and these are compared with those found in disorders already familiar to the diagnostician or recorded in the medical literature. Confirmation by laboratory or other testing is not often available, and the final diagnosis most commonly rests entirely on the "goodness of fit" between the observed clinical and historic features and those of a recognized syndrome.

Obviously, this diagnostic technique consumes a great deal of time, both in the data-gathering phase and in the often extensive search of medical literature necessary to identify rare syndromes. Furthermore, as in the Dr. Watson model, its success depends heavily on the pattern recognition abilities of the diagnostician. Countering these disadvantages, the Sherlock Holmes strategy permits diagnosis of exceedingly rare disorders, even in the face of confusing variability in their clinical presentation.

From the terminology chosen to describe these diagnostic techniques, the reader may detect a prejudice toward the third model for use in dysmorphologic diagnosis. In fact, the remainder of this chapter will be devoted to further description of the Sherlock Holmes method and some examples of its practical application.

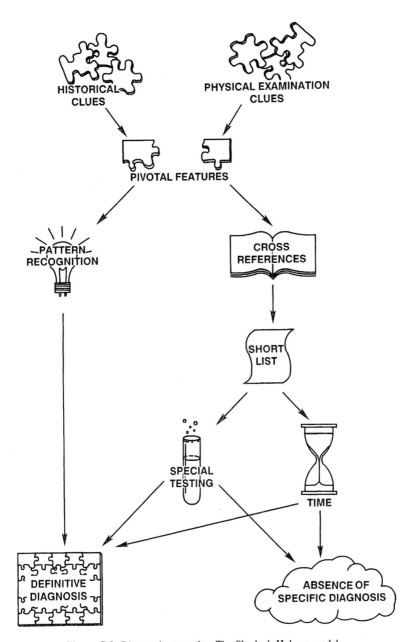

Figure 5.3. Diagnostic strategies: The Sherlock Holmes model.

5.3. PRINCIPLES OF DYSMORPHOLOGIC DIAGNOSIS

> *The ideal reasoner would, when he has once*
> *been shown a single fact in all its bearings,*
> *deduce from it not only all the chain of events*
> *which led up to it, but also all the results which*
> *would follow from it.*
> —"The Five Orange Pips"

Although no theoretical construct can do more than approximate what happens in the real world, it is easier to discuss the various steps of the Sherlock Holmes model as if they consisted of four separate activities: data gathering, analysis, synthesis, and definition. Each of these functions actually does take place in the diagnostic process, but they intermingle and overlap a great deal. With increasing experience, each person will develop his or her own approach, but in almost every diagnostic encounter these elements appear in some form. None of what follows is intended as a prescription for orthodox diagnostic behavior, but rather as a "tool kit" from which may be selected those techniques most useful in a specific situation.

5.3.1. Data-Gathering Phase

> *It is a capital mistake to theorize before you*
> *have all the evidence. It biases the judgment.*
> —"A Study in Scarlet"

In Chapter 3, the process of obtaining a complete genetic and medical history was outlined. In principle, this simply involves the transfer of information between the historian and the examiner. In practice, any medical history should be considered incomplete, subjective, and indispensable. The examiner must cultivate patience as well as the ability to listen and ask the right questions, because whatever its faults, historical information provides the foundation for all that follows.

The physical examination offers evidence that is considerably more objective, but its value depends not only on the examiner's skill in observing and eliciting physical signs but, even more importantly, on an ability to discriminate the normal from the suspicious or the downright aberrant. Here, nothing can take the place of clinical experience and a solid grounding in gross anatomy.

During this phase of the diagnostic process, it is vital to keep an open mind. Preconceived notions about the diagnosis may interfere with the detection of those very clues that point toward an alternative explanation. This does not mean, however, that one should stop thinking while obtaining the history and performing the physical exam. Data gathering is an active, not a passive, process, and the discovery of one fact often prompts the search for related ones. Keep thinking.

5.3.2. The Analytic Phase

> *Never trust to general impressions, my boy, but*
> *concentrate yourself upon details.*
> — "A Case of Identity"

Analysis entails breaking down into its component parts the overall clinical picture presented by the patient. This stage of the diagnostic process unavoidably overlaps that of data gathering, as the diagnostician identifies significant individual elements of the history and discrete physical findings that will be used as the building blocks to construct a diagnosis. The key here is defining which facts are really significant. Data are sifted to separate the pertinent from the inconsequential: the mother's exposure to acetaminophen during the last trimester may be disregarded; normal variants in the physical exam are identified and set aside. Here again, the examiner's knowledge, experience, and judgment come into play.

Some of the individual facts ascertained in this phase will prove to be more diagnostically helpful than others. These pivotal findings form the basis for differential diagnosis, providing a means for fairly rapid and efficient weighing of a vast number of rare syndrome entities. Selection of physical signs for this purpose is largely an art in which there is no substitute for experience and wide familiarity with the literature, but a few hints may be of help.

The best clues are the rarest. The physical features that will be the most helpful in differential diagnosis are those which are infrequently seen either in isolation or as a part of syndromes. Quite often, these are not the most obvious anomalies nor even the ones that have the greatest significance for the patient's health. It is easy to become distracted by the presence of a major anomaly, such as a large omphalocele, and miss the diagnostic importance of a seemingly negligible feature such as a large tongue. As another example, a small midline cleft of the upper lip is found in only a handful of dysmorphic syndromes, whereas a classic cleft lip is a feature of over 200.

Some anomalies may occur only sporadically as part of a larger pattern of malformation and therefore are of less value for diagnostic purposes. For example, a dysmorphic syndrome may include some type of congenital heart disease, but this feature may be present in less than half of the reported cases. By and large, any of the multifactorial abnormalities that are commonly seen as isolated defects (clubfoot, cleft palate, congenital hip dislocation, etc.) are poor choices as pivotal clues because their relationship to syndrome diagnoses is facultative rather than definitive.

All things being equal, it is better to choose as a pivotal finding that anomaly which has the earliest embryonic origin. Some of the structural anomalies arising later in intrauterine life may prove to be secondary effects of an earlier malformation, such as aberrant palmar crease patterning resulting from bone dysplasia or a cleft palate caused by micrognathia.

In most cases, only three or four key features need to be designated before one begins the synthesis phase. This number is usually sufficient to eliminate most of the "impossible" diagnoses, and more than this makes the search cumbersome.

5.3.3. The Synthetic Phase

> *It is of the highest importance in the art of detection to be able to recognize, out of a number of facts, which are incidental and which vital.*
> — "The Reigate Squires"

Information may be obtained piecemeal, but the value of each fact lies in its relationship to other facts. The next step, then, is to try to find relationships among the individual elements ascertained by analysis. The first level of synthesis is simply to decide whether the patient displays any features of dysmorphogenesis at all. If not, a final diagnosis of "absence of dysmorphic disorder" has been achieved, and the evaluation is completed. This conclusion is not infrequent in children referred primarily because of vague concerns about unusual facial appearance, growth discrepancies, or neurologic or behavioral disorders. Of course, this "diagnosis" is only part of the answer in such cases, and the patient may need further evaluation or therapy to deal with the actual problems present.

The next level of synthesis is reached if the patient does have one or more congenital anomalies. Here, a decision must be made concerning the underlying nature of the abnormalities. Malformations, disruptions, deformations, and statistical variants have widely differing implications for the patient and his family. At this stage, the examiner's knowledge of embryology plays a major role. For example, recognizing that two seemingly unrelated defects have the same embryologic origin may provide the key to an understanding of the entire clinical picture. Increasing experience in this phase of the process leads to more rapid, accurate, and "automatic" clustering of isolated facts into meaningful associations.

The third level of decision making involves the discrimination of isolated anomalies from syndromic patterns. Some single-system defects may produce a cascade of related phenomena, such as the hydrocephalus, sphincter paralysis, and limb weakness found in open neural tube defects. These sequences must be differentiated from true syndromes, and the decisions are often difficult. Characteristically, dysmorphic syndromes either show widespread abnormalities of a single body system, such as the skeletal defects in bone dysplasias, or multiple malformations of structures derived from different embryologic tissues, as seen in chromosomal anomalies. Deformations and disruptions may involve diverse body areas, but their distinctive effects are usually easy to recognize.

The final stage of synthesis takes place if no specific diagnosis can be achieved at one of the earlier steps. The pivotal clues defined in the analysis phase serve as points of entry for a search of the dysmorphology literature. In this case, the final product of the synthesis phase is the generation of a short list of possible diagnoses.

The best starting place for a search is the index or differential diagnosis section in such classic texts as Jones (1988). The simplest strategy is to list separately all conditions in which the first pivotal clue is found, then those having the second anomaly, and so on. The lists are then compared, and any syndromes appearing on all or most of them become the leading candidates for the syndrome definition phase. If no good diagnostic possibilities are found, additional pivotal clues are defined, and the procedure is repeated. On the other hand, if a dozen or more candidates are found, the diagnostic criteria are usually too broad and nonspecific. It is then worthwhile to try to shorten the list by defining one or more new pivotal findings.

This may seem a rather mechanical approach to diagnosis, but it actually replicates the mental processes used by clinicians in recognizing more common disorders. It is a bit slow and laborious, however, and for this reason several computer programs have been devised to handle the same task (see References).

5.3.4. The Syndrome Definition Phase

> *It is an old maxim of mine that when you have*
> *excluded the impossible, whatever remains,*
> *however improbable, must be the truth.*
> —"The Beryl Coronet"

When the short list of possible diagnoses has been drawn up, the next step is to refer to the brief summaries in books such as Jones (1988) to determine the other anomalies characteristic of each disorder still under consideration. Here, it is important to take into account the inherent clinical variability of dysmorphic syndromes. Very few patients will have all of the features mentioned in the texts. Therefore, the absence of some specific anomalies may not rule out a particular condition, but the presence of discordant features often can. Compare the syndrome descriptions with the findings in the patient not only in terms of physical anomalies but as to age of onset, natural history, and possible genetic factors as well.

Often this process will allow confirmation of a specific diagnosis. If it does not, and the search has been narrowed to two or three remaining possibilities, it is worthwhile exploring these further in the dysmorphology literature. Information in original articles, monographs, and specialized texts will help establish the spectrum of variability of each disorder, potential laboratory aids to diagnosis, and other manifestations that could be sought in the patient. Such references may also bring to light other diagnostic possibilities to be considered as well as details of genetic transmission, prognosis, and potential treatment.

Before a final diagnosis is attained, it may be necessary to see the patient again, to search for confirmatory findings in the history or physical exam, or to perform some special testing. As mentioned earlier, such testing can be used to confirm only a few congenital syndromes at present, although current research into the biochemical basis of genetic disease holds great promise for clinical application in the future. Diagnostic tests should be selected carefully to avoid needless discomfort, cost, and duplication and to provide the best possible discrimination between competing diagnoses.

On occasion, the best means of differentiating among several diagnostic possibilities may be monitoring the patient's clinical course over months or years. The development or disappearance of physical signs, pace of intellectual progress, and statural growth all may provide helpful clues pointing to a specific diagnostic entity. Rarely, the final definition of a diagnosis occurs through serendipity, as when the birth of another affected relative reveals a clear inheritance pattern that clinches the identity of the syndrome.

Inevitably, the diagnostic process is sometimes unsuccessful. (In fact, most dysmorphology units report that less than half of all children with unrecognized multiple malformation syndromes receive a definite final diagnosis.) In such cases, there may arise a temptation to force the patient into an inappropriate diagnostic category, if only to have something to tell the parents or the referring physician. It is far better to provide a qualified diagnosis (see below) or no diagnosis at all and schedule the patient for reevaluation at a later time. In the interval, new clinical clues may emerge, "new" syndromes may be described, or specific diagnostic tests may be developed that will allow definitive diagnosis.

Thus, the definition process may have three different outcomes. If it is successful (or if a syndrome has been recognized at an earlier stage), a final diagnosis results. Inability to differentiate among several known conditions may lead to a deferred diagnosis, and if *all* recognized dysmorphic disorders have been eliminated from consideration, a "bookmark" designation such as "unknown syndrome" or "provisionally unique malformation complex" may be assigned.

Each of these categories has different implications for further action. If a final diagnosis has been achieved, counseling can be provided concerning prognosis, recurrence risk, and any available options for treatment. A deferred diagnosis implies the prospect of further testing or surveillance to allow differentiation among the remaining diagnostic possibilities. A child with an unknown syndrome also may require follow-up visits and further testing, but in the absence of other recognized cases to provide guidance, meaningful counseling is difficult or impossible.

5.3.5. The Pattern Recognition Shunt

> *As a rule, when I have heard some slight indication of the course of events, I am able to guide myself by the thousands of other similar cases which occur to my memory.*
> — "The Red-Headed League"

The highest level of synthesis of dysmorphologic information is the recognition of a pattern of physical and historical features that defines a specific syndrome diagnosis. This process is more complicated than it sounds and probably involves quite sophisticated reasoning methods that are not yet well understood. For example, each of the letters in Fig. 5.4 is immediately and easily recognizable despite wide variation in typographic style, size, and orientation. Humans easily process subtle visual cues to accomplish such pattern recognition, but even the most sophisticated computer programs are still unable to duplicate this feat. In some instances, a dysmorphologic diagnosis can snap into focus suddenly, like the hidden image in an optical illusion. In fact, many dysmorphic conditions, such as Down syndrome, have features familiar enough to allow diagnosis virtually at a glance. In such cases, the diagnostic process can be "short-circuited" from the analysis stage directly to the definition stage.

Disparaging remarks have been made about the "Aunt Minnie" school of diagnosis, the implication being that simple familiarity, rather than rigorous analysis, is a weak foundation for a diagnostic conclusion. It is true that those who rely heavily on this technique run the risk of jumping to unsubstantiated conclusions and diagnostically mis-

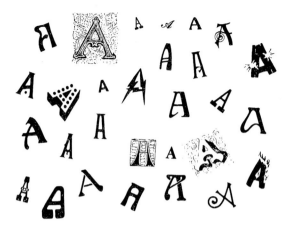

Figure 5.4. Instantly recognizable variations of a single meaningful pattern—the letter "A."

labeling their patients. Most dysmorphic syndromes, however, show considerable variation even in their most characteristic features. The real value of pattern recognition, therefore, is the ability to identify Aunt Minnie even when she is wearing a wig or playing the bagpipes. Used with caution and appropriate safeguards, this intuitive recognition of a diagnostic entity can be useful and efficient.

Sometimes the first clue to a diagnosis will come from recognizing a subtle resemblance between a patient and a photograph in a paper or book. This requires good visual memory and is rather haphazard, but it occasionally produces satisfying results. Unfortunately, retrieval of a pertinent reference is much more difficult by using pictorial clues than by the pivotal findings method.

Pattern recognition obviously becomes easier and more dependably accurate with both broadening experience and a deepening fund of knowledge. The more patients one has seen with a particular diagnosis, the more likely that the next will be correctly identified. Similarly, acquaintance with a wide variety of congenital syndromes allows more accurate categorization of the specific constellation of anomalies in a given patient. Experience, of course, has its own set of disadvantages, the primary one being a tendency to make the same mistakes over and over again.

5.3.6. Qualifying the Diagnosis

To a logician, all things should be seen exactly
as they are . . . .
— "The Greek Interpreter"

The most desirable outcome of the dysmorphology evaluation is the establishment of an unequivocal diagnosis. There are many occasions, however, when this is impossible, and the diagnosis must be qualified in some manner. If there is evidence for a certain syndrome but not enough to define the diagnosis with absolute certainty, modifiers such as "possible" and "probable" can be used. In such cases, reevaluation should be planned in the hope of removing any uncertainty as soon as possible.

Sometimes, multiple birth defects are present but the pattern cannot be identified as a known dysmorphic condition, even after pursuing the entire diagnostic protocol outlined above. In such instances, it is best to use a term such as "unknown syndrome" or "provisionally unique pattern of multiple malformations." To this can be added any additional information that may be available, such as evident inheritance patterns or suspected teratogenic influences. It is also good practice to record three of the pivotal clinical features to aid in later retrieval of the case record. Thus, a diagnostic entry might read "trigoncephaly, blepharophimosis, and hypoplastic nails: unknown syndrome, probable autosomal dominant." The objective is to specify the diagnosis only to the level of certainty and to record enough information to allow comparison with "new" syndromes that may eventually come to light.

5.3.7. When No Diagnosis Fits

> *There is nothing more stimulating than a case*
> *where everything goes against you.*
> *—The Hound of the Baskervilles*

The emphasis of this chapter has been on arriving at an accurate, timely, and specific diagnosis. Unfortunately, even under the best of circumstances, this may not be possible. Do not panic. The absence of a diagnosis may be distressing to the diagnostician and the family, but it is much less dangerous than the possibility of assigning the wrong diagnosis, with the risk of erroneous genetic and prognostic counseling and possibly hazardous treatment. Except in real emergencies, in which life-threatening anomalies demand immediate therapeutic intervention, there is almost always time to see the patient again, to pursue the pertinent literature, and to follow the clinical course. Moreover, in most instances the therapy that we have to offer, such as surgical repair, physical therapy, and intellectual testing, is directed toward obvious problems that can still be addressed even without a specific diagnosis. If in doubt, wait and be sure.

On the other hand, it is equally important not to defer judgment to the point that important aspects of counseling are neglected. For example, in many instances an unknown constellation of congenital anomalies could be caused by homozygosity for a recessive gene. Under these circumstances, the parents need to know of the potential one-in-four recurrence risk in order to make informed decisions about their future reproduction. It is equally important not to create a false sense of security in the parents when no definitive diagnosis can be reached. When told that their child "does not have a recognized diagnosis," the family may conclude that there is nothing really wrong and thus neglect his very real needs.

The Golden Rule is: Be sure the family understands everything you know (and don't know) about their child's condition.

5.3.8. Envoi

Come, Watson, Come!
The game is afoot!
— "The Abbey Grange"

A final diagnosis is just the beginning. Now the emphasis changes from *gathering* information to *providing* information—from reasoning to action. The first order of business is explaining the diagnosis and its implications in understandable terms to the parents and, if possible, to the patient. Next comes mobilization of whatever resources may be necessary to initiate treatment, define associated problems, and provide appropriate testing and rehabilitation. Finally, arrangements will be needed for longterm follow-up and support for the family. With the rapid pace of progress in the field, future contacts may be necessary because of new developments in therapy, the discovery of previously unrecognized complications, or new methods for genetic screening of family members.

An accurate dysmorphologic diagnosis may provide an intellectually satisfying explanation of a child's pattern of abnormalities, but much more importantly, it forms the basis for taking action to help the child and family. It can bring relief for parents' feelings of guilt or blame, and may even prevent a groundless lawsuit. But there is one thing a diagnosis does *not* do: it does not convert a child into a label. He or she is still a unique individual with physical and emotional needs which must be met. The diagnosis may, however, change *our* perceptions and expectations, ideally in ways leading to the most appropriate care, guidance, and counseling for our patient.

Appendixes

A

Special Examination Techniques

While general examination methods for each body region were outlined in Chapter 4, there are several other aids to diagnosis that have too low a "return" or are too cumbersome or time consuming to use routinely but may be valuable in special cases.

USE OF A MAGNIFYING LENS

In true Sherlockian fashion, the dysmorphologist often can make use of a low-power magnifying glass (3–5×). Although the 4-inch-diameter, brass-bound version bears a certain aura of authenticity and antique charm, a smaller lens with a built-in illuminator is more efficient and portable. Several inexpensive models made for stamp or coin collectors are sold in hobby stores. In a pinch, an otoscope or ophthalmoscope can be used for magnification. These have the advantage of a good light supply, but their field of view is severely limited.

Most frequently, a hand lens will be used to examine fine details of skin anatomy such as dermatoglyphic patterns or nevi. The iris also can be inspected with a simple magnifier, although the use of an ophthalmoscope set at +10 diopters provides better illumination and is less threatening to younger patients.

USE OF THE WOOD'S LAMP

A source of low-frequency ultraviolet radiation, the Wood's lamp finds its chief use in dermatology, where it makes certain lesions fluoresce in characteristic colors. Dysmorphologists use this instrument to help in the detection of the hypopigmented skin zones commonly seen in tuberous sclerosis. The examination should be carried out in the darkest room available, with the lamp help quite close to the skin, and special attention should be directed to the trunk, where most of the lesions appear. Genuine *ash-leaf* spots stand out rather clearly with this technique as pale patches on dull surrounding skin but they do not glow brightly.

A number of substances found on the skin may show unexpected and confusing fluorescence under ultraviolet light. Hand creams, medicinal ointments, and some cosmetics often produce areas of a light blue color. The edges of such zones will be poorly defined, and the materials can be removed with an alcohol pledget. Calluses, nails, and dead skin fluoresce yellow-brown. Additives in detergents and some other household products can impart a startling blue-white glow to clothing, and the dyes in some fabrics and food products reflect a dull red hue.

Another helpful sign revealed by examination under ultraviolet light is fluorescence of the teeth. A yellow-orange glow under a Wood's lamp suggests dental staining by prenatal exposure to tetracycline, while a dull red fluorescence of the teeth may be seen in porphyria.

SWEAT PORE ANALYSIS

Sweat glands are distributed over the entire skin surface but show variations of spacing in different regions. Some types of ectodermal dysplasia are marked by a paucity of these glands, and a quantitative estimate of sweat pore distribution can help in the differential diagnosis of such conditions. Furthermore, female carriers of the gene for X-linked hypohidrotic ectodermal dysplasia have diminished numbers of sweat glands, a fact helpful in genetic counseling.

Estimates of sweat pore distribution can be obtained in several ways. The easiest is counting the pits that surmount the dermal ridges on the fingertips, either by direct inspection with high power (10×) magnification or from a good fingerprint (see Appendix B). Normally these sweat gland orifices are evenly spaced, averaging 10 to each centimeter of ridge length. Markedly wider spacing or uneven distribution suggests a carrier state for X-linked ectodermal dysplasia, whereas virtual absence of pores indicates involvement with one of the hypohidrotic forms of the disorder.

Sweat pores also may be mapped by using chemical methods. In the time-honored technique, the skin is washed and dried and then painted with tincture of iodine. When the iodine has thoroughly dried, the area is dusted with starch powder. Moisture from the sweat glands permits the two substances to react to produce a tiny blue-black dot over each sweat pore. A more elegant and faster method uses a plastic compound dissolved in a volatile organic solvent to form a flexible film on the skin. This can then be peeled away and analyzed under a dissecting microscope for the number and distribution of the sweat pores.

EXAMINATION OF HAIR SHAFTS

In children with sparse or fragile hair, the configuration of the hair shafts may be of help in diagnosis. A few dozen hairs are clipped from an inconspicuous area of the scalp and placed on a microscope slide, where they are held in place by using either immersion oil and a cover slip or transparent plastic tape. Under a low- to medium-power lens, the hair shafts are examined for uniformity of caliber, breakage, or unusual structural features.

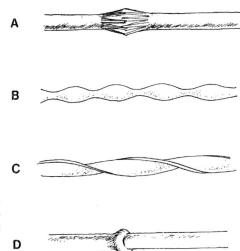

A

B

C

D

Figure A.1. Microscopic appearance of hair shafts in conditions causing fragility of hair. (All drawings magnified approximately 30×) (A) Trichorrhexis nodosa. (B) Monilethrix. (C) Pili torti. (D) Trichorrhexis invaginata.

Hair fragility may be caused by several different pathological processes that produce characteristic changes in the structure of hair. In trichorrhexis nodosa (Fig. A.1A), localized zones of dysplasia produce an appearance resembling two paintbrushes whose bristles are pushed together end to end. Abrupt angulation or fracture of the hair occurs through these zones, often accompanied by longitudinal splitting. Monilethrix (Fig. A.1B) produces evenly spaced regions of narrowing along the hair shaft, giving a beaded appearance. Fracture occurs in the constricted zones. *Pili torti* is the term used for kinky, brittle hair that is irregularly twisted on its long axis (Fig. A.1C). Trichorrhexis invaginata (Fig. A.1D) produces a microscopic appearance resembling a stalk of bamboo. At intervals along the length of the hair, the distal hair shaft seems to be pushed down into the proximal portion, resulting in a distinct bulge where breakage is likely to occur.

TESTING FOR STRABISMUS

In cooperative older children and adults, the position of the corneal light reflex is a helpful indicator for small degrees of fixed strabismus. The patient looks toward a bright window, room light, or flashlight held several feet away. The light will be seen reflected from a point centered over the pupil in the "fixing" eye but will be displaced in the deviant eye—medially in exotropia and laterally in esotropia. The standard "cover test" also can be used to assess strabismus. The patient is asked to focus on a distant object, and one eye is occluded with a card or the examiner's hand. When the cover is quickly removed, any lateral movement of the uncovered eye is noted. The process is repeated several times on each side. A consistent readjustment of one eye when the other is covered and uncovered suggests weakness of the extraocular muscles on that side.

In younger children, the Brueckner test is helpful in defining strabismus. The internal lenses of an ophthalmoscope are set at 0 diopters, and the widest light beam is shined on the patient's face from a distance of about 3 feet. The position of the bright, white corneal reflexes can then be judged. In addition, the yellow-red retinal reflex will appear in each pupil. The color and intensity of this reflection should be equal on the two sides. When strabismus is present, the deviant eye will show a slightly brighter and yellower reflex and an apparently larger pupil than the fixing eye. This is because of the slightly different path traveled by the light beam through the ocular lens and the more reflective nature of the retina in areas outside the macula.

MEASUREMENT OF JOINT RANGE OF MOTION

In some instances, documentation of the range of movement of one or more joints may be helpful, especially in long-term follow-up joint contractures. Accurate determination of the joint angles is best accomplished with a goniometer, which is simply a protractor with an extended base and a long rotating indicator arm. Simple goniometers often can be obtained from orthopedic appliance manufacturers. The zero point on the instrument is centered over the joint in question, which is then moved to one extreme of its range of motion. The two arms of the goniometer are lined up with the axes of the limb on either side of the joint, and the included angle is read directly from the protractor scale. This technique is not well suited to evaluation of some joint movement, such as rotation at the elbow or flexion and extension of the phalanges, but with a little ingenuity, the protractor scale still can be used to obtain a rough approximation of angular distances in these regions (see Table 4.19.1).

B

Dermatoglyphics

> *"Look at that with your magnifying glass, Mr. Holmes."*
> *"Yes, I am doing so."*
> *"You are aware that no two thumb-marks are alike?"*
> *"I have heard something of the kind."*
> — "The Norwood Builder"

In humans, dermal ridges are found only on the palms and soles, where they form patterns of greater or less complexity, from simple fields of parallel lines to intricate swirls and arabesques. The term *dermatoglyphics* (literally, "skin carvings") is used to distinguish these patterns from the flexion creases found in the same areas. The final configuration of dermal ridge patterns is influenced by the contours of the soft tissue pads underlying the volar and plantar skin during the first half of gestation (Fig. 4.20.2). The dermal ridges seem to be arranged around these pads in much the same way that furrows plowed in a field follow the contours of a hill. Dermatoglyphic patterns can be found on the hands by week 19, and once they have been laid down are fixed for life.

In the 1890s, criminologists first recognized that each individual's fingerprints are virtually unique and therefore can be used for purposes of identification. Much of the information on the fine structure of dermatoglyphics and the population distributions of various types of print patterns has come from the field of criminology. More recently, medical interest in dermatoglyphic analysis was kindled by the discovery that some genetic and dysmorphic syndromes often showed characteristic arrangements of dermal lines on the palms and soles. Further investigation, however, revealed that no specific array of dermal ridge patterns is actually pathognomonic for a particular congenital disorder, and for this reason the role of dermatoglyphics in dysmorphologic diagnosis has come to be peripheral rather than central. This appendix briefly outlines some of the principles and techniques of medical dermatoglyphic analysis.

EMBRYOLOGY AND ANATOMY

As mentioned above, the configuration of dermal patterns seems to be determined by the size and shape of the soft tissue mounds found on the digits, palms, and soles during the middle trimester of gestation (see Fig. 4.20.2). Vestiges of these mounds sometimes persist after birth, and their apices can be seen to coincide with the center of the overlying dermatoglyphic formations. High, symmetrically conical mounds give rise to concentric whorl patterns; asymmetric pads induce loops, while very low or absent tissue mounds produce arches or open-field configurations.

Along the crests of the dermal ridges, sweat pores appear as tiny, evenly spaced dimples that can be seen as white dots on a good print. The fine structure of individual ridges may vary considerably, producing features such as interruptions, islands, and branches. These minutiae are helpful for the forensic specialist but usually are of negligible help in medical diagnosis.

Dermal ridge patterns can be disrupted, distorted, or obliterated by trauma but are only locally obscured by the flexion creases that they traverse.

The most important landmarks in dermatoglyphic analysis are the central points of the patterns and the triradii formed when three ridge systems meet. Loops will be flanked by a single triradius, whorls by two or more, and simple arches by none. Normally, triradii are also found on the palm at the base of each finger and are designated as points a–d from the radial to the ulnar side. An axial triradius (t) appears near the midline distal to the wrist crease at the base of the palm. The size of a dermatoglyphic pattern may be defined numerically by counting the number of ridges cut by a line drawn between the center of the pattern and any adjoining triradii. By definition, the ridge count of a simple arch is zero, while that of a whorl is the sum of two or more counts, one for each flanking triradius.

EXAMINATION METHODS

In older children and adults, the dermatoglyphic patterns often can be studied easily with the naked eye, but a low-power magnifying glass, preferably with a built-in light source, may be of great help. In examining dermal patterns in newborns and young children, such magnification is indispensable. Neonates, and especially premature babies, often have macerated palmar skin and quite indistinct dermal ridges. In such instances, a higher-power glass, oblique lighting, and considerable patience may allow an adequate dermatoglyphic inspection, but in some cases nothing works and the examination must be deferred. Evaluation of the dermal patterns of a stillborn fetus sometimes can be accomplished by use of a binocular dissecting microscope, unless sloughing of the palmar skin has taken place.

The results of the visual inspection can be recorded in detail or simply summarized in the written report, depending on the circumstances. In rare instances, it may be desirable to obtain a permanent record of the dermatoglyphic patterns. This can be done by a number of methods, including the use of wet or dry ink on paper, latex molds, or even an electrostatic copying machine. One technique that provides adequate results even in young or uncooperative children (but not newborns) makes use of broad pieces of transparent plastic tape. The volar surface of the hand is first dried and then rubbed with crumpled carbon paper or a stick of solid graphite, to coat the skin with a thin but even layer of dry pigment. The tape is then smoothed over the palm from the wrist crease to the fingertips, including the sides of the fingers and thumb as much as possible. When the tape is peeled away, again starting at the wrist, it will bear a positive image of the dermatoglyphic patterns, outlined in dark pigment. The tape can be placed on a siliconized backing paper or a sheet of clear acetate for analysis and storage.

INTERPRETATION OF DERMATOGLYPHIC PATTERNS

The configuration of dermal ridge patterns is strongly influenced by genetic factors that seem to act primarily on formation of the fetal soft tissue pads. Both the types of patterns (arches, loops, or whorls) and their size are inherited in a polygenic fashion. Large population studies have revealed that total ridge counts on the fingertips of children lie close to the mean of the ridge counts of their parents. Monozygotic twins usually have very similar but not completely identical dermal ridge distributions. Some ethnic groups show characteristic distributions of dermatoglyphic patterns. For example, American Indians and Eskimos display a predominance of whorl patterns on the fingertips, which produces a higher average ridge count for members of these groups. These genetic influences must be taken into account when dermatoglyphic patterns are used for diagnostic purposes, and the prints of parents or other close relatives should be examined before one accepts a specific pattern as evidence of a dysmorphic disorder.

The configurations of dermal ridges on the fingertips are the most diagnostically helpful, followed by those of the palm. Toetip patterns are too small and variable to be of much value, but the hallucal area over the ball of the foot has been used in conjunction with digital and palmar patterns in the diagnosis of Down syndrome.

In most populations, the commonest fingertip patterns are loops, which are categorized as ulnar or radial by the direction in which their "open" ends point. A loop may be composed of a single recurved ridge. Next most frequent are whorls, which may form a concentric, "bull's-eye" system, a spiral, or a complex pattern consisting of two interlocked loops. Arches are composed of fields of parallel ridges that begin as a horizontal array at one edge of the finger, curve outward toward the tip, and then curve back to exit horizontally again at the other side. A single vertical ridge may be present in the center of the pattern, forming a tented arch.

Mixed patterns of radial and ulnar loops, whorls, and arches are found in most people, and the presence of any one pattern on all 10 fingertips is quite unusual. A predominance of ulnar loops is frequently seen in Down syndrome, while 10 simple arches is a hallmark of trisomy 18 syndrome. In Turner syndrome, complex whorls are often found on the fingertips, producing a high total ridge count. A rare genetic condition has been reported in which the ridges are arranged vertically and run off the tips of the fingers. Even rarer is the total absence of fingerprints, an autosomal dominant trait.

The most diagnostically helpful feature in palmar dermatoglyphics is the location of the axial triradius. Normally located within 2 cm of the wrist crease, the triradius may be displaced distally and laterally in Down syndrome and a number of other chromosomal disorders. Of equal significance is the presence of secondary axial triradii (t', t'', etc.) located distal to t. The relative position of these features can be specified by measuring the vertical distance of each from the proximal wrist crease, expressed as a ratio to the length of the palm. Placement of the t triradius at a distance less than 15% of palm length is normal. A more common measurement uses as landmarks the a and d triradii at the base of the index and fifth fingers, respectively. Lines drawn from these points to the axial triradius form the atd angle, which is normally 45° or less. A distal axial triradius will produce a high atd angle and is again a feature of Down syndrome and several other chromosomal anomalies.

The skin over the thenar and hypothenar areas of the hand normally bears an open-field pattern of parallel ridges. Loops or whorls in these regions may be familial features but are also seen in conditions such as Rubinstein-Taybi syndrome. Dermal ridge patterning is often disrupted, hypoplastic, or absent in the hypothenar zone in Cornelia de Lange syndrome, and aberrant patterns may be seen on either side of the palm in cases of radial or ulnar aplasia.

Even in the most severe instances of limb hypoplasia, a small zone or ridged skin often may be found at the distal terminus of the limb, often surmounting nubbins of tissue representing incompletely formed digital rays (Fig. 4.20.19). The presence of these abortive dermatoglyphic patterns is helpful in discriminating intrinsic limb deficiencies from congenital amputations.

SUMMARY

The extremely broad range of normal variability in dermatoglyphics is the result of polygenic effects on inherently complex structural patterns. At present, there are no recognized dermatoglyphic configurations that are pathognomonic of any congenital syndrome, but some unusual patterns of dermal ridges may provide supportive evidence for syndrome diagnosis.

C

Amniotic Bands

*Circumstantial evidence is a very tricky thing; it
may seem to point very straight to one thing,
but if you shift your own point of view a little,
you may find it pointing in an equally
uncompromising manner to something entirely
different.*

— "The Boscombe Valley Mystery"

The most common cause of disruptional abnormalities in humans is early rupture of the amnion. This membrane arises as a single layer of cells overlying the embryonic plate and encloses the fluid-filled *amniotic space*. The embryo and amniotic space are surrounded, in turn, by the much larger *chorionic cavity*. With continuing embryonic growth, the amnion gradually distends with fluid, enlarging at the expense of the chorionic space much like one balloon being blown up within another (Fig. 4.11.1A). Eventually, the chorionic and amniotic membranes touch and become loosely adherent, and the chorionic cavity is obliterated. By this time (20–22 weeks), the avascular amnion has been strengthened by fibrous tissue but is sufficiently permeable to allow passage of amniotic fluid through to the chorion, where it is absorbed to pass into the maternal circulation.

The cause of early amniotic membrane rupture remains unknown, although trauma has been implicated in a few cases. No genetic or other predisposing factors have been found, and neither amniocentesis nor maternal connective tissue disease seems to increase the risk. Interestingly, several unexplained "epidemics" have been reported, with an unusual number of affected fetuses detected in a limited geographic area over a period of months to years.

Premature rupture of the amniotic membrane leads to a wide variety of effects on the fetus, depending on the gestational period during which it occurs. Apparently, when the amnion is perforated in very early gestation, the defect rapidly widens, often extending all the way to the placental attachment of the umbilical cord. The embryo is exposed to the inner surface of the chorion, to which it may become adherent, and local breakdown of embryonic tissue follows. Shreds and strands of the membrane are left attached to the placenta, their free ends floating in the remaining amniotic fluid. These amniotic bands can adhere to the gelatinous surface tissues of the embryo, entangling and encircling the developing limbs. With continuing growth, the relatively tough and inelastic fibrous bands gradually cut through yielding fetal tissues, producing constriction rings or frank amputation of limbs. Furthermore, the normal intrauterine breathing and swallowing

283

movements of the fetus may carry the end of a strand into the oropharynx, where it becomes anchored, later slicing through adjacent facial structures.

Amniotic fluid leaking into the space between the amnion and an intact chorion is absorbed faster than it can be replaced, resulting in oligohydramnios. (If the chorion also is ruptured, the mother will experience vaginal leakage of fluid, and the risk of ascending infection becomes very high.) Unless the leak seals spontaneously, the chorion itself gradually becomes less absorptive, and amniotic fluid gradually accumulates again to a more or less adequate volume. In the last weeks of pregnancy, however, there is not enough time for completion of this process, and the resulting intrauterine constraint produces varying degrees of deformation and related problems, including lung hypoplasia.

Amniotic bands produce a wide spectrum of anatomic abnormalities, as might be predicted from the random nature of potential attachments to fetal parts. The most commonly recognized effects are constricting rings and amputations occurring at various sites on the limbs. When such anomalies are multiple, their common basis is quite clear. A deep constricting ring may extend almost to the underlying bone, with severe edema of distal elements. When two or more digits are encircled by the same band, pseudosyndactyly may result (Fig. 4.20.13B). Sites of complete amputation are usually well healed, sometimes with scarring, and there is no evidence of persisting distal structures (Fig. 4.20.13A). Dermal ridges of the hands, feet, or digits will be truncated by the lesions.

Facial disruption from swallowed bands takes the form of deep clefts that do not follow the usual embryonic planes of fusion and may involve the eye or even extend into the forehead. Very early amnion rupture can cause anencephaly, often characterized by fusion of remaining neural structures to the placenta. Cranial meningoceles and encephaloceles may also be produced by this mechanism at a somewhat later stage of neural tube closure. Large defects of the abdominal or thoracic wall, again with placental adhesion, have been reported, and massive transection of a lower limb and the adjoining pelvis with eventration of the abdominal contents has occurred. Amniotic rupture during week 5 of gestation has been implicated in the causation of polydactyly, true syndactyly, and limb reduction abnormalities that mimic intrinsic limb dysplasias.

Any of these disruptive lesions can be combined with various types of mechanical deformation in affected fetuses, yielding bizarre and confusing patterns of abnormality that make diagnosis difficult. The majority of severely affected fetuses are lost by spontaneous abortion, stillbirth, or neonatal death. In milder cases, where survival is not imperiled, the prognosis may be quite good. When the disruptions are few and localized, occult complications are rare and the outlook for general growth and intellectual function is excellent. Furthermore, the recurrence risk for this condition seems to be negligible, in contrast to those genetic disorders that can cause clinically similar anomalies. For these reasons, it becomes important to differentiate the effects of early amnion rupture from other dysmorphic conditions.

By definition, disruptions cause destruction of previously normal tissue. The most helpful physical clues in the differential diagnosis of amniotic band disruptions are features that point to such tissue degeneration rather than failure of some normal embryogenic process. Examples include facial clefting that does not coincide with the usual sites of cleft lip, defects of the body wall that do not correspond with the normal planes of ventral closure, and encephaloceles or meningoceles that do not lie over the midline. In cases of transverse hemimelia, the terminal portion of the limb should be examined closely for anything that might represent rudiments of distal structures. Even a small mound of tissue bearing dermal ridges, for example, would indicate intrinsic dysplasia rather than amniotic amputation as a cause for truncation of the midforearm. The pseudo-syndactyly caused by bands is usually a distal fusion, with the digits still separated proximally. In the newborn, deep constriction rings or zones of amputation sometimes bear adherent remnants of amniotic tissue in the form of strings or fibrous tags, but more frequently the bands will be resorbed or incorporated in fibrous scars before birth.

Examination of the placenta probably is the most useful method of confirming early amnion rupture. Shreds and fragments of the amniotic membrane will usually be found adhering near the base of the umbilical cord. These can best be seen by submerging the placenta in water, allowing the amniotic remnants to float free.

Since the consequences of early amnion rupture can take so many forms, this diagnosis at least needs to be considered in any child with multiple structural defects. The detection of even a single lesion compatible with disruption should prompt a search for others, because such circumstantial evidence may provide an explanation for the whole picture and form the basis for rational counseling concerning prognosis and recurrence risk.

D

Dysmorphology Evaluation

NAME: _____ DATE: _____

DIAGNOSIS: (1) _____ (2) _____

PEDIGREE:

GESTATION: Duration _____wk; Weight gain _____lb; Fetal activity began _____mo;
Vigor _____
Problems during pregnancy _____
_____
_____

BIRTH: Mode _____ Birth weight _____ Length _____ FOC _____
Problems at birth _____

POSTNATAL: Growth _____
Developmental progress: _____
_____

OTHER HISTORY: _____
_____

PHYSICAL EXAMINATION

Age _____   Ht. _____, _____%;   Wt. _____, _____%;   OFC _____, _____%

Other measurements _____

_____

Developmental age or IQ _____

Mental status and behavior _____

Neurological _____

Cranium _____

Face: General _____

Ears _____

Eyes _____

Nose _____

Mouth _____

Neck _____

Thorax _____

Heart _____

Abdomen _____

Back _____

Pelvis, hips, anus _____

Genitalia _____

Arms _____

Hands: General _____

Creases _____

Dermal patterns _____

Legs _____

Feet _____

Skin _____

Hair _____

Other/Comments _____

PREVIOUS STUDIES DONE _____

*Also present in other family members.

References

Athreya B, Silverman B: *Pediatric Physical Diagnosis*. Norwalk, Appleton-Century-Crofts, 1985.
Butterworth T, Ladda RL: *Clinical Genodermatology*. New York, Praeger Scientific Publishers, 1981.
Conan Doyle A: *The Complete Sherlock Holmes*. Garden City, Doubleday & Co, 1930.
Dyken PR, Miller MD: *Facial Features of Neurologic Syndromes*. St. Louis, CV Mosby Co, 1980.
Goodman RM, Gorlin RJ: *The Face in Genetic Disorders* (ed 2). St. Louis, CV Mosby Co, 1977.
Goodman RM, Gorlin RJ: *The Malformed Infant and Child*. New York, Oxford University Press, 1983.
Gorlin RJ, Cohen MM Jr, Levin S: *Syndromes of the Head and Neck*. New York, Oxford University Press, 1989.
Graham JM (ed): *Smith's Recognizable Patterns of Human Deformation* (ed 2). Philadelphia, WB Saunders Co, 1988.
Gray SW, Skandalakis JE: *Embryology for Surgeons*. Philadelphia, WB Saunders Co, 1972.
Hall JG, Froster-Iskenius UG, Allanson JE: *Handbook of normal physical measurements*. Oxford, Oxford Medical Publications, 1989.
Jirasek JE: *Atlas of Human Prenatal Morphogenesis*. Boston, Martinus Nijhoff Publishers, 1983.
Jones KL (ed): *Smith's Recognizable Patterns of Human Malformations* (ed 4). Philadelphia, WB Saunders Co, 1988.
Langman J: *Medical Embryology* (ed 5). Baltimore, Williams & Wilkins Co, 1969.
Lowrey GH: *Growth and Development of Children* (ed 8). Chicago, Year Book Medical Publishers Inc, 1986.
McKusick VA: *Mendelian Inheritance in Man* (ed 8). Baltimore, Johns Hopkins University Press, 1988.
Mehes K: *Minor Malformations in the Neonate*. Budapest, Akademiai Kiado, 1983.
Moore KL: *The Developing Human* (ed 3). Philadelphia, WB Saunders Co, 1982.
Moore KL: *Essentials of Human Embryology*. Toronto, BC Decker Inc, 1988.
Nishimura H, Okomoto N (eds): *Sequential Atlas of Human Congenital Malformations*. Baltimore, University Park Press, 1976.
O'Doherty N: *Inspecting the Newborn Baby's Eyes*. Lancaster, MTP Press Ltd, 1986.
Saul RA, Skinner SA, Stevenson RE, et al: Growth references from conception to adulthood. Supplement Number 1, *Proceedings of the Greenwood Genetic Center*. Greenwood, South Carolina, Greenwood Genetic Center, 1988.
Schaumann B, Alter M: *Dermatoglyphics in Medical Disorders*. New York, Springer-Verlag, 1976.
Schinzel A: *Catalog of Unbalanced Chromosome Aberrations in Man*. Berlin, de Gruyter, 1984.
Sedano HD, Sauk JJ, Gorlin RJ: *Oral Manifestations of Inherited Disorders*. Boston, Butterworths, 1977.
Smith DW: *Growth and Its Disorders*. Philadelphia, WB Saunders Co, 1977.
Spranger JW, Langer LO, Wiedemann HR: *Bone Dysplasias*. Philadelphia, WB Saunders Co, 1974.
Temtamy SA, McKusick VA: *The Genetics of Hand Malformations*. New York, Alan R Liss Inc, 1978.
Tunnessen WW: *Signs and Symptoms in Pediatrics*. Philadelphia, JB Lippincott Co, 1983.
Wiedemann HR, Grosse KR, Dibbern H: *An Atlas of Characteristic Syndromes*. Chicago, Year Book Medical Publishers Inc, 1985.
Winter RM, Knowles SAS, Bieber FR, Baraitser M: *The Malformed Fetus and Stillborn*. New York, John Wiley & Sons, 1988.
Wynne-Davies R, Hall CM, Apley AG: *Atlas of Skeletal Dysplasias*. Edinburgh, Churchill Livingstone, 1985.

Computerized Data Bases On Birth Defects

(All of these software systems operate under MS-DOS on IBM-compatible microcomputers, using English language prompts and data display. Further information about the capabilities of each system can be obtained from the distributors or sponsors at the addresses given.)

Micro BDIS (Dr. Mary Lou Buyse, Center for Birth Defects Information Services, Inc., Dover Medical Building, Box 1776, Dover, MA 02030)

The London Dysmorphology Data Base (Dr. Robin Winter, Syndrome Office, The Clinical Research Centre, Northwick Park Hospital, Harrow, Middlesex, England, *or* Dr. Michael Baraitser, Department of Clinical Genetics, Institute of Child Health, 30 Guilford Street, London WC1, England)

POSSUM (Pictures of Standard Syndromes and Undiagnosed Malformations); makes extensive use of photographs recorded on videodisk and requires a videodisk player and monitor) (C. P. Export Pty. Limited, 613 St. Kilda Road, Melbourne 3004, Australia)

TERIS (The Teratogen Information System) (Dr. Janine E. Polifka, TERIS WJ-10, Department of Pediatrics, University of Washington, Seattle, WA 98195)

Index

Page numbers in italics refer to illustrations.

Printed in the United Kingdom
by Lightning Source UK Ltd.
112328UKS00001BB/7